A Springer Publishing

Public Health and Aging
Second Edition

Physical Change and Aging
Fifth Edition

SPECIAL EDITION

Steven M. Albert, PhD, MSc, MSPH
Vicki A. Freedman, PhD

Sue V. Saxon, PhD
Mary Jean Etten, EdD, GNP, FT
Elizabeth A. Perkins, PhD (c), RNMH

SPRINGER PUBLISHING COMPANY
NEW YORK

A Springer Publishing Company Custom Book

Springer Publishing Company
11 West 42nd Street
New York, New York 10036
www.springerpub.com

Copyright © Springer Publishing Company LLC
ISBN: 978-0-8261-0809-8
All Rights Reserved.

This custom publication retains the page numbers of the original works to allow accurate citation and referencing, and new page numbers (at the bottoms of the pages) to facilitate classroom use.

> Special discounts on bulk quantities of our books are available to corporations, professional associations, pharmaceutical companies, health care organizations, and other qualified groups.
> If you are interested in a custom book, including chapters from more than one of our titles, we can provide that service as well.
>
> **For details, please contact:**
> Special Sales Department, Springer Publishing Company, LLC
> 11 West 42nd Street, 15th Floor, New York, NY 10036-8002
> Phone: 877-687-7476 or 212-431-4370; Fax: 212-941-7842
> Email: sales@springerpub.com

Contents

Public Health and Aging, Second Edition

1   Introducing Public Health and Aging   15
2   Population Aging: Demographic and Epidemiologic Perspectives   55
4   Chronic Disease in Older Adults   83
5   Disability and Functioning   125
6   Cognitive Function: Dementia   167
7   Affective and Social Function: Suffering, Neglect, Isolation   219
9   Aging, Public Health, and Long-Term Care   247

Physical Change and Aging, Fifth Edition

1   Perspectives on Aging   289
2   Theories of Aging   297
4   The Musculoskeletal System   309
7   The Sensory Systems   333
8   The Cardiovascular System   361

17	Health Promotion and Exercise 389
19	Nutrition 405
20	Medications and the Elderly 439

Public Health and Aging

Maximizing Function and Well-Being

Second Edition

STEVEN M. ALBERT, PhD, MSPH
VICKI A. FREEDMAN, PhD, MA

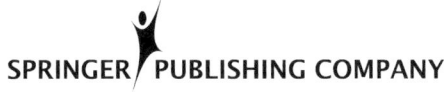

SPRINGER PUBLISHING COMPANY

New York

A Springer Publishing Company Custom Book

Springer Publishing Company
11 West 42nd Street
New York, New York 10036
www.springerpub.com

Copyright © Springer Publishing Company LLC
ISBN: 978-0-8261-0809-8
All Rights Reserved.

This custom publication retains the page numbers of the original works to allow accurate citation and referencing, and new page numbers (at the bottoms of the pages) to facilitate classroom use.

Special discounts on bulk quantities of our books are available to corporations, professional associations, pharmaceutical companies, health care organizations, and other qualified groups.
If you are interested in a custom book, including chapters from more than one of our titles, we can provide that service as well.

For details, please contact:
Special Sales Department, Springer Publishing Company, LLC
11 West 42nd Street, 15th Floor, New York, NY 10036-8002
Phone: 877-687-7476 or 212-431-4370; Fax: 212-941-7842
Email: sales@springerpub.com

Steven M. Albert, PhD, MSPH, is Professor of Behavioral and Community Health Sciences at the Graduate School of Public Health at the University of Pittsburgh. He is trained in anthropology (PhD, University of Chicago) and epidemiology (MS, Columbia University) and completed postdoctoral fellowships in aging and health policy (Rutgers University) and aging and cognition (Columbia University). Dr. Albert has 20 years of research in aging and public health, with completed projects investigating disability transitions in old age, mental health at the end of life, cross-cultural variation in health and chronic disease, home health care, family caregiving, and medication adherence. He conducted fieldwork in Papua New Guinea as a Fulbright Scholar. Current projects include studies of medication review in senior housing, dynamic computational modeling of health behavior, worksite health promotion for chronic disease management, and assessment of home care technologies. He cofounded the Aging and Public Health MPH Program at Columbia University and teaches courses in aging and public health and research methods in aging research. Dr. Albert is the author or editor of 3 books and over 100 peer-reviewed articles. He has served as an officer in the Behavioral and Social Sciences section of the Gerontological Society of America and the Gerontological Health Section of the American Public Health Association.

Vicki A. Freedman, PhD, MA, is a Research Professor at the Survey Research Center of the Institute for Social Research at the University of Michigan. Dr. Freedman has published extensively on topics related to population aging, disability, and long-term care. Her recent research focuses on the causes and consequences of late-life disability trends; measuring disability, time use, and well-being among older couples; evaluating the population-level effects of interventions to maximize functioning; and neighborhoods and late-life health and functioning. She has served on over a dozen national advisory panels for federal agencies, including the Institute of Medicine's Committee on the Future of Disability in America, and currently serves as Co-Principal Investigator for the National Health and Aging Trends Study and the Panel Study of Income Dynamics. She earned her doctorate in Epidemiology from Yale University and master's in Demography from Georgetown University.

Contents

Preface 9

1 Introducing Public Health and Aging 15
Essential Services of Public Health 16
What Is Aging? 19
   Chronological vs. Biological Aging 19
   Senescence vs. Disease 20
   Aging and "Social Age" 22
Five Faces of Aging 28
   The Robust Elder 29
   The Frail Elder 30
   The Elder With Dementia 31
   The Dying Elder 32
   The Compensating, Adaptive Elder 33
Healthy vs. Successful vs. Optimal Aging 35
How the First 50 Years Matter for Health Risks
   in the Second 50 Years: Three Illustrations 38
   Entry Into Late Life With Lower Cognitive Reserve 40
   Entry Into Late Life With Differences in Physical Reserve 42
   Early and Midlife Influences on Late-Life
      Disability Trends 44
The Domains of Public Health and Healthy Aging 46
Population Aging and the Goals of Public Health: Beyond
   Disease Prevention and Health Promotion 48
Summary 52

2 Population Aging: Demographic and Epidemiologic Perspectives 55
Measures of Population Aging 56
The Demographic Transition 63
   The Demographic Transition and Declining Death Rates 64
   The Demographic Transition and Increasing Life Expectancy 68

The Epidemiologic Transition and Shifting Causes
    of Death   76
Why Population Aging Matters   77
    Shifting Health Care Needs of the Population   78
    Emergence of the Oldest Old in America   80
Summary   81

4   Chronic Disease in Older Adults   83

Common Population-Based Measures of Illness
    and Disease   84
    Prevalence   84
    Incidence   85
Comparing Prevalent, Debilitating, and High-Mortality
    Conditions   88
Comorbidity, Multimorbidity, and Self-Care   90
The State of Health Promotion and Chronic Disease
    Prevention for Older Adults   92
    The U.S. Preventive Services Task Force   93
    Older Adults and the Influenza Vaccine   101
    Criteria for a Public Health Program   103
Medicare and Financing of Preventive Care in an
    Aging Society   104
    Medicare's Basic Benefit Structure   104
    Growing Emphasis on Prevention   107
    *Medicare's Fiscal Health and Disability and Disease
        Prevention   109*
Promoting Chronic Disease Management in Later Life   111
    Geriatric Evaluation and Management   113
    Making Patients and Families Partners in Medical Care   117
    *Avoiding Inappropriate Medication Use and Managing
        Polypharmacy   120*
Summary   122

5   Disability and Functioning   125

The Language of Disability   126
    *The International Classification of Functioning,
        Disability and Health (ICF)   127*
    The Nagi Model of Disablement   130
The Measurement of Disability   133
    *Centrality of the Activities of Daily Living in Measuring
        Late-Life Disability   133*
    *Difficulties in Measuring Activity Limitations Among
        Older Adults   137*

Contents   ix

     Measuring Capacity: Performance-Based Tests   142
     Measuring the Environment   142
  Trends in Disability Prevalence and Active Life Expectancy   143
     Trends in Prevalence   143
     Trends in Active Life Expectancy   145
     Disparities in Trends and Causes   146
  The Epidemiology of Disability: Risk Factors for Functional Decline   148
  A Clinical Perspective: Identifying Disablement Pathways   151
     The Link Between Capacity and Performance   152
     The Role of Accommodations   155
  Public Health Interventions to Maximize Late-Life Functioning   159
     Preventing Falls   159
     Comparing Potentially High-Impact Interventions   162
  Summary   164

6   Cognitive Function: Dementia   167

  What Is Dementia?   169
  Making and Receiving the Diagnosis of Alzheimer's Disease   171
  Cognitive Decline With Age: Distinct From Alzheimer's Disease?   177
  Cognitive Decline Prior to Frank Dementia   180
     Insight on Declining Cognitive Ability   182
     Mild Cognitive Impairment and Disability   183
  Prevalence and Incidence of Alzheimer's Disease   185
  Risk Factors for Alzheimer's Disease   189
     Genetic Risk Factors   189
     Socioeconomic Factors: Education, Lifelong Occupation, Cognitive Reserve   190
     Medical Morbidity: Hypertension and Vascular Disease, Diabetes, Bone Mineral Density Loss, Estrogen Deficiency, Depression   191
  Outcomes Associated With Alzheimer's Disease   195
     Mortality   195
     Nursing Home Care   198
     Hospitalization and Primary Care   199
     Disability and Psychiatric Morbidity   200
     Family Caregiving   202
     Quality of Life in AD   206
     Dementia and the End of Life   208
  Non-Alzheimer's Dementias   209

Interventions to Prevent Cognitive Decline 210
Interventions to Support Family Caregivers 211
Summary 214

7 Affective and Social Function: Suffering, Neglect, Isolation 219
Burden of Mental Illness 220
Presentation of Mental Health Symptoms in Late Life 223
Prevalence of Mental Illness at Older Ages 226
Mental Health in a Disabled Older Population 229
Outcomes Associated With Mental Illness in Late Life 231
Treatment of Depression in Late Life 233
Reducing the Risk of Depression and Associated Morbidity in Seniors 234
Neglect and Abuse 236
Social Isolation 238
Broader Considerations of Environmental Influences on Health 239
Summary 244

9 Aging, Public Health, and Long-Term Care 247
What Is Long-Term Care? 248
Overview: Trends in Long-Term Care Use and Spending 249
Home- and Community-Based Services 251
Personal Assistance Services and Public Health 253
Family Caregiving 257
Long-Term Residential Care Arrangements 260
Enhancing Long-Term Care 263
   Recognizing and Taking Older People's Care Preferences Seriously 265
   Upgrading Home Attendant and Nursing Assistant Care 267
   Special Care Units for People With Alzheimer's Disease 272
   Expansion of Options for Supportive Care and Housing 273
Summary 275

Preface

Cultural conceptions of the aging experience are many and often recognize a long arc of development followed by decline in later life. Consider Shakespeare's "seven ages of man" (*As You Like It,* II, 7). "One man in his time plays many parts, his acts being seven ages." The seven stages include infancy, "whining schoolboy . . . creeping unwillingly to school," lover, soldier ("seeking the bubble reputation even in the cannon's mouth"), judge or administrator, retirement based on frailty ("his big manly voice, turning again towards childish treble"), and finally "second childishness and mere oblivion . . . sans teeth, sans eyes, sans taste, sans everything."

Religious traditions also provide guidance on approaches to old age. Through a series of anecdotes, for example, the Talmud (i.e., Jewish law) teaches the obligation of honoring elderly parents. Stories feature parents who are physically frail and in some cases senile. Honoring parents involves what is now recognized as help with activities of daily living: offering food, helping with dressing, and assistance in getting around (*Bavli, Kiddushin* 31b). This obligation is traced back to an unusual source: the treatment of the first tablets of commandments, which were broken by Moses in anger upon seeing the Golden Calf. The fragments of the broken tablets were not discarded but rather kept alongside the new tablets that replaced them. Both were carried by the Israelites as they wandered through the desert (*Berakhot* 8b). The old shattered tablets were considered valuable by the community, not only in their own right, but also because they were linked to the newer tablets.

When the first edition of this book appeared in 2004, it noted that age is a dominating factor in health, as it is in so many social, psychological, and economic spheres. To see the centrality of age, consider these comments from our university alumni magazine (Cornell University, Spring, 2002). The 1995 graduate (age 30 or so) exhorts his classmates in this way: "May all your weddings be perfect, babies brilliant, exams easy, jobs fun, and friends true." The 1945 graduate (age 77 or so) makes this report: "Nothing to do and not enough time to do it." The 1938 graduate (age 84 or so) reports, "Angina in April, pacemaker in July, angioplasty in August. Otherwise, fine." And the 1934 graduate reports this: "My theme song now at 94 is 'Don't get around much any more!'" The same issue reports on the oldest living graduate of the college, a man from the class of 1916, aged 108. This long-time gardening columnist resides in an assisted living facility. Four generations of descendents attended his birthday party, which he remarked was "just a lot of fuss over me." This man's age puts him near the oldest-oldest old; the 2000 U.S. Census reported just 1,400 people over age 110 (of some 285,000,000).

Today aging poses a number of challenges for both individuals and the societies in which they live. The biomedical challenge is to develop ways to delay, prevent, or remediate much of the frailty and dementia that we observe in late life. The epidemiologic challenge is to identify risk factors that affect the incidence and progression of the chronic conditions that characterize old age, and that accordingly increase the prevalence of disability. The sociological challenge is to understand why different segments of populations experience old age and aging so differently, with groups defined by socioeconomic status or race already entering old age with very different resources, including cognitive and physical resiliency and social capital. The ethical challenge is to understand when to shift the goals of medical treatment from maximizing care to minimizing suffering.

These challenges have taken on a new urgency in the face of the imminent demographic change facing the United States and countries around the world. Over the next few decades older adults will reach numbers—and proportions—never before seen in human history. As we discuss in Chapter 5, longer life does not necessarily mean worse health and functioning. But the shift toward older ages is not simply a temporary phenomenon, but likely a permanent structural change with which public health must grapple.

Indeed, these different approaches to the challenges of aging come together in the public health approach to aging, the focus of this book. Unlike in Shakespearean or Biblical times, today, public health and aging must address a much more heterogeneous aging experience. Rather than only focusing on the prevention of disease and its debilitating effects, we argue in this volume that a broader lens is needed to address the many faces of aging, whether robust, physically frail, living with dementia, approaching death, or compensating and adapting to changes in capacity.

The public health challenge is to promote the development and maintenance of optimal physical, mental, and social function, irrespective of acquired disease and with due recognition of the senescent changes that accompany late life. In the case of public health and aging we argue that "health promotion and disease prevention," the mantra of public health, needs to be broadened to stress *maximizing function and well-being*. Hence, the subtitle of this book.

We also call for greater appreciation of the earlier-life origins of many features of health in old age. What happens in the first 50 years of life matters a great deal for the second 50 years. For this reason we prefer "public health and aging" over "public health gerontology" to describe the field.

In the first edition of this book, we sought to define the field of public health and aging and to identify the research tools and designs most fruitful in this area. We noted that public health and aging was still a developing field that lacked a unified treatment or overarching framework. The first edition of the book applied such a framework to a series of large questions that are still with us: How can we ensure a healthy old age? Why are some segments of society able to enter old age with greater physical and cognitive resources than others? To what extent can physical and cognitive disability be prevented? To what extent can they be remediated? Does it make sense to speak of the prevention of frailty or other forms of primary prevention in late life? These issues have become more pressing with population aging. By 2050, we can expect to see 15–20% of the world's population over age 65, in both more and less developed economies, and in some countries (such as Japan) as many as a third.

But in the half decade or so that separates the two editions of this book, the field of public health and aging has also changed. The Administration on Aging (AoA), state health departments, the CDC, the Centers for Medicare and Medicaid Services (CMS), as well as managed care organizations, corporate employers, and advocacy organizations, have all started, in their own ways, to *practice* public health and aging. For example, in collaboration with CDC and AoA, state health departments are developing community-wide health promotion and disease prevention efforts in the areas of chronic disease self-management, care management, physical activity, nutrition, environmental modification, and falls prevention. CMS has added a preventive health care visit and additional screening to Medicare's basic package of services. Many state governments now have integrated blueprints for healthy aging, and communities increasingly seek "elder-friendly" impact assessments for planning and development.

These developments, we would argue, make this new edition even more valuable. It is still unclear how best to link current public health efforts for seniors to the many other services they may require, such as medical care, pharmacy management, long-term and end-of-life care, allied health services, and supportive aging services. Too narrow a focus on promoting health may miss opportunities for promoting function. As we argue in Chapter 1, in the real world of imperfect screening tests, invasive diagnostic technologies, and difficult decisions about treatment in the context of declining health and the approach of death, promoting health and promoting function may not always correspond. In public health and aging, supportive care and services are often as important as medical treatment once we recognize that function and disability, rather than diagnosis, should guide population-focused policies. For this insight, we thank M. Powell Lawton, who came to this realization in the 1960s, long before either of us considered research on aging as a possible career.

The second edition of this book expands the first considerably, with fully a third more pages. We have added new chapters on the aging services network and public health (Chapter 3), chronic disease (Chapter 4), long-term care (Chapter 9), and ethical issues in public health and aging (Chapter 11). Other chapters have been substantially revised to reflect advances in thinking about population aging (Chapter 2), physical functioning and disability (Chapter 5), and cognitive disability (Chapter 6). We have updated the remaining chapters to reflect the explosion of knowledge and interest in the years between the editions and provide updates on demographic and epidemiologic perspectives (Chapter 2), affective and social function (Chapter 7), quality of life (Chapter 8), and mortality (Chapter 10). Our overall perspective begins with the "compensating, adaptive elder," who alters daily tasks, relies on spared abilities to compensate for deficits, and selectively invests physical, cognitive, and affective effort to maximize the likelihood of social participation and activity despite health-limiting conditions (Chapter 1).

The current volume reflects our understanding of public health and aging as a field today. Inevitably, important topics have been omitted, and, in places, classic references have been retained in place of newer studies. These choices reflect our desire to present a balance of breadth and depth.

We crafted this new edition with reviews of the first edition in mind. These reviews were favorable, but suggested that our focus on the tools of public health and aging should include, as well, discussion of how public health efforts are actually delivered to older people. We have tried to address this earlier gap in several chapters, which now examine development of "healthy aging networks" (Chapter 3), the growing preventive services emphasis of Medicare (Chapter 4), national efforts to reduce falls and make communities elder-friendly (Chapter 5), interventions to support family caregivers (Chapter 6), evidence-based depression management programs (Chapter 7), and efforts enhancing long-term care (Chapter 9).

We have designed this book to serve as the main text for an undergraduate or graduate class in aging as it relates to the core fields of public health: epidemiology, population studies, health systems and policy, and health behaviors. It may also be used as a supplementary text in gerontology and geriatrics, population studies, the allied health sciences, and sociology. An accompanying teaching guide is available for use of the book in the classroom. Beyond the classroom, this book represents an integrated treatment of one of the greatest challenges of our time, how to maximize functioning in later life, which we hope will be of interest to researchers across the clinical, behavioral, and population sciences.

We thank Sheri W. Sussman of Springer Publishing for her encouragement and patience, as well as the many colleagues who have helped us think through these issues. To our families, young and old, we add special thanks, for this revised edition would not have been possible without their support.

Steven M. Albert, PhD, MSPH
Vicki A. Freedman, PhD, MA
June 2009

1 Introducing Public Health and Aging

What is public health and aging? Although we understand each component reasonably well, this burgeoning interdisciplinary field is clearly more than the sum of its parts. Thus, the field of public health *and* aging has not been well defined. It draws on the more well-known population sciences of epidemiology and demography but often focuses on subpopulations, such as frail elders, healthy elders at risk for disability, or elders whose health is surprisingly robust. It requires an understanding of health behaviors and prevention, health systems and policy, research methods and statistical analysis, and social and environmental risk factors, but favors no single disciplinary approach. It not only draws on geriatric medicine to promote health outside the clinic and beyond the clinician-patient encounter, but also shares an affinity with gerontology more generally as a multidisciplinary study of aging. Nevertheless, it is distinct from these disciplines in its focus on populations rather than patients and its proactive recognition that health and functioning in later life are rooted in much earlier experiences.

To better demarcate the domains of this emerging field, we first provide an overview of what constitutes public health. We then provide a primer on aging, highlighting the most common archetypes of later life. Next, we introduce the life course perspective, providing examples particularly germane to public health and aging. We end the chapter with a discussion of healthy aging as a key goal and the corresponding domains of public health and aging.

ESSENTIAL SERVICES OF PUBLIC HEALTH

Open any introductory textbook on public health and you will inevitably find lists of what public health does, how public health serves, and what tools public health uses. In the mid-1990s, the Public Health Service, the U.S. agency responsible for public health at a national level, developed a consensus document in collaboration with other major public health organizations that outlined what constitutes public health practice. The lists have been adopted as a framework for identifying the responsibilities of local public health systems and evaluating public health efforts.

As shown in Box 1.1 public health has responsibilities in six distinct areas, summarized broadly as health promotion and disease prevention. What you will not see on this list is explicit mention of older adults, aging, or aging communities. In part, this reflects the tradition in public health of being concerned with communities at large without respect to age. Although any of these functions could easily be extended to an older population (e.g., from preventing epidemics and the spread of disease among older adults to assuring the quality and accessibility of health services for seniors), no explicit aim in this list of what public health does speaks directly to aging.

Box 1.1

WHAT PUBLIC HEALTH DOES

1. Prevents epidemics and the spread of disease
2. Protects against environmental hazards
3. Prevents injuries
4. Promotes and encourages healthy behaviors and mental health
5. Responds to disasters and assists communities in recovery
6. Ensures the quality and accessibility of health services

Source: http://www.health.gov/phfunctions/public.htm

A second common "to do" list explicitly addresses how public health serves communities. These 10 bullets constitute the essential services of public health (Box 1.2). The list includes critical tasks such as monitoring and investigating health, educating and mobilizing communities, developing policies and plans, evaluating services and programs, ensuring safety, linking people to services, assuring a competent workforce, and conducting research to solve public health problems. Together these essential services support public health's overarching goal: "assuring conditions in which people can be healthy" (Institute of Medicine [IOM], 1998).

> **Box 1.2**
>
> ### THE 10 ESSENTIAL SERVICES OF PUBLIC HEALTH
>
> 1. Monitor health status to identify and solve community health problems.
> 2. Diagnose and investigate health problems and health hazards in the community.
> 3. Inform, educate, and empower people about health issues.
> 4. Mobilize community partnerships and action to identify and solve health problems.
> 5. Develop policies and plans that support individual and community health efforts.
> 6. Enforce laws and regulations that protect health and ensure safety.
> 7. Link people to needed personal health services and ensure the provision of health care when otherwise unavailable.
> 8. Ensure a competent public and personal health care workforce.
> 9. Evaluate effectiveness, accessibility, and quality of personal and population-based health services.
> 10. Research for new insights and innovative solutions to health problems.
>
> Source: http://www.health.gov/phfunctions/public.htm

Again, although there is no explicit mention of aging, certainly each of these services can be readily applied to an older population. For example, "monitor the health status *of older adults*" would clearly fall within the first essential service and "inform, educate, and empower *older* people about health issues" fits squarely within the third function. But public health and aging is clearly more than the application of these essential services to older people.

The distinctive yet varied tools of public health stem from the core areas of study found within schools of public health. The names and scope of these core areas may vary slightly across teaching institutions, but each offers methods and materials for investigating populations, prevention, and policy.

- *Population sciences* provide demographic and epidemiologic tools to study population dynamics and the health of populations. These tools help describe population-level phenomena and identify risk factors for disease and disability.
- *Behavioral sciences* (also health education and community health programs) emphasize methods to design and implement programs to influence health and health behaviors. Essential tools from this subspecialty include evidence-based health behavior modification programs and community participatory research.
- *Environmental health sciences* are concerned with measuring and manipulating factors in the environment to influence health. Understanding the environment is critical to disease prevention, but it is also key for tertiary prevention of disability. That is, people with physical or cognitive deficits may remain above the threshold of disability in supportive environments. Environment is thus a malleable component of disability.
- *Health systems and policy* draws on policy analysis and economics to understand and improve health service delivery, including health planning, organization, and policy formulation. This subspecialty recognizes that public health programs do not operate in isolation but require linkage to existing systems and policies if they are to be sustained.
- *Biostatistics* draws on statistical tools and research methodology to characterize or investigate health problems and programs.
- *Public health genomics, infectious disease microbiology, global health, public health informatics, public health law, and emergency preparedness* represent emerging areas of public health

that will likely grow in importance as the field matures and adopts methods from adjacent fields.

As we will discuss in this chapter, researchers and practitioners in public health and aging bring to bear these varied and powerful toolkits to promote what we will call "healthy aging." *The aim of public health and aging is healthy aging: to balance prevention of disease and injury with promotion of behaviors and environments in a way that maximizes functioning and well-being across the life span.* The emphasis is decidedly population based rather than patient focused and recognizes that early and midlife status have implications for health in later life. Just how are the tools of public health implemented to achieve these ends? To answer this question requires a deeper understanding of the phenomenon that we call aging and a basic understanding of changes that individuals encounter as they age.

WHAT IS AGING?

All individuals, whether young or old, are aging. Annual birthday celebrations mark the passage of chronological age. But aging also occurs at the cellular level according to a biological clock. Changes that occur because of cellular aging are often difficult to discern from those caused by disease processes. Here, we discuss the distinctions between chronological and biological aging and between senescence and disease.

Chronological vs. Biological Aging

Aging is the maturation and senescence of biological systems. "Maturation" and "senescence" imply time-dependent changes: with time, our minds and bodies change in a variety of ways, and these changes are what we mean by "aging." With each additional decade of life, adults will see a decrease in reaction time, psychomotor speed, and verbal memory; declines in strength and walking speed; a decreased rate of urine flow; loss of skeletal muscle; and greater mortality, among many other changes. They will also see declines in addictive behaviors and crime, reduction in severe psychiatric disorders, and stability in psychological well-being; continuing increases in vocabulary; greater selectivity in friendship and increased contact with close family; less need for novel stimuli; and increases in leisure time and altruistic behaviors, among many other changes. The popular understanding of aging mostly stresses the first set, the negative changes; but a more complete and accurate understanding would more profitably stress both kinds of change, because both are relevant to a public health perspective on aging.

These changes, positive and negative, occur with the longer life or greater age of the organism. It would be useful to distinguish the two meanings of "aging." The first is simply the number of years an organism has survived, that is, chronological aging. Chronological age is marked solely by the passage of time since birth. Hence, two persons born on the same day, by definition, are the same chronological age, although one may live to an older age. The second definition involves the ticking of some kind of mechanism that governs the "maturation and senescence" of biological systems, and may vary from person to person. One 84-year-old may be biologically vigorous, whereas another born on the same day may lack vitality; hence, despite identical chronological ages, their biological aging, the rate of maturation of their biological systems, may be quite different.

Declines in health may be more prevalent in later life because they are, in fact, expressions of senescence and maturation. Or these declines may be more prevalent simply because of the greater length of time older people have lived, and hence the greater opportunity they have had to experience the risks or exposures that produce these effects. This is a key distinction. It is more than likely that some combination of true senescence and greater exposure to risk factors is likely to be responsible for the changes we consider "aging." For example, the highest audible pitch people can hear declines with greater age, suggesting that this change is a senescent feature of the auditory system. But it is also likely that long years of occupational exposure to noise, untreated ear infections during childhood, neurological conditions, and an accumulation of minor injuries might also contribute to loss of hearing in old age. Senescent changes, long periods of exposure to disease risk factors, and the interaction between the two are confounded in the lay understanding of aging, but a successful public health approach to aging must distinguish between them.

Senescence vs. Disease

Senescence is the progressive, cumulative deterioration in function or loss of physiological capacity associated with greater chronological age. Current thinking suggests that senescence is a biological feature of many physiological systems and that it is best measured as decreased reserve and reduced resistance to stressors. It is evident in a "diminished availability of redundant systems necessary for physical and social well-being" (Crews, 1990). For example, research suggests that sarcopenia, loss of skeletal muscle and lean body mass (and greater infiltration of fat cells in muscle), is a universal, involuntary change that is distinct from pathological wasting syndromes (such as those common in cancer) and cachexia (seen in patients with rheumatoid arthritis, congestive heart failure, or end-stage renal disease). Nonetheless, these senescent changes put older people at risk for pathological changes and, in this sense, can be considered "the backdrop against which the drama of disease is played out" (Roubenoff & Castaneda, 2001). A senescent change, such as sarcopenia, puts the body at risk for disease and poor recovery from disease; for example, "a body already depleted of protein because of aging is less able to withstand the protein catabolism that comes with acute illness or inadequate protein intake" (Roubenoff & Castaneda, 2001).

Hence, senescence and disease are related but distinct. We only see senescence in organisms that have lived a long time, but a longer time alive also means a greater opportunity to develop disease or suffer health insults that are actually distinct from these senescent changes.

Consider cancer. It is often said to be a disease of aging. This presumption is probably based on the higher death rate from malignant neoplasms evident among older adults. Indeed, the mortality rate from cancer among adults aged 85 and older in 2005 was 1,637.7 per 100,000, much higher than the rates of 118.6 among people aged 45–54 and 326.9 among people aged 55–64 (Arias, 2007, Table 38). Of the 512,894 deaths due to cancer in the United States in 2005, 388,322, or 69.4%, involved older adults (Arias, 2007, Appendix Table 32). But the larger number of cancer deaths in older adults does not mean that cancer is a feature of aging. In fact, cause-specific mortality from cancer is actually higher in the 45–64 age group; 32.6% of deaths in this group were due to cancer, compared with 21.7% of deaths in the older age group. Cancer incidence is also lower in the 7th and 8th decade of life, compared with the 5th and 6th decades (Hadley, 1992). Here again, we see confounding between old age as a time for longer exposure to disease agents that may lead to cancer, and old age as an expression of senescent changes that may lead to cancer directly (i.e., dysregulation of cellular processes, such as apoptosis), or that put one at risk for cancer (such as slower bowel motility, development of polyps, and onset of colorectal cancer).

This combination of disease- and senescence-determined factors complicates public health efforts for older adults. In the setting of late-life declines in physiological reserve, what is "normal" senescence and what is disease? Put another way, what is an age-determined relationship (senescence) and what are age-related phenomena (disease)? Wallace (1997) describes some of the different ways disease and senescence may be related. First, the pathogenesis of some diseases is likely to be altered with age. Declines in immune response, for example, a feature of aging, may turn a viral infection into pneumonia rather than a less complicated respiratory tract infection. Second, an age-determined change in one physiological system (which may not cause overt disease in that system) may increase susceptibility to disease in another system. An example mentioned by Wallace is an increase in stroke related to age-determined hypotension. Third, age-determined changes can make older people more susceptible to disease when exposed to environmental challenges. Older adults develop reductions in glucose tolerance, for example, that may lead to frank diabetes under certain conditions. Wallace also points out that some age-determined changes may actually retard development of disease. Lactose intolerance, an age-determined change to the extent that it increases with age, may lead to less fat intake and reduced risk of atherogenesis.

Why make the distinction between age-determined and age-related phenomena? Whether age-determined or age-associated, if changes in later life lead to loss of reserve and put one at risk for disease, are they not appropriate targets for intervention? They may be, but distinguishing changes that are due to senescence from those that are due to external risk factors may help sharpen the appropriate intervention strategy. Moreover, science has made great strides in understanding the risk factors for many of the common diseases of later life, but has yet to identify the specific biological mechanisms responsible for senescence.

Aging and "Social Age"

When people think of old age, they first think of years or some other indicator of the passage of time (for example, in societies where people do not use year-based calendars, these indicators might include the number of harvests completed, the number of ritual cycles conducted, or the number of relocations of dwellings). But even in contemporary American culture, "old age" is not simply a matter of chronological age or the biological expression of senescence. Fry (1980) used a technique drawn from cognitive anthropology to show that cultural dimensions, such as productivity, vulnerability, and reproductive potential, underlie judgments of "young," "middle-aged," and "old." In her pile-sort study, respondents were asked to group hypothetical age-linked social statuses according to similarity. Multidimensional scaling analyses revealed a clear chronological age dimension, but also second- and third-order dimensions, showing, for example, that respondents also grouped older people and children together as opposed to people of middle age. This finding is consistent with research on the "infantilization" of older people (Albert & Brody, 1996; Ryan, Bourhis, & Knops, 1991). "Baby talk" is often applied to older people with cognitive impairment or other disabilities, and terms typically reserved for children are often applied to older people. For example, older people are often spoken of as "cute" and elicit a protective urge seen with infants, such as a desire to hug or comfort.

The reverse is also true. Younger adults who are not active, not interested in new experiences or travel, not willing to switch careers, or who are slow, deliberate, or narrow-minded, are often called "old." They are said to be "old before their time." These negative features of aging—negative, at any rate, when applied to younger people—are meant to criticize or embarrass young people. This use of language also suggests a social component in our understanding of aging. People are old not only because of their age, but also because of their behavior, their health, their attitudes, their choices, and even their politics.

More generally, evidence from cross-cultural studies suggests that the defining characteristics of old age include chronological age, as well as many other criteria, such as achieved social status, having grandchildren, holding political office, oratorical skill, and physical changes. In societies with high mortality and short life expectancy, having children reach adulthood is associated with a change in status to "elder" and associated honorific terms (Albert & Cattell, 1994). Again, the other side to social age needs to be mentioned. In American society, adults can refuse to "grow up," and people can insist on "not acting their age." This can take a variety of forms: not leaving a parent's home, not marrying at an appropriate age, refusing to establish clear career goals, marrying someone much younger than you are, and even buying consumer products associated with a different age stratum.

Thus, old age has a social dimension. For public health efforts, this social component is most relevant in its bearing on expectations for health and function in later life. Even this brief discussion of the use of age criteria to label behaviors suggests that attitudes toward aging and old age are mostly negative. Old age is seen as a time of decline, withdrawal, and vulnerability. In this view, aging is not welcome, and little should be expected of older people; instead, we are expected to ease their decline, provide care, and protect them from exploitation or danger related to their increased vulnerability. These are the elements of "ageism" (Butler, 1969; Palmore, 1999): assumptions of disability, lack of ability, or vulnerability (and, hence, need for protection) based on age, rather than on actual competencies.

The pervasiveness of ageism should not be underestimated. Older persons who miss a word because of a hearing problem are considered too old for conversation and patronized with simplified language. Words may be put in their mouths and their opinions ignored. Older people who forget a name are called "senile," dissatisfaction with illness-related activity restrictions is called "crankiness," and expressions of sexual interest make one a "dirty old man or woman." Even medical personnel are not above recourse to ageist stereotypes.

This sort of ageist thinking has consequences for public health. If missing a word is considered a feature of "getting old," families (and older people themselves) may not take advantage of tertiary treatments available to manage hearing loss, such as hearing aids. Losing track of names may indicate mild cognitive impairment, not just aging; and people with mild cognitive impairment may benefit from cognitive prostheses, environmental modification, antidementia drugs, or increased supervision by family members. "Crankiness" may be depression, or genuine dissatisfaction with unpalatable symptoms, a complaint against undesirable housing, or simply a bad mood, any of which would otherwise be understood as features of daily life for people of any age. From a public health perspective, these expressions of ageism are doubly damaging. They falsely label potentially treatable medical conditions (such as memory or hearing loss) as "aging," and also turn everyday complaints, dissatisfactions, interests, and behaviors into pseudomedical aging syndromes ("crankiness," "childishness," "the dirty old man").

Ageist thinking is revealed for what it is when one compares preconceptions about older people with the facts at hand. For example, younger people mostly imagine old age as a time of sickness, disability, and loss of autonomy. In fact, nearly 80% of people aged 65 and older have no disability of any sort and less than 5% reside in nursing homes. For all our fears of cognitive decline and Alzheimer's disease as invariant features of aging, it is mainly a disease of the very old; most surveys find an Alzheimer's disease prevalence of 6% for people aged 75–84 and 20% for people aged 85 and older (Brookmeyer, Gray, & Kawas, 1998; GAO, 1998). A recent prevalence survey for a nationally representative sample of Americans aged 71+ puts the prevalence of Alzheimer's disease at 9.7% and any dementia at 13.9% (Plassman et al., 2007). Evidence also suggests that the prevalence and incidence of both physical and cognitive limitations in later life may be declining (Schoeni, Freedman, & Martin, 2008). Clinical depression is also not more common in older people (see Chapter 9); it is often a comorbid feature of physical illness and bereavement and, for this reason, seems more common among older people.

Myths About Aging

Many of these ageist attitudes have been elicited by use of questionnaires, such as "What Is Your Aging IQ?" (Special Committee on Aging, 1991). The questions present typical preconceptions about aging and in this way highlight ageist thinking. One version of the questions is shown here, with suggested correct answers:

True or False?

1. Baby boomers are the fastest growing segment of the population. *False.*
2. Families don't bother with their older relatives. *False.*
3. Everyone becomes confused or forgetful if they live long enough. *False.*
4. You can be too old to exercise. *False.*
5. Heart disease is a much bigger problem for older men than for older women. *False.*
6. The older you get, the less you sleep. *False.*
7. People should watch their weight as they age. *True.*
8. Most older people are depressed. Why shouldn't they be? *False.*
9. There's no point in screening older people for cancer because they can't be treated. *False.*
10. Older people take more medications than younger people. *True.*
11. People begin to lose interest in sex around age 55. *False.*
12. If your parents had Alzheimer's disease, you will inevitably get it. *False.*

13. Diet and exercise reduce the risk of osteoporosis. *True.*
14. As your body changes with age, so does your personality. *False.*
15. Older people might as well accept urinary accidents as a fact of life. *False.*
16. Suicide is mainly a problem for teenagers. *False.*
17. Falls and injuries "just happen" to older people. *False.*
18. Everybody gets cataracts. *False.*
19. Extremes of heat and cold can be especially dangerous for older people. *True.*
20. You can't teach an old dog new tricks. *False.*

These questions elicit ageist stereotypes well. They reflect unrealistic fatalism and therapeutic nihilism ("everybody gets cataracts," "falls and injuries just happen to older people," "there's no reason to treat older persons with cancer," and "most older people are depressed"), false assumptions about the aging process ("you can't teach an old dog new tricks," "people begin to lose interest in sex after age 55," and "the older you get, the less you sleep"), overestimates of the heritability of late-life disease ("If your parents had Alzheimer's disease, you will inevitably get it"), sociological naïveté ("American families have by and large abandoned their older members"), and underrecognition of the truly negative aspects of aging, such as the increased risk of suicide among older White men and the greater use of prescribed medicines. Sometimes the problem is a misplaced recognition of a problem, such as the claim of less sleep with greater age. It is true that older people sleep for shorter durations, and this is related to poorer quality of sleep. However, older people also nap more during the day, resulting, in fact, in greater amounts of sleep overall than younger people have.

Together, these prejudices suggest that aging is mostly misunderstood. Overall, the negative features are exaggerated and the positive features ignored. This social or cultural component of aging should be recognized as a potential obstacle to successful public health interventions for older people.

When Does Old Age Begin?

So far, we have examined aging and older persons without specifying when someone is old. From what we have said already, we see that the question is unreasonable. There is no single age at which we can say that people cross the threshold into "old age." People age at different rates; hence, for any given age, there will be great variation in all proposed biomarkers of aging or phenotypes of healthy aging. "Old age" does not have a biological definition, only a social one. For example, in the United States, establishment of the Social Security system linked old age to age 65. This definition of old age was more a product of social perceptions and economic necessity than anything else.

But people do have an idea of when people become old. A number of surveys have asked at what age someone is old. The start of "old age" can be assigned to a wide range of chronological ages. This assigned age may reflect attitudes toward aging and older persons. For example, assigning the start of old age to increasingly older ages means that many aspects of aging, once considered hallmarks of old age, now fall short of making someone old. It also stands to reason that many of the characteristics of the respondents, such as age and social status, are likely to be related to judgments regarding the start of old age. One may imagine that minority groups with a shorter life expectancy might date the onset of old age to earlier ages than other more advantaged groups.

Someone who reports that old age begins at age 55 clearly has a different attitude toward aging than someone who asserts that it begins at age 75. In the one case, a larger portion of the life span is considered the period of "old age," with the physical and psychological changes of the 5th and 6th decade already considered signs of senescence. In the other, only changes typical of the 7th decade and beyond qualify as "old age," and senescence is pushed ahead to a point closer to death and the maximum biological life span. Respondent choices of an age for "old age" tell us the decade when people are expected to slow down, retire, and focus on self-maintenance rather than new careers or goals.

Figure 1.1 shows the age at which respondents consider women to be old. These data are drawn from the National Council on Aging *Myths and Realities of Aging* survey, conducted in 2000 in a national probability sample of the United States. The data are weighted to reflect the sampling scheme and overrepresentation of older people and minorities. The figure plots the mean age that "the average woman" is said to be old by respondent's age and sex.

Note the strong relationship between a respondent's age and his or her report of when women are old. Young people clearly consider the start of old age to be much earlier than older people do. For people at about age 20, women are old at age 45. By the time people reach the

14   Public Health and Aging

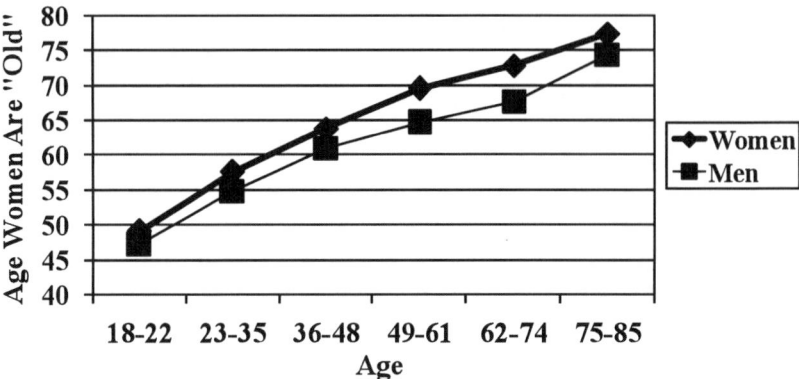

Figure 1.1 Age at which women are "old," by respondent age and sex (United States).
Source: From National Council on Aging (NCOA), 2001; weighted data.

6th and 7th decade, old age is pushed back to the late sixties and early seventies. Note too that women date the start of old age to a later age than men do, whatever the respondent's age. Women consider old age to begin 2–4 years later than men do. They push old age further back than men do, not only for themselves, but also in their reports of the start of old age for men (Albert, O'Neil, Muller, & Butler, 2002d). Moreover, the age at which old age is said to begin now seems to be far more correlated with one's own age than in earlier surveys.

FIVE FACES OF AGING

The experience of late life is varied and complex. To better understand the aims of public health and aging, it is useful to delve into some of the most common experiences of aging. Gillick (1994), a clinical geriatrician, has provided an excellent account of the most common faces of aging. As a geriatrician with a primary care focus, one of the few physicians who still make home visits, her experience offers important guidance on what it is like to be old, ill, and in need of medical care. She begins her account with an overriding principle: "Only if we start with a deep understanding of what being sick is like can we hope to reach a consensus on what kind of health policy is appropriate for the elderly" (Gillick, 1994, p. 10). In her account, Gillick identifies four types of elder and has provided clinical vignettes of the particular challenges and opportunities specific to each type.

The Robust Elder

The robust older persons are "physically vigorous, mentally acute, a fount of wisdom and experience for their families, [and] busy accomplishing all the things they never previously had the time to undertake." However, as Gillick reminds us, they typically have accumulated at least some chronic conditions in their 70 or 80 years of life, such as arthritis, hypertension, diabetes, hearing loss, glaucoma or macular degeneration, essential tremor, and other treatable but only minimally impairing conditions. Hence, "their date books are sprinkled with doctor's appointments; they carry a packet of their medicines in their pockets; their night tables are lined with containers for hearing-aids, glasses, and dentures." A defining feature of this type of elder is increases in health care use, but lack of disability.

An example of a robust elder described by Gillick was Mrs. Landsman (a pseudonym), who at age 96 was quite active until she developed anemia, which led to detection of an advanced colorectal cancer. As a competent adult, she had to choose between surgery (and a risk of immediate death) and symptomatic treatment, where the progression of the cancer would ultimately lead to increasing morbidity and disability and later death. Gillick (1994, pp. 55–56) describes Mrs. Landsman's response in this way:

> Mrs. Landsman thought long and hard about the various options. She had no illusions about her own mortality, and in fact was quite ready to depart from this world. But there was one thing she was quite clear about: she did not wish to be a burden to others, nor did she wish to be dependent on others, which she regarded as equivalent. The prospect of repeated visits to the hospital for transfusions or treatment for chest pain or fractures was dismal. The prospect of fading away over an extended period of time, becoming increasingly dependent, was even more unappealing.
>
> Mrs. Landsman opted for surgery. Ironically, an operation that would probably prove to be curative was performed because it provided the best palliation available. The simplest, most humane, and cheapest way to provide comfort for this very elderly woman was to perform major surgery.

Studies suggest that the robust senior is not an uncommon experience. Indeed, 20%–33% of older adults are robust without any chronic disease (Strawbridge, Wallhagan, & Cohen, 2002). An even greater proportion of older adults—perhaps as much as 40%—experience minimal interruption of usual activities and maintain social participation in the face of disease. Seventy-five to 80% of Americans over age 65 report no disability in personal self-maintenance activities, such as bathing or dressing.

The Frail Elder

Gillick (1994, p. 105) describes frail older people as "hav[ing] no one overriding health problem. Instead they suffer from impairments in multiple domains . . . that collectively render them vulnerable to the slightest perturbation."

She describes Mr. Schaeffer, age 83, who had diabetes, hypertension, congestive heart failure, psoriasis, and emphysema. Fatigue and weakness led him to live an increasingly less active life. He was unable to babysit for his grandchild on his own, could not go out unless he had a ride from someone, could not read the newspaper through without falling asleep, and employed a homemaker to do grocery shopping, cooking, laundry, and cleaning. He then developed repeated bouts of pneumonia, which led to repeated hospitalizations. At the hospital he was diagnosed with aortic stenosis, which was treated with a valvuloplasty, but he subsequently developed delirium, lost weight, acquired a nosocomial infection, and became increasingly less mobile. His family then recognized that he could not safely live independently and would not be able to return to his apartment. He became a candidate for the nursing home. He had a cardiac arrest, however, while still in the hospital, which led to the last of his three intubations. This time, however, he could not be revived and died.

These are the prosaic but important details of medical care for the frail elder. They are not glamorous. As Gillick writes, "autobiographical and fictional accounts of aging focus on the drama, but seldom on the prosaic details that make all the difference to the frail older person. I have yet to read a story in which the elderly protagonist describes his intense embarrassment upon suddenly developing incontinence, only to be rescued by a geriatric consultant who determines that his problem has been caused by the new blood pressure medicine he has been taking" (1994, p. 106).

Efforts to establish frailty as a phenotype have resulted in an explosion of research on this topic in recent years. One proposed operationalization consists of the following components: shrinking (unintentional loss of 10 lbs or more), weakness (scores in the lowest 20% of the distribution of grip-strength values), poor endurance (reports of exhaustion when performing daily activities), slowness (scores in the lowest 20% of the distribution of timed gait speeds), and low activity (scores in the lowest 20% of activity profiles, as determined by estimated expenditure of calories). Older adults with three or more of these characteristics are considered to be frail (Fried et al., 2001). This concept overlaps with, but is distinct from the notion of disability, more generally defined as a gap between an individual's capacity and the challenges of his or her environment. Estimates of frailty in clinically based samples have ranged from about 12% to 16% (Rockwood, Andrew, & Mitnitski, 2007).

The Elder With Dementia

Dementing disease is one of the central challenges of public health and aging. Although many diseases cause the global, progressive, irreversible impairment in cognitive function that we call "dementia," the most prevalent sources are vascular disease and Alzheimer's disease. These diseases of later life, for the most part, pose extreme challenges to caregiving families and medical providers. As Gillick remarks,

> The dilemma of when to stop treating, or when to provide less than maximally intensive care, is never more poignant than with the elderly person who has Alzheimer's disease or one of several types of dementia. Dementia, the gradual loss of multiple facets of the mind such as memory, language, and judgment, robs people of their ability to understand what is happening to them when they get sick. Illness becomes as incomprehensible to these patients as its treatment. Moreover, the future they are vouchsafed if they are successfully cured of pneumonia or appendicitis is one of relentless decline. If they live long enough, they will likely pass from a state of mild forgetfulness to apathy and incontinence, and ultimately to a bed-bound existence. (1994, p. 17)

Older adults with dementia have varied symptoms, which may include memory loss, difficulty understanding or using words, inability to carry out motor activities (despite physical ability to do so), and failure to identify or recognize objects. Dementia is often accompanied by behavioral disturbances (e.g., wandering, pacing, and repetitive questions). Although approximately 10% of adults aged 71 and older have frank dementia, as many as 22.2% in addition may have cognitive impairment short of dementia (Plassman et al., 2008; see Chapter 8). Most seniors who meet criteria for dementia are cared for in the home by relatives or paid caregivers and the remainder live in residential care settings (e.g., nursing homes, assisted living facilities).

The Dying Elder

"Late life," as the term implies, is the period of life closest to death. Although it is not always clear when the dying process starts (and, as a result, when medical care goals should shift further toward palliation), care of the dying elder is a key component of geriatric care and an important consideration in public health and aging.

One challenge in meeting the needs of the dying elder is the lack of realistic appraisal of the risk of dying by patients and their families, which, in some cases, unfortunately is encouraged by clinicians. These unrealistic appraisals may lead to poor choices in medical care, such as recourse to invasive procedures that have little or no chance of success. Clinicians may be as uncomfortable with end-of-life choices as patients, but with proper communication of risk, this situation can change. As Gillick (1994, p. 80) writes, "if instead of being told that they had a 10% or 20% chance of survival with ICU care, patients were told they had an 80% to 90% chance of dying with ICU treatment, and a 99% chance of dying without it . . . how many in fact would choose the ICU?" This is an interesting question worth a study in itself (see Chapter 10).

A second challenge for this type of elder is the issue of control and autonomy at the end of life, which may be complicated further by mental health issues. Gillick describes Mrs. Renan, who is dying of cancer. Mrs. Renan sought physician-assisted suicide and would not accept reasonable medical management of her condition, which included blood transfusions and easily available palliative treatments. "She accused me of abandoning her because I said I would not and could not give her a lethal injection." Gillick distinguishes reasonable medical care goals, such as strategies to reduce disability and relieve symptoms, and inappropriate goals, such as elimination of existential suffering.

> Was I a failure as a doctor if I could not cure . . . her overwhelming sadness and rage over aging? My role was supportive. I could try to make Claire as functional as possible during her final months or years. This entailed such things as blood transfusions to improve her strength and prescrib-

ing a wheelchair to help her maintain some degree of mobility. I could try to make her as comfortable as possible by treating her arthritic pain with medication and trying to regulate her bowels with a judiciously selected combination of stool softeners and cathartics. I could provide relief by simply being there, by acknowledging her misery and promising not to abandon her. But [I do not] think that physicians must at all costs obliterate suffering, if necessary by causing death. (Gillick, 1994, p. 90)

Nearly 2 million older adults die each year. So, liberally, 5%–7% of the older population faces end-of-life issues in a given year. Trajectories to death also vary widely. Lynn and Adamson (2003) describe three prototypical descents experienced by Medicare beneficiaries: a short period of decline, typical of many cancers; a longer period of limitations with multiple exacerbations and sudden death, typical of organ system failure; and a slow, prolonged decline typical of dementia, disabling stroke, and frailty. Lunney, Lynn, and Hogan (2002) have found that about one fifth of deaths in a given year occur in a manner consistent with the first trajectory, another one fifth follow the second profile, and as many as two fifths follow the prolonged trajectory.

Trajectories of dying are an active area of research. Could the type of trajectory influence the kind of dying one faces (such as death at home or in the hospital, or perhaps the likelihood of transitions between health care settings)? Or could the type of trajectory influence expectations for dying and decision making at the end of life? Both questions fall within a growing subdomain of public health and aging, namely, the public health impact of the end of life (Anderson & Smith, 2005; GAO, 1998).

The Compensating, Adaptive Elder

Cutting across these archetypes of aging is the reality of being old, the need to maintain function and accomplish daily goals in the face of declining abilities, often pressing symptoms of chronic disease, and awareness in some cases of impending death. As in people with disabilities or younger people facing life-limiting illness, older people alter daily tasks, rely on spared abilities to compensate for deficits, and selectively invest physical, cognitive, and affective effort to maximize the likelihood of social participation and activity. The psychological analog to such modification of daily life in the face of declining abilities is "selective optimization with compensation" (Baltes & Baltes, 1990).

Research in compensation is still in its infancy. Baltes and colleagues have shown for psychological processes that even quite frail older people are active in the management of dependency. They may accept personal self-maintenance care to allow them the physical strength or energy to accomplish more valued activities, such as social activity or leisure pursuits. Unable to go outside or even ambulate indoors, the elder with mobility limitation may seek a strategic position in a home, perhaps a chair with a commanding view. This too can be considered a selective investment of resources to compensate for a deficit and in this way optimize experience in the face of disability. Recourse to personal assistance equipment is a similar accommodation. The essence of selective optimization with compensation is development of strategies that allow older adults to retain control or accomplish some goal in the setting of declining ability.

Researchers are just beginning to generalize this paradigm to physical function (Agree & Freedman, 2000; Verbrugge & Sevak, 2002; Weiss, Hoenig, & Fried, 2007). For example, it stands to reason that the elder with lower extremity disability may rely more heavily on preserved upper body function to accomplish daily tasks. The elder able to do so will likely report less disability and perhaps better mental health, signs of effective adaptation. At the microscopic ergonomic level, people make such accommodations all the time, changing the way in which they reach or grasp in the face of arthritic pain, making lists or using elaborate mnemonics in the case of memory impairment, or avoiding hills or simply slowing down in the case of dyspnea. Compensatory processes may also cross physiological domains. In our experience, elders with severe physical deficits but preserved cognition manage to figure out ways to complete physical activities.

Studying compensation would probably be valuable, because it may be possible to teach such optimization strategies. In fact, Clark and colleagues have completed a series of occupational therapy interventions designed to do just this and have shown benefit in mental health, self-efficacy, quality of life, and range of activities accomplished. They have taken the research further to examine the physical and neuroendocrine effects (Clark et al., 1997) of such compensatory efforts.

Table 1.1 summarizes these types of aging experience and goals of medical care and public health. We will return to these issues in later chapters.

Table 1.1

TYPES OF AGING EXPERIENCE AND GOALS OF MEDICAL CARE AND PUBLIC HEALTH

TYPE OF ELDER	GOAL OF MEDICAL CARE	GOAL OF PUBLIC HEALTH
Robust	Life prolongation, cure	Prevention of frailty and disability
Demented	Maximization of function, palliation	Prevention of excess morbidity; excellent custodial care
Dying	Palliation ("upstreamed")	Reduction of isolation, maximization of choice
Frail	Upper bound: maximum medically tolerable intervention Lower bound: medical care based on best interest of patient	Environmental modification to reduce task demand; rehabilitation to increase capacity by developing spared abilities
Compensating	Occupational, physical, speech therapy; rehabilitation; cognitive remediation	Provision of appropriate aging services; promotion of maximally integrated setting

HEALTHY VS. SUCCESSFUL VS. OPTIMAL AGING

It is salutary to try and explain the functions of public health and aging to the audience for our efforts, the people who have experienced old age and who confront the risk of frailty and chronic disease. One case will speak for many. Hannah is a 92-year-old Israeli. She has lived on a kibbutz, a collective settlement, for over 50 years, a hard but supportive environment for older persons that has been shown to confer important health advantages (Walter-Ginzburg, Blumstein, & Guralnik, 2004). At age 92, she was quite frail and required 24-hour personal care assistance, which was provided by the kibbutz. She used a walker for indoor mobility, left her small home to go outside only rarely, and required help with dressing, toileting, and meal preparation. She had given up housework, shopping, and travel. In contrast, she took medications and used the telephone independently, kept track of her affairs quite efficiently, and, despite pain from osteoporosis and some dyspnea from a heart condition, appeared to be active within her home.

She asked one of us (SA) what public health could do for her and whether she was an example of healthy aging. Put on the spot, I first asked her about her health. She explained that she suffered from many chronic conditions: heart disease, hypertension, osteoporosis, osteoarthritis, kyphoscoliosis, diabetes, and hearing and vision loss. She needed to take 10 different medicines daily, from digoxin to diuretics. What could I do for her, she wanted to know, and what could she do to promote healthy aging? I then asked if she found her days more or less satisfying and interesting. "Oh yes," she said, "I am always reading, I hear from my daughter and grandchildren on the telephone everyday, I make sure I check off medicines and meals on my chart throughout the day, and people come and visit all the time. I enjoy some of the shows on television, especially basketball, and make sure I watch the news everyday."

"You mean you find each day satisfying despite your poor health?"

"Of course."

"Well, then," I said, "I would say you are a very good example of healthy aging. Public health could learn from you. How is it that your days are so full and satisfying despite all the illness and pills?"

"My mind is clear, I have the help I need, and I still can appreciate books, friends and neighbors, and my children and grandchildren. But are you sure there is nothing else I should be doing?"

I demurred. Aside from checking for adverse effects from polypharmacy and perhaps some minor environmental modifications of the home, this 92-year-old serves as an excellent illustration of one kind of healthy aging: high risk of poor health and disability typical of very old age, but also engagement in daily projects, expert in self-care and disease management, maximally supported to promote independence in the face of frailty, well-connected to family and community, funny and feisty.

Indeed it is useful to contrast the notion of "healthy aging" with the perhaps more popularized notion of "successful aging." Rowe and Kahn (1987) define the latter as consisting of three elements: absence of disease and the risk factors for disease, maintenance of physical and cognitive abilities, and engagement in productive activities. They viewed the three elements as roughly hierarchical: absence of disease allows maintenance of physical and cognitive skill, and preservation of these skills in turn allows engagement in productive activity. Their key insight was recognition of variation in aging, which allows us to raise the bar for goals and expectations about health in old age. If successful aging is possible, then we can aim higher than "usual aging." They stress that aging is more than disease and disability, and that there is more to successful aging than avoiding disease and disability. In their view, successful aging includes avoiding disease and disability, which may involve interventions that enhance cognitive and physical function. This may also require that we develop a society that provides individuals opportunities of continuing engagement in life.

Rowe and Kahn (1987) did not specify what proportion of older people met this definition of successful aging, or, more critically, what proportion, given any particular age stratum, would be a reasonable goal for public health. Nor did they try to operationalize the three criteria. Attempts to use existing measures to partition the older population in this way (and relaxing criteria to stress minimal rather than absence of disease or disability) show that only 20%–33% of community-resident older Americans meet the criteria for successful aging (Strawbridge et al., 2002).

Other working definitions of successful aging have been proposed that are closer to the notion of healthy aging. An alternative approach stresses minimal interruption of usual activities and maintenance of social participation in the face of disease. By this criterion a majority of older adults, including the 92-year-old described earlier, could be considered successful agers. As we have seen, one mechanism for this preservation of activity and social participation is "selective optimization with compensation," that is, doing well with remaining strengths by recruiting preserved abilities to compensate, when possible, for areas of weakness (Baltes & Carstenson, 1996).

Most recently, researchers have recognized that neither "successful aging" nor "healthy aging" are the right terms. Elders who reach old age with chronic conditions or who develop disabilities would be considered examples of "failed" aging by using the first term. Likewise, because most seniors have some declines in function and chronic disease (or ultimately will develop them), the focus on "healthy aging" narrowly construed misses the point of maintenance of function and well-being despite these common features of old age. Perhaps the better term is "optimal aging," defined as a range of values for clinical indicators that we would expect more in people of younger ages. Thus, a 90-year-old with a gait speed typical of a 75-year-old can be said to have met the optimal aging criterion in this one key phenotype.

The focus on optimal aging is superior to prior approaches because it is norm-driven and uses chronological age as a criterion. It also allows an individual to age optimally in one area but perhaps not in another (although in practice these will be highly correlated). An elder at age 85 can have memory performance 1.5 SD above the norm for her age and education, making her equivalent in this domain to a 75-year-old. This is optimal aging in a cognitive domain. The same may be true for grip strength, light-touch pressure sensation, visual contrast sensitivity, insulin or glucose chemistries, bone mineral density, systolic blood pressure, or wound healing. We prefer this approach because it opens the door to more reasonable endpoints in clinical trials and better characterization of the health of older populations.

Such notions of optimal or healthy aging are important to keep in mind in articulating the boundaries of public health and aging. Assuring conditions for health promotion in late life must be considered along with conditions to foster successful adaptation to states of ill health. Both are reasonable goals for public health promotion, and the mix of emphasis on the two may change with age. That is, while assurance of the conditions for health should be the goal at all ages, with very old age the more critical goal may be assuring conditions to promote successful compensation in the face of disease and disability. Our 92-year-old *kibbutznik* failed all three of the Kahn and Rowe criteria but had successfully optimized her remaining abilities to live well.

HOW THE FIRST 50 YEARS MATTER FOR HEALTH RISKS IN THE SECOND 50 YEARS: THREE ILLUSTRATIONS

Gillick's portraits provide rich and varied snapshots of later life. Yet, as we explained earlier in this chapter, aging begins at birth and continues throughout the life course. How these earlier life experiences influence outcomes in later life is a growing area of interest. Hayward and Gorman (2004), for example, have referred to this phenomenon as the "long arm of childhood" in their study demonstrating important childhood influences on male mortality in later life.

It is challenging to study the ways in which health and risk behaviors in the first half of life may affect health in the second 50 years and even more difficult to generalize public health applications from such studies. Imagine the definitive cohort study that follows prospectively an entire birth cohort until each and every member dies or reaches very old age. Such a study would lend itself to precise measurement of risk factors in early life and allow researchers to relate them to outcomes in later life. Despite decades of gerontological research, we still do not have a prospective cohort study that has observed people from birth to death. Even if we did have such a cohort, what we could learn from studying such a cohort that would apply to today's public health system is unclear, because the members of the cohort would have been born over 100 years ago.

In practice, most gerontological research cohorts usually begin at age 65, or perhaps at preretirement, at age 50 or 55. Therefore, we often do not have direct evidence of health at earlier ages. As a result, we are forced to use proxy measures, or sometimes retrospective measures, to summarize health and risk experience in the first half of life. These proxy measures typically include such factors as:

- Occupation, to assess environmental exposures during work years
- Education and literacy, to assess cognitive engagement over the life span
- Parent occupation and education, to assess perinatal and childhood conditions
- Recollections of childhood health and experiences
- Household income, to assess access to health services over the life span
- Birthplace, to assess environment and access to health care in migrating populations
- Birth weight and stature, to assess pre- and postnatal nutritional status
- Race and ethnicity, to assess the effects of culture and potentially restricted access to health services

Recent progress in molecular genetics, environmental health, and imaging technologies now allows derivation of biological indicators, in some cases, for these lifelong factors. For example, some genes, such as APOE, are more common in particular racial or ethnic groups. If a sociocultural group is more at risk of a disease associated with this gene, such as a cardiovascular condition or Alzheimer's disease, we can now begin to separate sociocultural and genetic factors. Likewise, long-term environmental exposures leave a DNA signature, just as long-term cognitive engagement, evident in educational attainment and literacy, may be visible in functional magnetic resonance images.

We turn now to case studies that illustrate well the different legacies from the first 50 years that affect the health resources older adults have when they enter later life. These examples also show some of the difficulties involved in public health research, where biological and clinical factors are often confounded with socioeconomic status. The first two focus on relationships over the life course at the individual level, and the second brings a population-level perspective.

Entry Into Late Life With Lower Cognitive Reserve

African Americans face a higher risk of Alzheimer's disease (AD) than White Americans. This difference remains when we stratify samples by *APOE* e4 status, a well validated risk factor for Alzheimer's disease. Figure 1.2 compares the incidence of AD in Whites, African Americans, and Hispanic Americans living in northern Manhattan, New York City. Only people with the e3/e3 variant of *APOE* (the so-called wild type) are included, thus removing the effect of this genetic risk factor. The cumulative incidence curves in the figure plot the risk by age in the three race-ethnicity groups. As in all incidence studies, people included in the analysis were free of the disease initially, and all were followed up at regular intervals with a common cognitive assessment battery to identify the age at which people first met criteria for AD.

As the figure shows, minorities were significantly more likely to meet criteria for AD. By age 75, 2% of the Whites and 9% of the minorities developed the disease. By age 80, approximately 9% of the Whites and 21% of the minorities met AD criteria. These large differences in incidence persisted even with statistical control for differences between the race-ethnicity groups in a great variety of risk factors for AD, such as years of school, family history of AD, number of comorbid chronic disease conditions, and behaviors such as smoking and head injury. Tang and colleagues (1998) also recalculated incidence by use of a stricter definition of dementia to identify only clear and obvious cases of AD. This strategy eliminated more mild forms of AD as "cases" and, as a result, also should have helped to eliminate subtle diagnostic biases, either from clinicians interpreting cognitive tests or from the tests themselves, and in this way to reduce any differential misclassification. Even with this conservative approach to diagnosis, differences between the race-ethnicity groups persisted.

Chapter 1 Introducing Public Health and Aging 27

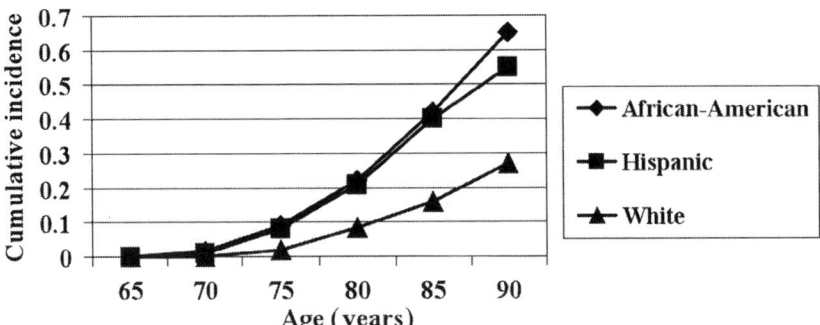

Figure 1.2 Cumulative risk of AD, by race-ethnicity, limited to APOE e3/3.

Source: From "The APOE-Epsilon4 Allele and the Risk of Alzheimer Disease Among African Americans, Whites, and Hispanics," by M. X. Tang et al., 1998, *Journal of the American Medical Association, 279*, Table 1. Copyright © (1998) American Medical Association. All rights reserved.

These differences in the risk of AD raise important questions. Do we overdiagnose minorities (and if so, why?), or do we underdiagnose Whites (and again, if so, why?). Graphically, is the cumulative incidence curve for the minorities too high, or is the cumulative incidence curve for Whites too low? Why should minorities be at greater risk for developing AD? Is it because they enter later life with previously poorer abilities, so that they start follow-up at age 65 or 70 closer to the threshold of the low cognitive ability used to define AD? Or do they enter late life with abilities similar to Whites, but decline at a faster rate in old age? The first factor suggests an effect in the first 50 years of life; the second implies an effect in the second half of life.

We investigated this issue in a related sample of 871 older adults drawn from the same community and assessed with the same clinical battery and diagnostic paradigm. We selected all people who had at least three cognitive assessments, where the AD diagnosis, if made for a respondent, was made at the last of the series of assessments. Of the 871 people, 138 met criteria for AD at their last assessment, whereas the remainder never met criteria for AD.

To assess whether the race-ethnicity groups entered old age with different cognitive resources, we examined scores on the Selective Reminding Test, a test of memory, at baseline, that is, when no one had yet met criteria for dementia. The test asks respondents to repeat a list of 12 words over six trials, for a maximum score of 72 and minimum of 0. Mean scores at baseline were significantly lower among minorities. If we divide the distribution into tertiles (upper third, middle third, lower third), the lower third included scores with a range from 8 to 34. Of Whites 16.3% scored in the lowest tertile, but 32.4% of African Americans and 44.4% of Hispanics scored in this range. This difference strongly supports the claim of earlier life events as a predictor of a key later life outcome. Minority elders enter later life with poorer memory scores and, hence, less cognitive reserve.

By contrast, the slope of memory score change over the serial assessments, that is, the mean rate of decline, was not significantly different across the three race-ethnicity groups. Age, education, and initial memory score were all independently associated with rate of decline in memory performance, but in a regression model that included these factors, race-ethnicity was not significantly associated with rate of decline. Thus, cognitive performance in minorities did not decline at a faster rate. Baseline differences, differences that predate old age, seem to be responsible for the higher risk of AD among minorities. Of course, poorer memory performance at baseline very likely reflects an early stage of disease progression, prodromal AD. But this too is consistent with earlier life experience as the source of greater risk of AD in later life.

Entry Into Late Life With Differences in Physical Reserve

Rantanen and colleagues (1999) examined a cohort of men aged 45–68 and found that grip strength at this age was a strong predictor of disability 25 years later. These men, all from the Honolulu Heart Program—Asia Aging Study, were first assessed in 1965–1968 and were reassessed between 1991 and 1993, when participants were 71–93 years old. Grip strength is correlated with strength in other muscle groups and for this reason is considered a good indicator of overall strength. Grip strength performance was assessed with a handheld dynamometer, and hand strength at midlife was categorized into low (<37 kg), middle (37–42 kg), and high (>42 kg) performance tertiles.

Men with low performance in midlife were significantly more likely to report disability in late life. These men reported nearly twice as much disability as men in the upper tertile in doing heavy household work (25% vs. 14%), walking (26% vs. 15%), bathing (8% vs. 3%), as well as a variety of other indicators of disability and functional limitation (i.e., walking speed, ability to rise from a chair). Men in the middle tertile fell between these two groups in risk of disability in late life. The increased risk of disability in old age associated with low grip strength in midlife persisted in regression models that controlled for age, height, weight, education, occupation, smoking, physical activity, and chronic conditions at the examination in which disability status was established.

This finding is extremely important. "Muscle strength is found to track over the life span: those who had higher grip strength during midlife remained stronger than others in old age" (Rantanen et al., 1999). For this reason, these men entered late life with a greater reserve in strength, and this reserve helped forestall onset of disability. Rantanen and colleagues mention a number of alternative hypotheses for this finding, which are also of note: (1) grip strength may be a marker of physical activity, which may itself prevent disability; (2) low grip strength may reflect early disease processes that later progress and cause disability; and (3) grip strength may be related to motivation to stay fit and through this mechanism lower the risk of disability in late life. Each of these hypotheses merits investigation, but all suggest the critical role of health factors in midlife as predictors of late-life outcomes.

It turns out, as well, that grip strength in midlife is related to birth weight. In the UK Medical Research Council National Survey of Health and Development, 2,815 men and 2,547 women born in 1946 were observed through 1999, when they were 53 years old (Kuh et al., 2002). Men and women in the highest fifth of the distribution of birth weight had 10% greater grip strength at age 53, compared with people in the lowest birth weight group. A 1-kg increase in birth weight was associated with a 1.9-kg increase in grip strength for men and a 1.2-kg increase for women 53 years later. This relationship persisted even with control for weight and height and "suggest[s] the importance of prenatal influences on muscle development that have persisting consequences through to later adulthood."

Thus, grip strength in middle age is related, at least in part, to prenatal environment. And grip strength in midlife is related to disability in late life. These investigations represent a rare case in which a single important risk factor or health indicator has been investigated across the whole life span and related to outcomes at different points in the life span. They suggest the unity of the life span, where a risk factor acquired at the earliest ages is expressed in different ways across the life span. More research of this type will be required if we are to understand health outcomes in late life.

Early and Midlife Influences on Late-Life Disability Trends

The prevalence of activity limitations in later life has declined in the United States over the past 25 years. Efforts to understand why this is so have been hampered until recently by the inability to sort out factors that occur in the early, intermediate, and late phases of the life course (Schoeni, Freedman, & Martin, 2008). A study analyzing survey data from the 1995–2004 Health and Retirement Study (HRS) sheds light on this question by sorting out the influence of early and midlife factors on recent late-life activity limitation trends (Freedman, Grafova, Schoeni, & Rogowski, 2008).

The HRS is a national study designed to provide both snapshots of the experience of adults aged 50 and older in the United States and dynamic assessments of changes as individuals age. Respondents are selected in such a way (with a known probability of selection) that responses can be weighted to reflect national experience. More than 20,000 individuals aged 50 and older are observed over time, with individuals newly turning 50–55 years of age added every 6 years.

In this analysis, the samples were limited to between 4,500 and 4,700 persons aged 75 and older in 1995, 1998, 2000, 2002, and 2004. Measures of activity limitations included both difficulty with activities of daily living (ADLs, e.g., bathing, dressing, grooming, using toilet) and with instrumental activities of daily living (IADLs, e.g., managing money, using the telephone, light cleaning, managing medications). Early-life measures included self-reported race-ethnicity; recollections of region of birth, mother's education, childhood socioeconomic status, and childhood self-rated health; and an estimate of having lower than average peak stature, obtained by adjusting initial reports of current height. In addition, three indicators of midlife were included: completed education; whether the respondent was a veteran; and lifetime occupation.

Between 1995 and 2004, the profile of the older population changed in many ways. Reports of difficulty with ADLs declined significantly from 30.2% in 1995 to 26.0% in 2004. There were also fewer reports of smoking, increases in reports of many common chronic conditions, including obesity and hearing problems, and improvements in self-rated vision. In addition, more older adults were classified in the highest levels of income and wealth.

The profile of early and midlife factors among those very old adults also shifted during this period. For example, older adults in 2004 reported more years of school completed for themselves and their mothers and better health in childhood. In 2004 they were also more likely to have worked in a white-collar or pink-collar occupation, and to be a veteran. The question is whether these shifts in early and midlife factors can account for the changes observed in the prevalence of activity limitations in late life.

With use of multinomial logistic regression techniques our study demonstrated that early-life factors were independent predictors of late-life disability. For example, respondents who rated their childhood health as fair or poor had an increased odds (1.3 times) of reporting limitations in ADLs in later life compared with those who reported excellent childhood health. And respondents who had service sector and secretarial occupations had an increased odds of IADL limitations compared with those in white collar professional and managerial positions. These findings persisted even after controlling for other early-life, midlife, and contemporaneous factors.

Moreover, shifts in the older population with respect to education, mothers' education, health during childhood, and lifetime occupation all contributed to the declines in the prevalence of ADL limitations. Improvements in late-life vision and increases in wealth also appeared to contribute to the declines, but reports of increased chronic conditions in late-life offset these gains. Analysis of changes in ADL onset and recovery over the time period suggested that early and midlife factors contributed, along with late-life factors, to U.S. late-life disability trends, mainly through their influence on the onset of, rather than recovery from, limitation.

As with any study, this analysis had limitations worth reviewing because they highlight the difficulty in conducting research on ways in which the first 50 years of life influence the latter 50 years. Although rich in details about current health and economic status, some of the earlier life measures used were less than ideal. For example, lifetime occupation (based on work histories) could not be ascertained for a significant portion of the sample, and measures of childhood socioeconomic status and health relied on long-term memory. Measures of midlife health were also not available. And because the HRS began in the 1990s, only a decade's worth of trends could be assessed (at least thus far).

What are the public health implications of such findings? One certainly cannot go back and intervene in the early-life circumstances of today's oldest members of society. Rather, the findings are instructive in what they suggest about the persistence of early and midlife effects on late-life activity limitations. The health and economic circumstances of today's children and adults can have a profound influence on the health and functioning of the nation's future elders. In other words, the target of public health and aging efforts is not just the older adults of today but the children and adults who are the future elders.

THE DOMAINS OF PUBLIC HEALTH AND HEALTHY AGING

We are now ready to address the domains of public health and aging. As mentioned earlier, the majority—although certainly not all—of older adults have already developed chronic disease and many have developed disability, frailty, and cognitive impairment. Hence, the aims of public health in an aging society arguably go well beyond creating circumstances that support health and prevent disease and injury. Instead, the overarching aim of public health and aging is to promote the development and maintenance of optimal physical, mental, and social well-being and function, irrespective of acquired disease. Examples of what public health does to promote healthy aging are provided in Box 1.3.

The true test of this approach to public health and aging is whether it is broad enough to meet the needs of each of the illustrative faces of aging described earlier (see Table 1.1). Recall the robust elder with chronic disease. For those meeting the criteria of robust aging, health promotion and disease prevention may be ample, but those with chronic disease need additional attention to disease management and prevention of disability. For the frail elder, the public health goal is not solely to slow progression of disease but to maximize function and well-being. This typically takes two forms: environmental modification programs to reduce task demands and rehabilitation to increase capacity and adapt spared abilities. For the elder with dementia, the public health goals include excellent supportive care that addresses both quality of care and quality of life, support of informal caregivers, and, when possible, physical and cognitive remediation. For the subset of the population who are dying, public health goals may depend on the nature and course of the trajectory (Lynn & Adamson, 2003), but, in all cases, maximizing well-being and providing the opportunity for patient and family to experience a "good death" are of interest. For all groups, support for compensatory strategies is appropriate. These draw on the allied health and rehabilitation fields (occupational, physical, and speech therapy; physical medicine), nursing, social work care management, and new specialties such as certified driving rehabilitation specialists, doula support for dying, and cognitive remediation for patients with Parkinson's and stroke.

Box 1.3

EXAMPLES OF WHAT PUBLIC HEALTH DOES TO PROMOTE HEALTHY AGING

1. Prevent epidemics and the spread of disease
   - Influenza immunization
   - Screening for chronic disease
2. Protect against environmental hazards
   - Recognition and reduction of environmental health risks in the homes of older adults
   - Development of aging-friendly communities that promote physical activity in later life
3. Prevent injuries
   - Fall prevention programs
   - Wander prevention programs for dementia care
   - Interventions to reduce motor vehicle crashes among older adults
4. Promote and encourage healthy behaviors and mental health
   - Promotion of later life engagement (senior centers, life-long learning, volunteerism)
   - Enhancement of self-management of chronic disease
5. Respond to disasters and assist communities in recovery
   - Development and implementation response strategies that address unique concerns of older adults
6. Ensure the quality and accessibility of health services
   - Development of quality indicators for aging experiences (home care, assisted living, end-of-life care, nursing home care, etc.)
   - Training of medical professionals about aging experiences.

How does all this differ from current approaches? How does the field of public health and aging, as we envision it, differ from clinical geriatrics and gerontology? These differences should now be clear. Clinical geriatrics stresses medical management of chronic disease and rehabilitation in the face of disabilities related to these conditions (and now, increasingly, "prehabilitation" to delay the onset of disability due to disease and frailty) (Gill et al., 2002). Wallace and Gutierrez (2005) explain that, unlike clinical geriatrics, public health and aging places emphasis on prevention, proactive measures to preserve and promote health, rather than on the reactive treatment of disease. Moreover, public health focuses on the population rather than on the individual, and its programs and policies therefore address the community as a whole.

Public health and aging also overlaps with social and clinical gerontology. Like public health and aging, gerontology is concerned with the study of human aging, and involves attention not just to health, but also to the social and policy context of aging. Like geriatrics, gerontology mostly focuses on individuals rather than the experience of populations. Moreover, public health and aging is explicit in its use of population-based public health tools to address primary and secondary prevention of frailty, disease, and disability in later life. For these reasons, public health and aging represents an emerging field with a distinct focus, along with developing tools and study designs that we describe in later chapters.

POPULATION AGING AND THE GOALS OF PUBLIC HEALTH: BEYOND DISEASE PREVENTION AND HEALTH PROMOTION

As we have discussed, the goal of public health is to create circumstances under which a population is likely to achieve health. More commonly, this aim is referred to as "health promotion and disease prevention." Here, we review this goal and take up a question that is implicit in our approach to public health and aging. In an aging society, where an increasing proportion of the population survives into older ages, is the goal of health promotion and disease prevention sufficient? We argue that the focus in some cases should be broader to encompass *promotion of function*. Promoting health and promoting function may not always correspond in the real world of imperfect screening tests, invasive diagnostic technologies (whose harm is often underappreciated), otherwise successful treatments that may yet put patients at risk for new medical challenges (such as methicillin-resistant *Staphylococcus aureus* [MRSA] or *Clostridium difficile* infection in the hospital setting), and a variety of other tough calls. These challenges may go in the other direction too, as when an apparently more invasive attempt at preserving health may actually offer greater palliative and functional benefit for the person at the end of life (see Chapter 11). Reframing the challenge as "maximizing function and well-being" broadens the goals of public health but is critical, we would argue, in the case of aging populations.

Another way to frame the question is to ask how well public health's concern for people with disabilities subsumes the needs of older people. Are current approaches to disability a reasonable model for public health approaches to aging (or for thinking about aging more generally)? In this approach, aging can be seen as an accumulation of disabilities, and public health would accordingly aim to reduce the probability of disability at every age and lessen its impact on the quality of life. As we examine sources of disability in old age (in later chapters devoted to physical, cognitive, and affective function), the relevance of disability will become apparent. The difference between current public health approaches to disability and aging viewed as an accumulation of disabilities may lie in the type and generality of disability in old age (produced, for example, by slowing across multiple physiological domains) and the challenge of separating primary sources of disability and secondary conditions related to such disability among older people.

To think through these issues in light of population aging, it is helpful first to return to the elements of public health. "Health promotion" refers to activities that are not specific to any particular diseases but contribute to lowering the likelihood of disease. For example, maintaining a healthy weight, getting regular physical activity, eating a balanced diet, maintaining cognitive vitality, and managing stress would all be considered health promotion activities. These activities reduce the risk of disease and offer more immediate benefits for function. At the community level, cleaning up toxins in a neighborhood and putting in a park or walking paths would also be considered health promotion activities because they allow health-promoting behaviors, such as physical activity. Mounting evidence suggests that older adults benefit from health promotion activities, just as middle-aged and younger adults do. The gain is in lower risk of future disease and more immediate benefit in function.

"Disease prevention" includes primary, secondary, and tertiary efforts. Primary prevention efforts seek *to arrest disease processes by reducing or eliminating risk factors for disease*. Efforts of this kind include vaccination (for flu and pneumonia and now zoster), drug therapies (statins, anti-inflammatory agents, chemoprophylaxis for heart disease and possibly dementia), smoking cessation, physical therapy "prehabilitation," and assistive technology (hip protectors, grab bars, and other environmental modifications to prevent falls, for example).

Secondary prevention involves *early detection and treatment of disease to minimize morbidity and risk of disability*. These efforts involve increasing appropriate screening to detect disease at an early, asymptomatic stage. Examples of screening include checks for bone mineral density for osteoporosis, glucose metabolism for diabetes, cognitive assessment for dementia, mental health assessment to detect depression, and hypertension screening.

Tertiary prevention seeks *appropriate disease management to reduce disability*. Examples of tertiary prevention include education to support patient self-care, telemedicine to monitor clinical chemistries or heart rhythm, "lifeline" devices that allow elders to report medical emergencies, podiatry in diabetics, inhalers for pulmonary disease, and perhaps most critically a single medical provider to coordinate care.

These health promotion and disease prevention goals have been extended to people with congenital or degenerative conditions who may already face disease and disability. Here, the public health goal is to minimize the risk of "secondary conditions," conditions that may come about as the result of disability. For example, the Centers for Disease Control and Prevention (CDC) *Healthy People 2010* states:

> The health promotion and disease prevention needs of people with disabilities are not nullified because they are born with an impairing condition or have experienced a disease or injury that has long-term consequences. People with disabilities have increased health concerns and susceptibility to secondary conditions. Having a long-term condition increases the need for health promotion that can be medical, physical, social, emotional, or societal. (CDC, 2009)

How do we apply disease prevention and health promotion goals to the older adult with frailty, dementia, or terminal illness? Promoting function is a major goal of *Healthy People 2010*, which explicitly aims to increase years of healthy life, that is, disability-free years. This emphasis is carried forward in the draft vision for *Healthy People 2020,* which seeks "a society in which all people live long and healthy lives." This vision is echoed in the CDC *State of Health and Aging in America 2007,* which adopts the goal of increasing "the numbers . . . who live longer, high-quality, productive, and independent lives."

Yet, when one looks specifically at elder-specific public health recommendations beyond clinical prevention services, these documents do not say much about promoting function. The *State of Health and Aging in America 2007* offers the following additional calls to action: (a) increase physical activity among older adults by promoting environmental changes, and (b) encourage people to communicate their wishes about end-of-life care. The *Healthy People 2020* Older Adult Workgroup suggests a variety of additional goals and indicators that could be considered:

- Increase the quality of life for those with multiple chronic illnesses
  - Measure frequency and intensity of community supportive services
  - Measure participation in self-management programs
  - Measure use of Medicare prevention benefits and health utilization services
- Increase the percentage of individuals reporting good physical functioning
  - Measure frequency and type of exercise, including regular physical activity, vigorous physical activity, strength and endurance, flexibility, walking for transportation, bicycling for transportation
- Decrease the rate of pressure ulcers and physical restraints in nursing homes
- Decrease preventable hospitalizations of individuals receiving home health care
  - Measure efficiency and effectiveness of transition between levels of care

These are extremely important advances in setting goals for public health and aging. They take us beyond the use of clinical prevention services and a narrow focus on disease prevention to health promotion in the fullest sense as maximization of function and well-being. However, they do not fully connect with the supportive services older adults also need for maximization of function and which, to date, have not made a bridge to public health. We turn to these in Chapter 3.

SUMMARY

Definition of Public Health and Aging. Public health and aging uses the methods and materials of public health to promote healthy aging—that is, to ensure conditions that promote the development and maintenance of optimal physical, cognitive, affective, and social well-being and function in later life. In addition to promoting primary and secondary prevention in old age, and facilitating older adults' adaptation to disease and disability, a central goal for public health and aging is to ensure conditions in the first 50 years of life that will predispose people to live a healthy second 50 years.

Defining Aging. Chronological aging is the passage of time, whereas biological aging or "senescence" involves maturation of cells and physiological systems. Senescence reflects changes that are age dependent, whereas disease represents changes that are age associated because of longer exposures to risks. In practice, senescence and disease are often difficult to distinguish, although public health interventions are currently more readily implemented to address the latter.

Types of Older Adult and Public Health Goals. It is useful to identify different types of "old age." Prominent types in geriatric care include the robust, frail, demented, and dying elder, as well as the compensating, adaptive elder. Just as the goals of medical care will be different for each type of elder, so too will the goals of public health. In the case of robust elders, the majority of whom have some chronic disease, public health goals include preventing frailty and disability. The public health goal for the frail elder is to maximize function. This typically takes two forms: environmental modification to reduce task demand, and rehabilitation to increase capacity and adapt spared abilities. The public health goals for the elder with dementia include excellent supportive care, support of informal caregivers, and, when possible, physical and cognitive remediation. For the dying patient, public health goals include a good death for both patient and family. To support compensation, the allied health specialties are critical.

How the First 50 Years Matter for Health in the Second 50 Years. It is difficult to study the ways in which health and risk behaviors in the first half of life may affect health in the second 50 years. Grip strength illustrates well the unity of the life span with respect to risk factors and later health outcomes. This is a measure of general muscle strength, easily obtained with a hand dynamometer. Grip strength in midlife is related to prenatal environment, and grip strength in midlife is related to disability in late life. These investigations represent a rare case in which a single important risk factor or health indicator has been investigated across the whole life span and related to outcomes at different points in the life span.

Successful vs. Healthy Aging. Rowe and Kahn suggested that successful aging consists of three elements: absence of disease and the risk factors for disease; maintenance of physical and cognitive abilities; and engagement in productive activities. About 20%–33% of older adults meet this definition. In contrast, the aim of public health and aging is healthy aging, that is, ensuring the conditions that allow older adults to develop and maintain optimal physical, mental, and social well-being and function across disease states and across the life span.

The Domains of Public Health and Aging. In practice, the field of public health and aging encompasses a wide variety of programs, services, and research activities. Some are aimed at health promotion and disease prevention in later life and others at self-management among those who have already developed chronic disease. Behavioral interventions that complement clinical care are of interest as are enhancements of the social context of older adults, including those geared to people living in residential or skilled nursing care settings. Development of quality indicators for particular kinds of aging experiences and settings, such as dementia care, nursing home residence, assisted living, home care, and end-of-life care, are important contributions. Programs to promote independence, through use of assistive technologies, and to maximize functioning and well-being more generally also fall in the purview of public health and aging.

Aims of Public Health in an Aging Society. In an aging society, where an increasing share of the population survives into older ages, traditional public health goals may be too narrow to meet the needs of the aged population. Instead, the aim of public health in an aging population is to maximize function and well-being of older adults irrespective of the level of disease or disability.

2 Population Aging: Demographic and Epidemiologic Perspectives

Chapter 1 defined public health's mission as promoting the conditions under which a population can be healthy (IOM, 2002). Although many individuals experience loss of health and functioning as they age, *populations* that age do not necessarily experience worsening health. To comprehend this paradox requires an understanding of what it means for a population to age, under what conditions this phenomenon occurs, and the implications of population aging for a population's health and for the aims of public health.

Population aging occurs when the age distribution of the population shifts toward older ages. The fields of demography and epidemiology offer complementary perspectives on this process. Demography is the study of population dynamics; and an increasingly important subfield, referred to as the demography of aging, emphasizes determinants and consequences of a population's age structure shifting toward older ages (Preston & Martin, 1994). Like demography, epidemiology is a population-focused science, but it emphasizes the distribution of diseases in populations, along with their causes and consequences. The subspecialty known as the epidemiology of aging has a distinctive focus on diseases among older populations (Satariano, 2006). Here, we provide both demographic and epidemiologic perspectives on critical aspects of population aging.

MEASURES OF POPULATION AGING

Projections based on the last Census suggest that in 2010, approximately 40 million people in the United States will be aged 65 or older, accounting for about 13% of the U.S. population (U.S. Census Bureau, 2004a). Over 6 million Americans, 2% of the total population, will be age 85 or older. The centenarian population—individuals ages 100 or older—reached 50,000 in 2000 (Hetzel & Smith, 2001), and given current mortality rates this figure is projected to nearly double approximately every 10 years (Krach & Velkoff, 1999). The median age, defined as the age at which half the population is older and half younger, will be about 37 in 2010. Compared with the world's "oldest" countries (with at least 10% of their population age 65 and older), the United States ranked 41st in 2006 (see Table 2.1). At the top of the list are Japan, Italy, Germany, and Greece, all with at least 19% of the population aged 65 and older.

Table 2.1

POPULATION OF COUNTRIES WITH AT LEAST 10% OF POPULATION AGE 65 AND OVER, 2006

REGION OR COUNTRY	TOTAL	65 AND OVER NUMBER	65 AND OVER PERCENT
Japan	127,464	25,535	20.0
Italy	58,134	11,450	19.7
Germany	82,422	16,018	19.4
Greece	10,688	2,027	19.0
Spain	40,398	7,170	17.7
Sweden	9,017	1,588	17.6
Belgium	10,379	1,809	17.4
Bulgaria	7,385	1,279	17.3
Estonia	1,324	228	17.2
Portugal	10,606	1,822	17.2
Austria	8,193	1,401	17.1

(Continued)

Table 2.1

POPULATION OF COUNTRIES WITH AT LEAST 10% OF POPULATION AGE 65 AND OVER, 2006 (*Continued*)

REGION OR COUNTRY	TOTAL	65 AND OVER NUMBER	PERCENT
Croatia	4,495	754	16.8
Georgia	4,661	768	16.5
France	60,876	9,998	16.4
Latvia	2,275	373	16.4
Ukraine	46,620	7,628	16.4
Finland	5,231	846	16.2
United Kingdom	60,609	9,564	15.8
Slovenia	2,010	315	15.7
Switzerland	7,524	1,171	15.6
Lithuania	3,586	554	15.5
Denmark	5,451	828	15.2
Hungary	9,981	1,518	15.2
Serbia	10,140	1,544	15.2
Belarus	9,766	1,462	15.0
Norway	4,611	683	14.8
Romania	22,304	3,275	14.7
Luxembourg	474	69	14.6
Czech Republic	10,235	1,481	14.5
Bosnia and Herzegovina	4,499	647	14.4
Netherlands	16,491	2,349	14.2
Russia	142,069	20,196	14.2
Malta	400	55	13.7
Montenegro	692	95	13.7
Canada	33,099	4,407	13.3
Poland	38,537	5,128	13.3
Uruguay	3,432	455	13.3
Australia	20,264	2,649	13.1

(*Continued*)

Table 2.1

POPULATION OF COUNTRIES WITH AT LEAST 10% OF POPULATION AGE 65 AND OVER, 2006 (*Continued*)

REGION OR COUNTRY	TOTAL	65 AND OVER NUMBER	PERCENT
Hong Kong S.A.R.	6,940	890	12.8
Puerto Rico	3,928	504	12.8
United States	298,444	37,196	12.5
Slovakia	5,439	653	12.0
New Zealand	4,076	481	11.8
Iceland	299	35	11.7
Cyprus	784	91	11.6
Ireland	4,062	470	11.6
Virgin Islands (U.S.)	109	12	11.2
Armenia	2,976	332	11.1
Macedonia	2,051	225	11.0
Moldova	4,326	465	10.7
Argentina	39,922	4,244	10.6
Cuba	11,383	1,206	10.6
Martinique	436	46	10.6

From Federal Interagency Forum on Aging-Related Statistics, 2006.

Such statistics suggest that the United States has a sizeable population living into what has traditionally been considered old age; however, these statistics say little about whether the population is aging. Demographers define population aging as a *shift in the age distribution of the population toward older ages.* The phenomenon is most often measured by increases in the percentage of the population reaching old age, but can also be captured by changes in a population's distribution across age groups (illustrated by age and sex in a population "pyramid") and by changes in ratios of the older to younger population ("age-dependency" or "support" ratios). By all three standards, the U.S. population is aging and has been for over a century, but the pace has accelerated over the past several decades.

Although some demographers have argued against use of a chronological age to indicate late life (Robine & Michel, 2004), reaching the threshold of normal retirement age—in the United States still age 65 for those born before 1938—is most often synonymous with reaching old age. At the turn of the century only 3 million people—less than 4% of the total population—were age 65 (Federal Interagency Forum on Aging-Related Statistics, 2008). Today, approximately 13% are considered old, and by 2030 the proportion of people in the United States aged 65 and older will approach 20% of the total population (Table 2.2). Other age cutoffs indicate a similar increase. For example, the percentage of the total population aged 85 or older is projected to reach 2.6% (nearly 10 million) in 2030 (U.S. Census Bureau, 2004a).

Population pyramids for the United States in 2010 and 2030 are shown in Figure 2.1. The pyramids depict the number of men (left) and women (right) in millions in each 5-year age group, ordered from lowest to highest. By comparing shapes across the two pyramids, the shifting age distribution toward older ages is readily apparent. These age-sex pyramids are perhaps less of a pyramid than an emerging rectangle or pillar, a typical shape for countries that have already undergone the demographic transition, in which a regime of high mortality and fertility is replaced by

Table 2.2

ESTIMATES AND PROJECTIONS OF THE NUMBER AND PERCENTAGE OF THE U.S. POPULATION AGES 65 AND OLDER AND 85 AND OLDER: 2000–2050 (U.S. CENSUS BUREAU, 2004A)

YEAR	65 AND OVER		85 AND OVER	
	NUMBER	PERCENT	NUMBER	PERCENT
2000	35.0	12.4	4.2	1.5
2010	40.2	13.0	6.1	2.0
2020	54.6	16.3	7.3	2.2
2030	71.5	19.6	9.6	2.6
2040	80.0	20.4	15.4	3.9
2050	86.7	20.6	20.9	5.0

one of low mortality and fertility (see below). The left-hand figure has a bulge in the center, with age groups between 45–49 and 60–64 clearly the most populous. These age strata correspond to the aging baby boom generation, people born in the years 1946–1964. Lower fertility after this period, which continued over the next three decades, has led to fewer people at younger ages and hence absence of a wide base for the pyramid. By 2030, the pyramid will be even more rectangular, with age groups 65 and older nearly as populous as the nonelderly age groups. Projections of developed countries portend that by 2040 the pyramid shape will begin to invert as the age group 80 and older outnumbers all other age groups (Kinsella & He, 2009).

Both pyramids also show the strong preponderance of women over men in later life. Among people aged 65 and older, the sex ratio (number of women for each man) is 1.4; for people aged 85 and older it is 2.5, and for people 100 and older it is 4.0. This asymmetry affects living arrangements and marital status in important ways, leaving older women more likely to live alone, depend on children when frail, and enter assisted living and nursing homes at higher rates than men (for further discussion of long-term care, see Chapter 9).

A shift in age structure is also occurring in many less developed countries. Figure 2.2 shows the projected transformation in age structure underway in Pakistan for the years 2000, 2025, and 2050. In the 25 years separating the first two panels of the figure, the proportion of the population aged 65 and older will rise from 4.1% to 5.6%, 5.8 to 12.0 million people. In this period, life expectancy will also rise from 61.1 to 69.8 years. The major engine of this demographic transformation is declining fertility. In the same period, the number of births per 1,000 women will decline from 32 to 6; and completed fertility will drop from 4.6 children per woman to 2.3 (U.S. Census Bureau, International Data Base, 2002). With fewer children born, the base of the age-sex pyramid shrinks and the mean (or median) age of the population must rise, because people already alive continue to age. If this trend continues, as is expected, most of the world's countries will eventually have an age distribution shaped more like a pillar and less like a pyramid (Kinsella & He, 2009).

Aggregating across the strata of the pyramid gives the size of the older (aged 65 and older) population, or the combined young (ages 0–18) and older populations, relative to people of working age (ages 18–64). These so-called "support" ratios do not actually measure dependency, either in health or economic terms. In fact, only a minority of people

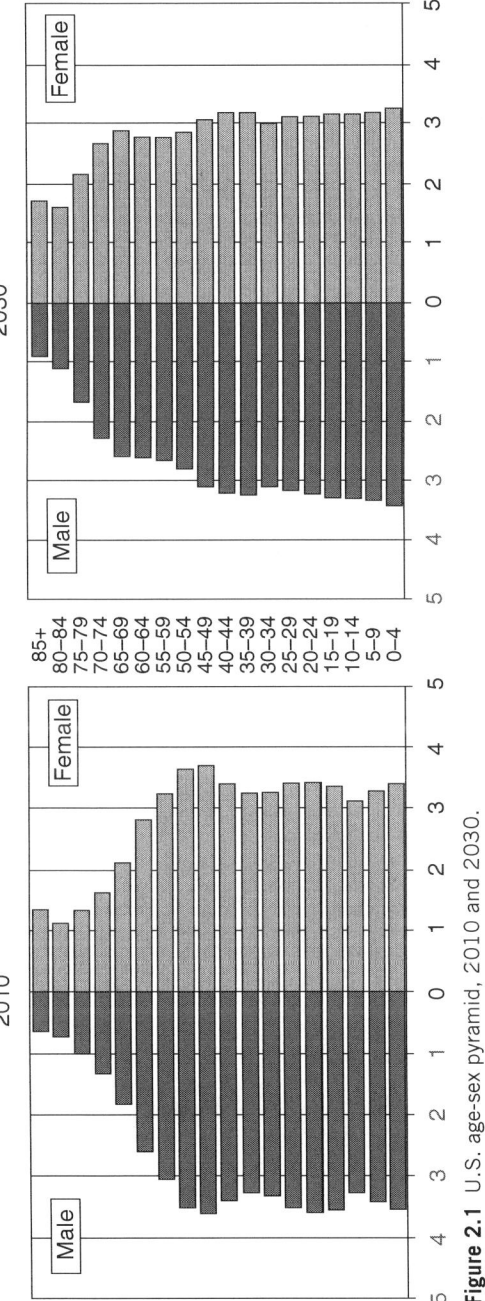

Figure 2.1 U.S. age-sex pyramid, 2010 and 2030.

Source: From "Population Projections. Interim Projections Consistent With Census 2000. Population Pyramids and Demographic Summary Indicators for U.S. Regions and Divisions," by U.S. Census Bureau, 2004b. Retrieved March 23, 2008 from http://www.census.gov/population/projections/52PyrmdUS1.pdf and http://www.census.gov/population/projections/52PyrmdUS3.pdf.

47

Public Health and Aging

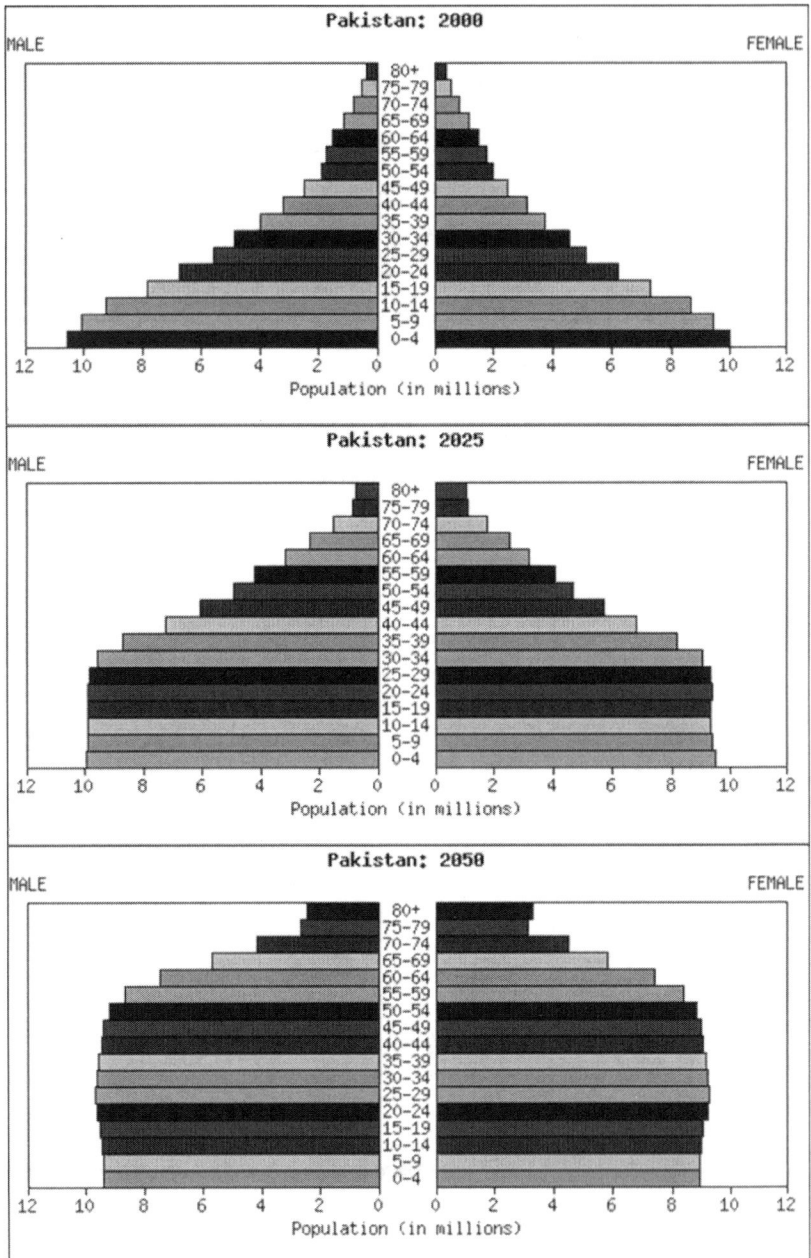

Figure 2.2 Age-sex pyramids, Pakistan, 2000, 2025, 2050.

Source: From http://148.129.75.3/ipc/www/idbnew.html (U.S. Census Bureau, International Data Base).

aged 65 and older, about 20%–25%, can be considered dependent, at least according to need for help in one or more of the personal self-maintenance activities, or ADLs (bathing, dressing, grooming, feeding, using toilet), and this proportion has declined over the past few decades (Spillman, 2004). Increasingly, people aged 65 and older delay retiring, provide intergenerational transfers of resources to their children aged 18–64, and contribute to child-rearing support for grandchildren. Instead, these ratios are more useful for providing insight into the age distribution of the population. Shifts in the elderly support ratio, in particular, indicate population aging. The elderly support ratio, obtained by dividing the number of elderly people per 100 working age population, was 21 for the United States in 2008 (Kinsella & He, 2009) and is projected to be 37 by 2030 (Kinsella & Velkoff, 2001).

Demographers have long recognized that the number of people in any given age group is influenced by births (or new entrants into an age group), deaths (or aging out of a given age group), and net migration (moving in or out of the geographic area of interest). Population aging cannot be attributed to high or low levels of fertility, mortality, or migration but to changes in such rates. The long-term downward trend in birth rates (the higher fertility of the baby boom cohorts notwithstanding) was the dominant factor driving population aging through the first half of the 20th century in the United States. During the 1980s, however, reductions in mortality at older ages were the dominant factor shaping population aging (Preston, Himes, & Eggers, 1989). Long-term shifts in birth and death rates are known more generally as the demographic transition.

THE DEMOGRAPHIC TRANSITION

The demographic transition is a model that describes sweeping changes that populations undergo from high to low rates of deaths and births (Population Reference Bureau, 2004). The model was initially developed based on data from the 19th century in Western Europe. It characterized the population's transition as an ordered sequence of four stages (Figure 2.3). In the first stage, a population has high birth rates, high death rates, and hence little or no population growth. The first stage is exemplified by agrarian, nonindustrialized societies, which historically averaged 35–45 deaths and births per 1,000 people. A population undergoing the second stage is characterized by high birth rates and falling death rates at younger ages as living conditions and nutrition improve, and hence rapid population growth. In the third stage, birth rates begin to decline while death rates remain low. As a result, population growth slows and the population begins to age.

The final stage was initially thought to consist of very low and relatively constant birth and death rates, and consequently very low or no population growth and a constant age distribution. Industrialized, urban societies in the 1980s, for example, with fertility and mortality rates of approximately 10–15/1,000, were thought to have reached the final stage (Mausner & Kramer, 1985). However, even "old" populations have experienced continued declines in mortality rates at older ages (see below), raising the possibility of a different fourth stage. In such a regime, birth rates are low and old-age death rates continue to decline, leading to low population growth, but, importantly, a continued shift toward older ages, or population aging.

The Demographic Transition and Declining Death Rates

The mortality side of this transition is clearly seen for death rates in Sweden over three centuries, summarized by Horiuchi (2003). Data for this

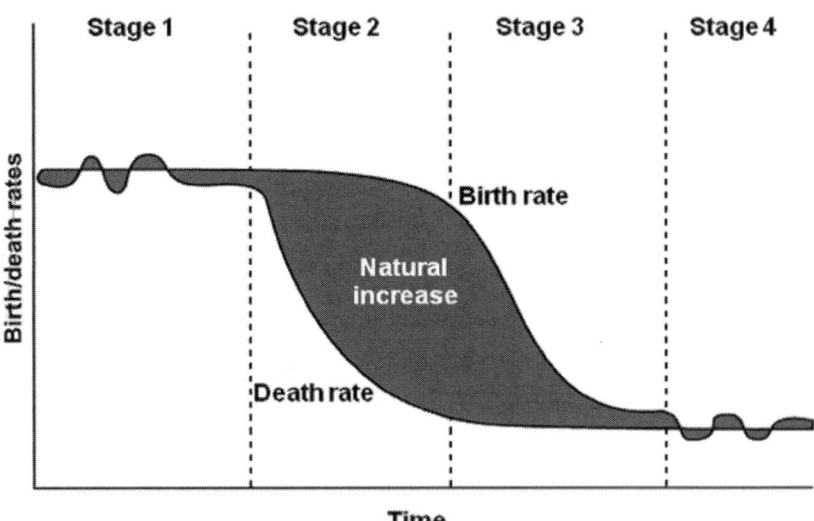

Figure 2.3 The demographic transition.

Source: From Population Reference Bureau, www.prb.org/LP/training_manual/DemoTrans.ppt. Reprinted with permission.
Note: Naturral incresase is produced from the excess of births over deaths.

Chapter 2 Population Aging: Demographic and Epidemiologic Perspectives

comparison are not easily available, because the comparison requires nearly 300 years of continuous, complete mortality data on a national scale. Sweden is one of the few countries with vital registration systems that have collected such data. Figure 2.4 shows death rates for three cohorts of Swedish women, the first born in 1751–1755, the second in 1876–1880, and the third in 1951–1955. The figure (which graphs mortality on a logarithmic scale) shows little difference in mortality risk for the first two cohorts. Mortality is well over 10% per person-year in the first 1–2 years of life, reaches its nadir (<1%) at about age 10, hovers around 1%–3% until age 35 or so, and then climbs exponentially (i.e., doubling every 7 years or so).

The mortality risk is completely different for the third birth cohort (1951–1955), born 100 years later. Mortality in the perinatal period for this cohort is <1%, the mortality nadir is again around age 10 (as it is in all human populations), but is well under 1/1,000, and mortality risk does not reach 1% until age 60 or so. At every age, except perhaps when people reach their eighties, mortality for the most recent birth cohort is vastly lower than it is in the prior cohorts.

It is useful as well to plot the distribution of deaths by age for the three cohorts. Figure 2.5 shows what proportion of deaths occurred at each age across the life span. For the 18th and 19th century birth

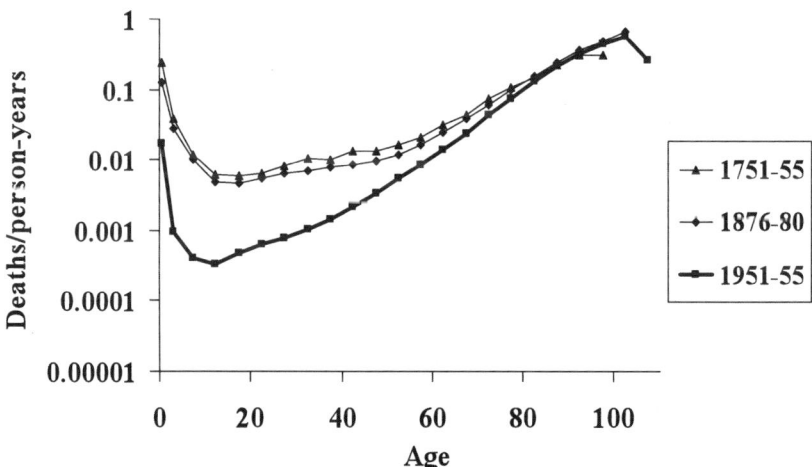

Figure 2.4 Death rates by age for Swedish females, three centuries.

Source: Prepared by Shiro Horiuchi, using Human Mortality Database (2003), http://www.mortality.org.

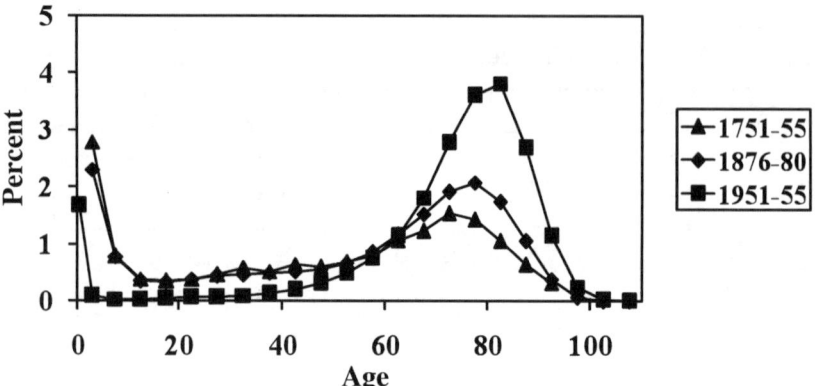

Figure 2.5 Distribution of ages at death: three cohorts of Swedish women, three centuries.

Source: Prepared by Shiro Horiuchi, using Human Mortality Database (2003), http://www.mortality.org.

cohorts, a relatively high risk of death prevails at all ages. Certainly, there are modes at both very young and very old ages, but high numbers of people are also dying at all ages across the life span. With the more recent 20th century birth cohort, the age distribution of deaths is quite different. Here, deaths are concentrated at the oldest ages, as shown in a large shift to the right in the distribution of deaths. The vast majority of deaths now occur in people over age 60.

If we add an even more recent birth cohort and plot its age distribution at death, as Figure 2.6 does, we see that this trend continues into our own era. The age distribution of death for Swedish women born 1996–1999 is pushed even further to the right and is even more clearly unimodal. Almost all deaths are concentrated in later life, with a mode above age 80.

These data should be kept in mind when examining the declining death rate in late life in the past half century. Although mortality rises with age, such that the annual risk of death approaches 15% for people in their early eighties, between 1950 and 2000 the rate of death for people over age 80 has actually declined. Declines in mortality for people aged 85 and older between 1950 and 2000 across a number of countries are shown in Figure 2.7. Between 1950 and 1990 death rates declined from 170 to 90 per 1,000 in the oldest old (Vaupel, 1997). Stratifying by age and plotting death rates by year shows that death rates fell even for people aged 90 and 95.

Chapter 2 Population Aging: Demographic and Epidemiologic Perspectives

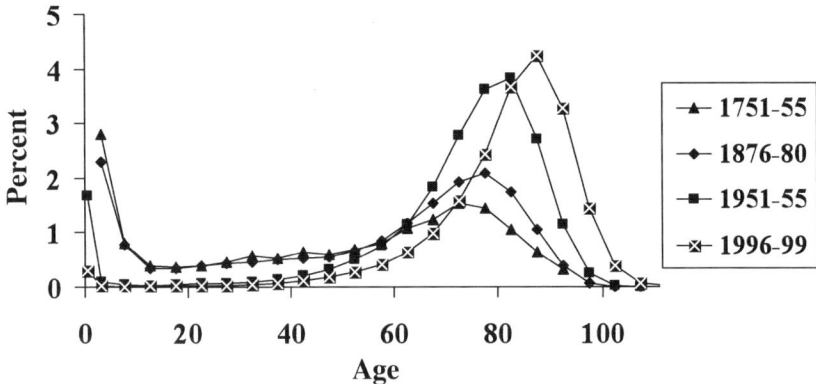

Figure 2.6 Age distribution of ages at death for Swedish females, selected periods, 1990s cohort.

Source: Prepared by Shiro Horiuchi, using Human Mortality Database (2003), available at http://www.mortality.org or www.humanmortality.de

Why should death rates among the oldest old population be declining? Some of the decline is probably due to medical advances applied specifically to the diseases of the very old. More of the decline is probably due to improvements in health and living conditions over the whole life course. The latter changes appear to have allowed a subset of people with some kind of long-life genetic endowment—"longevity genes"—to reach old age. While this genotype must have always been present in a subset of the human population, only in the 20th century have health and living conditions improved to the point where accidental mortality (such as death from trauma or infection) has been controlled well enough for substantial numbers to reach later life.

Will mortality rates continue to decline and life span continue to increase? The answer is hotly debated and depends in part on whether human populations have a limit to their life span—that is, a limit on the maximum number of years that can be lived—and, if so, whether humans have begun to reach such limits. Olshansky, Carnes, and Cassel (1990) have demonstrated that mortality rates would have to decline dramatically to very low levels for life expectancy to exceed 90 years in the 21st century. In contrast, Vaupel's findings that death rates for the oldest old have decreased over time and that mortality rates actually decelerate at approximately age 80, seem to suggest that continued declines are possible.

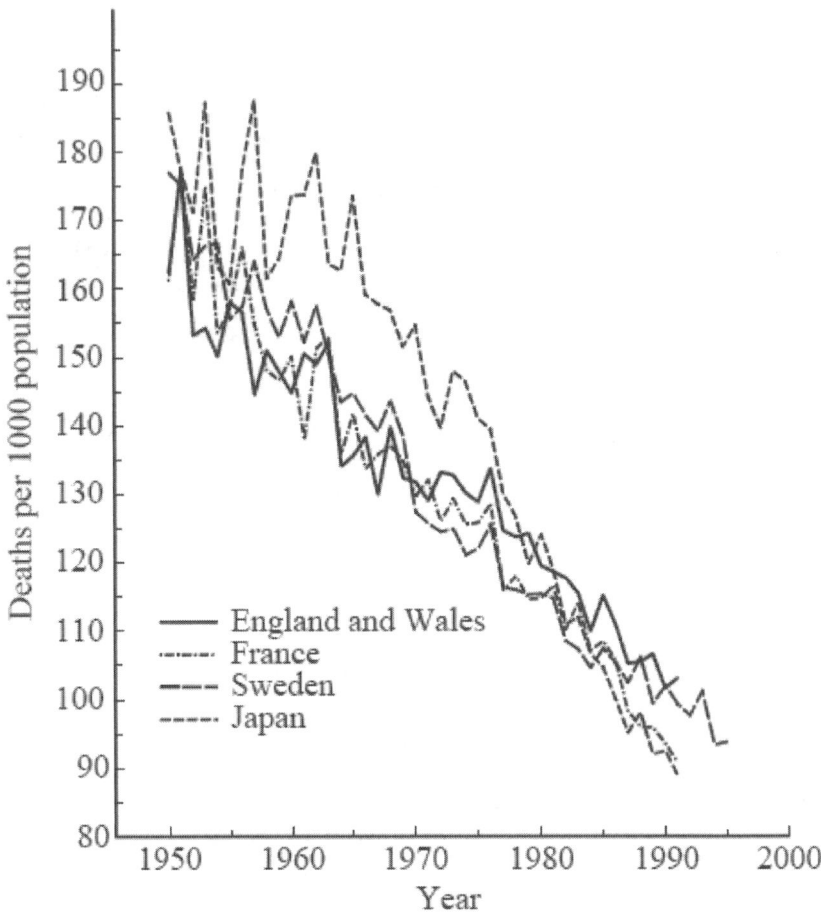

Figure 2.7 Mortality reductions in people aged 80 and older.

Source: From "The Remarkable Improvements in Survival at Older Ages," by J. W. Vaupel, 1997. *Philosophical Transactions of the Royal Society of London. Series B, Biological Sciences, 352,* 1799–1804; Figure 2, p. 1800.

The Demographic Transition and Increasing Life Expectancy

As mortality rates shift, populations experience changes in life expectancy. According to the National Center for Health Statistics, life expectancy at birth in the United States has nearly doubled in the past century to nearly 78 years in 2004 (Arias, 2007). Not everyone alive or

Chapter 2 Population Aging: Demographic and Epidemiologic Perspectives

born in 2004 can expect to live to this age. Instead, life expectancy is a hypothetical summary measure calculated by use of a demographic tool called the life table. The life table is a model of what would happen to a hypothetical birth cohort if age-specific death rates for a given period were to remain constant and were to apply throughout the experience of the entire generation.

Although we cannot give a full description of life table functions here, life expectancy cannot be fully understood without at least a basic familiarity with the life table. Essentially, the life table model applies the mortality risk prevailing at a given time to a hypothetical birth cohort, typically 100,000 in size. Mortality rates for each age (or age group, if abridged) are then applied to the cohort. An unabridged life table for the United States in 2004 (Arias, 2007) is shown in Table 2.3.

The function nqx is simply the mortality rate (proportion dying) for each age group in that year. Plotting nqx on the ordinate and age on the x-axis reveals the bathtub or j-shaped curve typical of mortality for human populations: a small but sharp upturn in the perinatal period, a decline that reaches its nadir at ages 5–15, and a slow but steady increase after this age.

The function l_x is the number of people entering each age interval; by convention, the starting number, or radix, is usually 100,000. The number of people entering each age interval reflects the number of deaths in the prior interval. The survival curve, or proportion of the population surviving to each age, is traced out by the l_x column. Fifty percent of the cohort is still alive at age 81.

The function ndx is the number of people dying in each age interval. If we multiply the mortality rate (nqx) by the number of people entering each age interval (l_x), we obtain ndx, the number of deaths. The number of people dying in each age interval is subtracted from the total and yields the number of people surviving to enter the next interval.

The function $_nLx$ is the number of person-years lived by the cohort in each age interval. The total number of person-years is the product of l_x and the number of years that define the age interval (1 year in a standard life shown in Figure 2.3; 5 years in an abridged life table). In calculating nLx we need to make an assumption about the timing of death. Did people die at the beginning or end of the age interval? This assumption clearly affects the total person-years contributed by the cohort in the age interval. By convention, we assume that people die in the middle of the age interval, except for the 0–1 age interval, which demands more sophisticated treatment because most deaths are concentrated near the time of birth.

Table 2.3

LIFE TABLE FOR THE TOTAL POPULATION: UNITED STATES, 2004

AGE	PROBABILITY OF DYING BETWEEN AGES X AND X+1 $q(x)$	NUMBER SURVIVING TO AGE X $l(x)$	NUMBER DYING BETWEEN AGES X AND X+1 $d(x)$	PERSON-YEARS LIVED BETWEEN AGES X AND X+1 $L(x)$	TOTAL NUMBER OF PERSON-YEARS LIVED ABOVE AGE X $T(x)$	EXPECTATION OF LIFE AT AGE X $E(x)$
0–1	0.006799	100,000	680	99,403	7,783,712	77.8
1–2	0.000483	99,320	48	99,296	7,684,309	77.4
2–3	0.000297	99,272	29	99,257	7,585,013	76.4
3–4	0.000224	99,243	22	99,232	7,485,755	75.4
4–5	0.000188	99,220	19	99,211	7,386,524	74.4
5–6	0.000171	99,202	17	99,193	7,287,313	73.5
6–7	0.000161	99,185	16	99,177	7,188,119	72.5
7–8	0.000151	99,169	15	99,161	7,088,943	71.5
8–9	0.000136	99,154	14	99,147	6,989,781	70.5
9–10	0.000119	99,140	12	99,134	6,890,634	69.5
10–11	0.000106	99,129	11	99,123	6,791,500	68.5
11–12	0.000112	99,118	11	99,112	6,692,377	67.5
12–13	0.000149	99,107	15	99,100	6,593,264	66.5
13–14	0.000227	99,092	23	99,081	6,494,164	65.5
14–15	0.000337	99,070	33	99,053	6,395,084	64.6

15–16	0.000460	99,036	46	99,014	6,296,031	63.6
16–17	0.000579	98,991	57	98,962	6,197,017	62.6
17–18	0.000684	98,933	68	98,900	6,098,055	61.6
18–19	0.000763	98,866	75	98,828	5,999,155	60.7
19–20	0.000819	98,790	81	98,750	5,900,327	59.7
20–21	0.000873	98,709	86	98,666	5,801,578	58.8
21–22	0.000926	98,623	91	98,577	5,702,911	57.8
22–23	0.000960	98,532	95	98,484	5,604,334	56.9
23–24	0.000972	98,437	96	98,389	5,505,850	55.9
24–25	0.000969	98,341	95	98,294	5,407,460	55.0
25–26	0.000960	98,246	94	98,199	5,309,166	54.0
26–27	0.000954	98,152	94	98,105	5,210,967	53.1
27–28	0.000952	98,058	93	98,012	5,112,862	52.1
28–29	0.000958	97,965	94	97,918	5,014,850	51.2
29–30	0.000973	97,871	95	97,824	4,916,932	50.2
30–31	0.000994	97,776	97	97,727	4,819,109	49.3
31–32	0.001023	97,679	100	97,629	4,721,382	48.3
32–33	0.001063	97,579	104	97,527	4,623,753	47.4
33–34	0.001119	97,475	109	97,420	4,526,226	46.4
34–35	0.001192	97,366	116	97,308	4,428,805	45.5

(Continued)

Table 2.3

LIFE TABLE FOR THE TOTAL POPULATION: UNITED STATES, 2004 (continued)

AGE	PROBABILITY OF DYING BETWEEN AGES X AND X+1 Q (X)	NUMBER SURVIVING TO AGE X L (X)	NUMBER DYING BETWEEN AGES X AND X+1 D (X)	PERSON-YEARS LIVED BETWEEN AGES X AND X+1 L (X)	TOTAL NUMBER OF PERSON-YEARS LIVED ABOVE AGE X T (X)	EXPECTATION OF LIFE AT AGE X E (X)
35–36	0.001275	97,250	124	97,188	4,331,497	44.5
36–37	0.001373	97,126	133	97,059	4,234,310	43.6
37–38	0.001493	96,993	145	96,920	4,137,250	42.7
38–39	0.001634	96,848	158	96,769	4,040,330	41.7
39–40	0.001788	96,690	173	96,603	3,943,562	40.8
40–41	0.001945	96,517	188	96,423	3,846,959	39.9
41–42	0.002107	96,329	203	96,227	3,750,536	38.9
42–43	0.002287	96,126	220	96,016	3,654,308	38.0
43–44	0.002494	95,906	239	95,787	3,558,292	37.1
44–45	0.002727	95,667	261	95,537	3,462,506	36.2
45–46	0.002982	95,406	284	95,264	3,366,969	35.3
46–47	0.003246	95,122	309	94,967	3,271,705	34.4
47–48	0.003520	94,813	334	94,646	3,176,738	33.5
48–49	0.003799	94,479	359	94,300	3,082,092	32.6

58

Age					
49–50	0.004088	94,120	385	93,928	2,987,792	31.7
50–51	0.004404	93,735	413	93,529	2,893,864	30.9
51–52	0.004750	93,323	443	93,101	2,800,335	30.0
52–53	0.005113	92,879	475	92,642	2,707,234	29.1
53–54	0.005488	92,404	507	92,151	2,614,592	28.3
54–55	0.005879	91,897	540	91,627	2,522,441	27.4
55–56	0.006295	91,357	575	91,070	2,430,814	26.6
56–57	0.006754	90,782	613	90,475	2,339,744	25.8
57–58	0.007280	90,169	656	89,841	2,249,269	24.9
58–59	0.007903	89,512	707	89,159	2,159,428	24.1
59–60	0.008633	88,805	767	88,422	2,070,269	23.3
60–61	0.009493	88,038	836	87,621	1,981,848	22.5
61–62	0.010449	87,203	911	86,747	1,894,227	21.7
62–63	0.011447	86,291	988	85,798	1,807,480	20.9
63–64	0.012428	85,304	1060	84,774	1,721,683	20.2
64–65	0.013408	84,244	1130	83,679	1,636,909	19.4
65–66	0.014473	83,114	1203	82,513	1,553,230	18.7
66–67	0.015703	81,911	1286	81,268	1,470,718	18.0
67–68	0.017081	80,625	1377	79,936	1,389,450	17.2
68–69	0.018623	79,248	1476	78,510	1,309,513	16.5

(Continued)

Table 2.3

LIFE TABLE FOR THE TOTAL POPULATION: UNITED STATES, 2004 (*continued*)

AGE	PROBABILITY OF DYING BETWEEN AGES X AND X+1 Q (X)	NUMBER SURVIVING TO AGE X L (X)	NUMBER DYING BETWEEN AGES X AND X+1 D (X)	PERSON-YEARS LIVED BETWEEN AGES X AND X+1 L (X)	TOTAL NUMBER OF PERSON-YEARS LIVED ABOVE AGE X T (X)	EXPECTATION OF LIFE AT AGE X E (X)
69–70	0.020322	77,772	1580	76,982	1,231,004	15.8
70–71	0.022104	76,191	1684	75,349	1,154,022	15.1
71–72	0.024023	74,507	1790	73,612	1,078,673	14.5
72–73	0.026216	72,717	1906	71,764	1,005,060	13.8
73–74	0.028745	70,811	2035	69,793	933,296	13.2
74–75	0.031561	68,776	2171	67,690	863,503	12.6
75–76	0.034427	66,605	2293	65,458	795,812	11.9
76–77	0.037379	64,312	2404	63,110	730,354	11.4
77–78	0.040756	61,908	2523	60,646	667,244	10.8
78–79	0.044764	59,385	2658	58,056	606,597	10.2
79–80	0.049395	56,727	2802	55,326	548,542	9.7
80–81	0.054471	53,925	2937	52,456	493,216	9.1
81–82	0.059772	50,987	3048	49,463	440,760	8.6
82–83	0.065438	47,940	3137	46,371	391,297	8.2
83–84	0.071598	44,803	3208	43,199	344,925	7.7

60

Age					
84–85	0.078516	41,595	3266	39,962	301,727	7.3
85–86	0.085898	38,329	3292	36,683	261,765	6.8
86–87	0.093895	35,037	3290	33,392	225,082	6.4
87–88	0.102542	31,747	3255	30,119	191,690	6.0
88–89	0.111875	28,491	3187	26,898	161,571	5.7
89–90	0.121928	25,304	3085	23,761	134,673	5.3
90–91	0.132733	22,219	2949	20,744	110,912	5.0
91–92	0.144318	19,270	2781	17,879	90,168	4.7
92–93	0.156707	16,489	2584	15,197	72,289	4.4
93–94	0.169922	13,905	2363	12,723	57,092	4.1
94–95	0.183975	11,542	2123	10,480	44,369	3.8
95–96	0.198875	9,419	1873	8,482	33,889	3.6
96–97	0.214620	7,545	1619	6,736	25,407	3.4
97–98	0.231201	5,926	1370	5,241	18,671	3.2
98–99	0.248600	4,556	1133	3,990	13,430	2.9
99–100	0.266786	3,423	913	2,967	9,440	2.8
100 or over	1.00000	2,510	2510	6,473	6,473	2.6

From "United States Life Tables, 2004," by E. Arias, 2007. *National Vital Statistics Reports* (Vol. 56). Hyattsville, MD: National Center for Health Statistics. Retrieved May 15, 2009, from http://www.cdc.gov/nchs/data/nvsr/nvsr56/nvsr56_09.pdf.

The function T_x is the sum of nLx. It is the total number of person-years lived by the birth cohort in the given age interval and in all subsequent ones. Thus, the T_x entry in the first row of the life table is the sum down the column of all nLx entries and gives the total number of person-years lived by the birth cohort, 7,783,712 years. The second row T_x value shows that cohort members who survived the first year of life lived a total of 7,604,389 years. People who survived to age 85 lived a total of 261,765 person-years in this and subsequent years until the last person died.

If we divide T_x by l_x in any given age interval, we obtain e^x, life expectancy at a given age. Thus, life expectancy at birth for the U.S. population in 2004 was 7,783,712/100,000, or 77.8 years. Life expectancy at age 50 was 30.9 years, and at age 80, 9.1 years.

Life expectancy at a given age, then, is simply the total number of person-years lived by persons reaching that age, divided by the number of people reaching that age. Life expectancy at birth (usually called simply "life expectancy") is the total number of person years lived by a birth cohort divided by the number of people in the cohort. It is the average number of years a person can expect to live—with, we must hasten to add, all the assumptions that go into the life table model. The major assumption in these models is a fixed mortality schedule; the models assume that prevailing mortality rates do not change over the lifetime of the cohort. They also assume a fixed birth cohort, with no loss or gain to migration.

How then does life expectancy (at birth) change with the demographic transition? In the first stage of the demographic transition, life expectancy is low, typically age 20–30. As mortality rates begin to fall at younger ages, life expectancy increases to the 30–50 range. In stage 3, as death rates reach very low rates, life expectancy exceeds age 50 and may reach as high as age 70. In stage 4, if death rates continue to drop at advanced ages, life expectancy can reach age 80 and beyond.

THE EPIDEMIOLOGIC TRANSITION AND SHIFTING CAUSES OF DEATH

Whereas the demographic transition emphasizes shifting birth and death rates, the epidemiologic transition, a theory first proposed by Omran in the 1970s, focuses on causes of death as a population shifts from high- to low-mortality regimes. (For more on mortality and how causes of death are identified, see Chapter 10.) The stages of the epidemiologic transi-

Chapter 2 Population Aging: Demographic and Epidemiologic Perspectives   **63**

tion correspond directly to the first three stages of the demographic transition, but the emphasis is on causes of death and the speed of change may vary. Stage 1 (high birth and death rates) was deemed the age of "pestilence and famine." Infectious and parasitic diseases such as pneumonia and influenza, tuberculosis, diarrhea, and enteritis dominated this period (along with deaths due to war, famine, malnutrition, and complications of childbirth). Stage 2 (falling death rates at younger ages and high population growth) was dubbed the "age of receding pandemics" and characterized by the emergence of degenerative diseases, notably heart disease, as a major cause of death. In stage 3 (declining birth rate, low death rates, and very low population growth), dubbed the "age of degenerative and man-made diseases" chronic degenerative diseases—heart disease, cancer, stroke, chronic obstructive pulmonary diseases—dominated as causes of death. Olshansky and Ault (1986) postulated the existence of a fourth stage, dubbed "the age of delayed degenerative diseases." In the proposed stage 4, the causes of death are similar to those in stage 3, but the age of death increases as a consequence of prevention and health promotion efforts.

Although not explicitly recognized by Omran's original theory, the epidemiologic transition also results in a fundamental shift in the morbidity profile of adults. As populations enter the 3rd and 4th stages of the transition, the prevalence of chronic conditions increases, although they may be less debilitating (Manton, 1989). In the United States, as in most developed countries, the two most common chronic conditions—arthritis and hypertension—are not among the most common causes of death (Table 2.4).

WHY POPULATION AGING MATTERS

According to demographers, "population aging will be one of the most important social phenomena of the next half century" (Preston & Martin, 1994). In the United States, population aging over the next few decades will be keenly felt in all major social institutions. Families will undoubtedly change in terms of composition and dynamics, work and retirement will be transformed, and the country's major social transfer programs—Social Security and Medicare—will be strained without major changes in financing or eligibility. Two additional consequences, the shifting health care needs of the population and the emergence of an oldest old population, are especially germane for public health.

Table 2.4

MOST COMMON CAUSES OF DEATH VS. MOST PREVALENT CONDITIONS

Cause of death	Prevalent conditions
Heart disease	Hypertension
Cancer	Arthritis
Stroke	Heart disease
COPD	Cancer
Unintentional injuries	Diabetes
Diabetes	COPD/Asthma
Alzheimer's disease	Stroke

From http://www.cdc.gov/nchs/products/pubs/pubd/hestats/finaldeaths04/finaldeaths04.htm and Older Americans 2008: Key Indicators of Well-Being.

Shifting Health Care Needs of the Population

For over three decades demographers have debated the implications of longer life for population health and health care needs. Gruenberg (1977) argued that longer life meant worsening health and warned of a pandemic of disease and disability. Fries' famous "compression of morbidity" hypothesis (Fries, 1980; Fries & Crapo, 1981) purported the opposite: as individuals, on average, lived longer and the population approached the limits to human life, the period of morbidity before death would be compressed into a shorter period. Manton (1989) offered a third perspective, dubbed "dynamic equilibrium," which explicitly recognized the complex interactions among morbidity, disability, and mortality processes. The three processes are interrelated so that interventions designed to affect one of the processes inevitably influence the other two as well. Years of life are gained through a combination of postponement of disease onset, reductions of severity of disease and speed of progression, and improved techniques for clinical management.

These differing perspectives can be illustrated with the World Health Organization's model (1981) of the relationship between morbidity, disability, and survival (Figure 2.8). The curves in the figure represent the proportion of the population surviving to each age without morbidity (or subclinical disability), disability, and death, respectively. The model assumes that the survival function from the 2004 life table holds and presents

Chapter 2 Population Aging: Demographic and Epidemiologic Perspectives

hypothetical curves for morbidity and disability under the assumption that these risks follow the pattern established for survival: an increasing, accelerating risk with age. Further, these risks are assumed to be nested: morbidity precedes disability, so that people develop disease before disability, and everyone with disability has passed through a period of morbidity. Similarly, states of disability, with varying duration, precede mortality.

In this model, the proportion of older people surviving to each age is shown in the outermost curve. In the figure, which is based on the 2004 life table described above, 50% of elders are still alive at age 81. The area under the survival curve indicates the total person-years lived by the cohort. Survival in this model is further partitioned according to functional status. The area under the remaining curves represent person-years spent by the population without morbidity (under curve C) and with morbidity but no disability (between curves B and C). Person-years lived with disability are represented by the area between the survival and disability curves (curves A and B).

Increases in life expectancy mean that the survival curve in Figure 2.8 is shifting upward and to the right. The key question is whether the disability curve is shifting in the same direction at the same pace. If the disability curve shifts at a slower pace than the survival curve, then an expansion of the number of person-years of disability will occur, and active life expectancy will decline as a share of life expectancy, as predicted by Gruenberg (1977). If the disability curve moves outward at a rate faster than the survival curve, person-years of disability across the life span will be reduced. Accordingly, active life expectancy will increase as a share of life expectancy, as predicted by Fries (1983). In contrast, Manton's

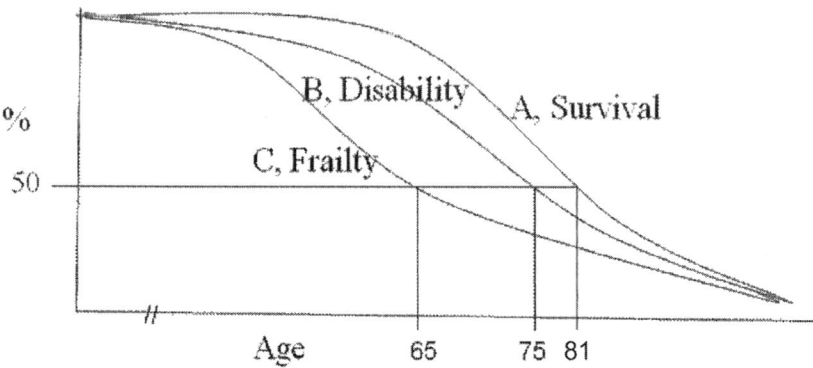

Figure 2.8 WHO model of observed survival and hypothetical morbidity and disability.

theory of dynamic equilibrium anticipates that all three curves will shift and change in shape with reduction in the incidence, prevalence, or severity of a disease. Thus, during one period a population may experience an expansion, and during another, a compression of morbidity. In fact, the evidence over the past 30 years for the United States is consistent with dynamic equilibrium, with expansion occurring during the 1970s and compression beginning in the 1980s (Crimmins, Saito, & Ingegneri, 1997a). As discussed in more detail in Chapter 5, evidence for more recent years is mixed, with some studies suggesting a continued compression and at least one finding a leveling off of active life expectancy.

Emergence of the Oldest Old in America

An additional consequence of population aging is the emergence of an "oldest old" population. The oldest old are typically defined as people aged 85 and older (Suzman, Willis, & Manton, 1992). Some of the characteristics of this group, now numbering 5.3 million (Federal Interagency Forum on Aging-Related Statistics, 2008), include:

- They are the fastest growing segment of older population in the United States; in fact, the United States will have the largest number of oldest old of any country in the next 50 years. This is a paradox because the United States will not have the most elderly, as defined by the proportion aged 65 and older.
- They are largely female (68% are women and 32% men), White, and widowed. Note, however, that people aged 65 and older are becoming increasingly more diverse racially. And women are twice as likely to be widowed as men (76% vs. 34%).
- In 2006, only 11% were living in poverty. This figure had declined steadily from 21% in 1982. The oldest old are also increasingly well educated. Educational attainment in this group has increased dramatically: 29.1% completed high school in 1985, and 63% of this age group is expected to have completed high school in 2015.
- Fewer women in this age group will be childless, compared with the young-old, although fewer will also have 5 or more offspring. This may affect the availability of family caregivers.
- The proportion of men aged 85 and older who are veterans is projected to increase from 33% in 2000 to over 60% in 2010.
- They are high consumers of supportive care. In 2005, 17% resided in a nursing home (a decline from nearly 25% in 1985) and an-

Chapter 2 Population Aging: Demographic and Epidemiologic Perspectives **67**

other 7% in community housing with services (sometimes called "assisted living"), such as meals, housekeeping, laundry, or medication management. Average annual Medicare costs were $22,000 per enrollee. Average nursing home costs were over $7,000.
- Sixty-two percent of people age 85 and older have trouble hearing, 27% have trouble seeing, and 32% are edentulous, that is, have lost all of their natural teeth; 19% report depressive symptoms.
- Thirty-eight percent of oldest old men and 56% of oldest old women are unable to perform common physical functions, such as stooping or walking 2–3 blocks. Forty-two percent report an activity limitation (difficulty with personal care activities such as dressing, bathing, or walking or activities necessary to live independently, such as doing housework, preparing meals, or managing money). Still, 66% rate their own health as good, very good, or excellent, and 10% engage in regular physical activity.

SUMMARY

Population Aging. Population aging is a *shift in the age distribution of the population toward older ages.* The phenomenon is most often measured by increases in the percentage of the population reaching old age, but can also be captured by changes in the population "pyramid" and by changes in ratios of the older to younger population ("age-dependency" or "support" ratios). By all three standards, the U.S. population is aging and has been for over a century, but the pace has accelerated over the past several decades.

Demographic Transition. The demographic transition is a model that describes sweeping changes that populations undergo from high to low rates of deaths and births. In the first stage, a population has high birth rates, high death rates, and hence little or no population growth. In the second stage, high birth rates are accompanied by falling death rates at younger ages as living conditions and nutrition improve, and hence rapid population growth occurs. In the third stage, birth rates begin to decline while death rates remain low; consequently, population growth slows as the population begins to age. In the fourth stage, the population experiences continued declines in late-life mortality and continued population aging.

Life Expectancy. Life expectancy at a given age is calculated from a life table. Life expectancy is the total number of person-years lived divided by the number of persons reaching that age. Life expectancy at birth is the average number of years a hypothetical person can expect to live under the assumption that that prevailing age-specific mortality rates do not change over the lifetime of a hypothetical cohort

Epidemiologic Transition. Whereas the demographic transition emphasizes shifting birth and death rates, the epidemiologic transition focuses on causes of death as a population shifts from high to low mortality regimes. Stage 1 was deemed the age of "pestilence and famine." Infectious and parasitic diseases, such as pneumonia and influenza, tuberculosis, diarrhea, and enteritis, dominated this period. Stage 2 is called the "age of receding pandemics" and is characterized by the emergence of degenerative diseases, notably heart disease, as a major cause of death. In stage 3, the "age of degenerative and man-made diseases," chronic degenerative diseases—heart disease, cancer, stroke, chronic obstructive pulmonary diseases—dominate as causes of death. Olshansky and Ault (1986) also postulated the existence of a fourth stage, "the age of delayed degenerative diseases."

Dynamic Equilibrium. The consequences of shifting disability and survival curves for health care needs are not clear and depend on the processes driving mortality declines. Several competing theories have been proposed to predict changes in population health as mortality declines. Evidence over the past 30 years for the United States has been most consistent with the theory of dynamic equilibrium, a theory that recognizes complex interconnections among morbidity, mortality, and survival curves (Manton, 1989). Expansion of active life expectancy occurred during the 1970s and a compression followed in the 1980s. More recent evidence is mixed with one study suggesting a continued compression and another suggesting no change overall despite shifting rates on onset, recovery, and mortality.

The Oldest Old. An additional consequence of population aging is the emergence of an "oldest old" population. The oldest old are typically defined as people aged 85 and older. They are the fastest growing segment of older population in the United States. They are largely female, White, and widowed. The percentage living in poverty in this group has declined, whereas the percentage completing high school has increased dramatically. Men in this age group are increasingly likely to be veterans. They are high consumers of supportive care and have high rates of functional loss. Still, 66% rate their own health as good, very good, or excellent, and 10% engage in regular physical activity.

4 Chronic Disease in Older Adults

Prevention has been identified as a key element of healthy aging, yet a substantial number of older adults are living with one or more chronic diseases. This chapter provides an introduction to common population-based measures of chronic illness and disease. Verbrugge and Patrick (1995) define chronic conditions as "long-term diseases, injuries with long sequelae, and enduring structural, sensory, and communicative disorders." They add, "their defining aspect is duration. Once they are past certain symptomatic or diagnostic thresholds, chronic conditions are essentially permanent features for the rest of life. Medical and personal regimens can sometimes control but can rarely cure them."

We also review the current state of health promotion and disease prevention aimed at older adults, including which preventive services are currently recommended for older adults and how scientific evidence is used in the process of setting these recommendations. A third section discusses the Medicare program and its role in financing preventive services. A final section offers an overview of existing chronic disease management programs.

COMMON POPULATION-BASED MEASURES OF ILLNESS AND DISEASE

Prevalence

One of the most common measures of illness and disease is referred to as disease prevalence. If you want to understand at a point in time, what a "snap shot" of the population looks like, you are probably interested in prevalence. Point prevalence refers to the number of persons who have a particular disease among the population at a given point in time. Most of the time true point prevalence is not available, because large surveys and epidemiologic studies take place over a period of time. Instead, epidemiologists count the number of people with illness (the numerator) and divide it by the average population during the study period (the denominator), yielding a measure of period prevalence. Prevalence measures in general give a useful cross section of what is happening, but the measure is influenced by at least two processes: the chance among those who do not have the condition of developing it (incidence) and the duration of the condition among those who develop it. The latter is a function of the probability of surviving with the condition and recovering from it.

Figure 4.1 shows reports of prevalent chronic conditions for men and women for 2005–2006 from the National Health Interview Survey, ordered from most to least prevalent. Note that, like most surveys, participants are asked whether a doctor ever told them they had a particular condition. For many conditions that approach is a reasonable way to ascertain prevalence, but for some conditions that are known to be underdiagnosed, such as diabetes or hypertension, these estimates will likely be lower than the true prevalence.

Although older men and women have a similar (within 2 percentage points) prevalence of hypertension, stroke, asthma, chronic lung disease, and diabetes, there are several important differences: women report higher levels of arthritis and depressive symptoms, whereas men report higher levels of heart disease and cancer.

Not shown in Figure 4.1 are important differences by race and ethnicity. According to the most recent chart book on older Americans prepared by the Federal Interagency Forum on Aging-Related Statistics (2008), in 2005–2006, among people age 65 and over, the prevalence of hypertension and diabetes was higher for non-Hispanic Blacks than for non-Hispanic Whites: 70% vs. 51% for hypertension and 29% vs. 16% for diabetes. Hispanics also reported higher levels of diabetes than

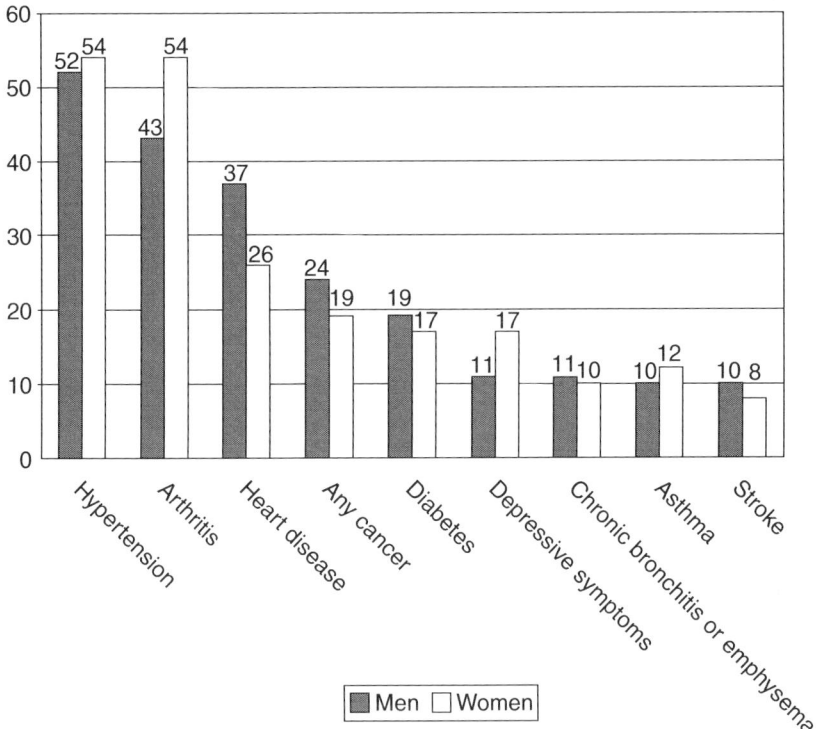

Figure 4.1 Percentage of people age 65 and over who report having selected chronic conditions, by sex, 2005–2006.

Source: From *Older Americans 2008: Key Indicators of Well-Being,* by Federal Interagency Forum on Aging-Related Statistics, March 2008. Washington, DC: U.S. Government Printing Office.

non-Hispanic Whites (25% vs. 16%), but similar levels of hypertension (54% and 51%, respectively) and lower levels of arthritis (40% vs. 50%).

Incidence

In contrast to prevalence, the incidence rate provides a measure of new events that occur during a specified period of time among a population at risk for getting the disease. Incidence rates are especially useful in establishing risk factors linked to the onset of conditions and for understanding whether prevention efforts are reducing the onset of new cases.

The difference between the numerator in a prevalence estimate and in an incidence rate is relatively straightforward: instead of including everyone with the condition in the numerator, as is done in calculating prevalence, only *new* cases found during the specified period of time are counted in the numerator for calculating incidence.

The denominator in an incidence rate also differs conceptually from that found in prevalence calculations. The denominator for an incidence rate ideally should exclude individuals who already have the condition of interest, because they are not at risk for becoming a new case. For rare conditions, this adjustment does not make much difference, but for common chronic conditions, like hypertension, heart disease, arthritis, and even some forms of cancer, these adjustments may be important. Because the incidence rate is calculated over a time period, the number of people at risk for developing a condition is likely to change over time. Sometimes the population at risk at the beginning of the period is used and then the rate is called a cumulative incidence rate. In other cases, the population that is at risk at the midpoint is used to represent the average size population that is at risk. If people are observed for different follow-up periods, the denominator may be expressed in terms of "person-time" units. That is, individuals contribute to the denominator, for instance, one month for each month they are alive, in the study, and have not contracted the condition. All new cases are then divided by this person-time denominator.

In practice, large surveys that monitor individuals at regular intervals (say, every 2 years) do not provide a true incidence rate. Instead, one can get an estimate of onset between waves if one limits calculations to those who did not have the condition at first contact, and reports the percentage that are alive, and report having the condition at follow-up. Onset differs from a true incidence rate because individuals who die or are lost from the study are not included in the calculations, but it is a reasonable approximation over short periods of time for conditions with relatively low mortality. For higher mortality conditions, onset calculations will probably be lower than true incidence.

Table 4.1 shows by sex the percentage of adults age 55 and older who reported having one of six common chronic conditions in 2002 and the percentage who reported a new condition in 2004 (among those without the condition in 2002). Consistent with the statistics from the National Health Interview Survey, women report higher levels of arthritis and whereas men report higher levels of heart problems. However, gender patterns are different in Table 4.1 than in Figure 4.1. Why might this be the case?

Two obvious possibilities come to mind. First, the populations are defined differently (65 and older in Figure 4.1 vs. 55 and older in Table 4.1).

Table 4.1

PERCENTAGE OF 55 AND OLDER POPULATION REPORTING CHRONIC CONDITIONS IN 2002, AND PERCENTAGE REPORTING ONSET OF CONDITION IN 2004, BY SEX

CONDITION	MEN		WOMEN	
	PREVALENCE: % REPORTING CONDITION IN 2002	*2-YEAR ONSET:* % REPORTING ONSET OF CONDITION IN 2004 (AMONG THOSE WITHOUT CONDITION IN 2002)	*PREVALENCE:* % REPORTING CONDITION IN 2002	*2-YEAR ONSET:* % REPORTING ONSET OF CONDITION IN 2004 (AMONG THOSE WITHOUT CONDITION IN 2002)
High blood pressure	50.2	10.2	52.5	12.3
Arthritis	49.8	11.2	64.8	15.2
Heart problems	27.1	6.3	21.9	5.4
Diabetes	17.9	3.5	15.0	3.3
Cancer	13.4	3.5	13.6	2.4
Stroke	8.3	1.9	7.7	2.1
No. in 2002	6,580	—	8,794	—

Analysis of the 2002 and 2004 waves of the Health and Retirement Study adapted from "Neighborhood Associations With Chronic Disease Prevalence and Onset in Later Life," by V. A. Freedman, I. B. Grafova, R. F. Schoeni, & J. Rogowski, November 16–20, 2007a. Paper presented at the annual meeting of the Gerontological Society of America, San Francisco, CA.

Second, and more subtle, the two surveys have different definitions of cancer. The National Health Interview Survey asks: "Have you EVER been told by a doctor or other health professional that you had . . . Cancer or a malignancy of any kind?" Whereas the Health and Retirement Study asks: "Has a doctor ever told you that you have cancer or a malignant tumor, excluding minor skin cancers?" It is possible that the exclusion of skin cancer results in a different pattern by gender. Because men are more likely than women to develop skin cancer, leaving minor skin cancers out of the calculations tips the scale toward women.

Another pattern evident in Table 4.1 is that high blood pressure and arthritis are the most prevalent conditions, but also have the highest rates of onset in this population, with higher rates of prevalence and onset reported by women than men. In contrast, diabetes, cancer, and stroke have much lower rates of onset (in the 2%–4% range over the 2-year period), with women reporting fewer onsets of diabetes and cancer, but not stroke.

It is noteworthy, based on Table 4.1, that greater onset does not always mean greater prevalence. In the case of cancer (excluding minor skin cancers), for example, men have a higher percentage experiencing onset (3.5% vs. 2.4%), but a similar, or slightly lower, prevalence than women (13.4% vs. 13.6%). Why might this be? The populations and definitions are the same, so we must consider other explanations. Recall that prevalence is influenced not only by incidence, but also by survival. The pattern we see for cancer suggests that men are not surviving as long with cancer as women are.

COMPARING PREVALENT, DEBILITATING, AND HIGH-MORTALITY CONDITIONS

To this point, we have focused on the most commonly reported chronic conditions. However, the most prevalent conditions among older adults are not necessarily the most debilitating, nor are they necessarily likely to result in death. An important distinction then is among conditions that are common, those that are debilitating, and those that are most likely to result in death. Table 4.2 shows the top six conditions falling into each category. The first two columns are based on analysis of the 2004 National Health Interview Survey (NHIS). Note that omitted from the NHIS analysis were two relatively debilitating conditions: unintentional injuries (such as hip fractures) and cognitive conditions such as Alzheimer's disease and related dementias. The last column comes directly from death certificate data, which are discussed in more detail in Chapter 10.

The only condition common to all three lists is diabetes. It is not only highly prevalent (17% in 2004) but also fairly debilitating (18% of those with diabetes in 2004 reported having an activity limitation). And in 2004 diabetes was the 6th leading cause of death. In contrast, hypertension and arthritis are highly prevalent but do not make the top six debilitating or common causes of death. Other conditions, such as stroke and lung conditions, are debilitating and have high mortality, but they are not prevalent enough to make the top-six list.

Why are these distinctions important? If the goal of public health is to prevent the onset of or to detect early highly prevalent chronic conditions (primary and secondary prevention), the six most prevalent conditions make excellent targets. At the other extreme, programs like Nixon's "war on cancer" are appropriate if the goal is to maximize life expectancy. However, if the aim is to maximize functioning, then conditions appearing in the middle of Table 4.2 become important to target: mental distress and hearing limitations, for example, do not appear on either of the other two lists, but clearly are important in maximizing the functioning and well-being of older adults.

Table 4.2

SIX MOST PREVALENT, MOST DEBILITATING, AND MOST COMMON CAUSES OF DEATH IN THE 65 AND OLDER POPULATION

MOST PREVALENT CONDITIONS[a]	MOST DEBILITATING CONDITIONS[b]	MOST COMMON CAUSES OF DEATH[c]
Hypertension	Mental distress	Heart disease
Arthritis	Stroke	Cancer
Heart disease	Vision limitation	Stroke
Cancer	Hearing limitation	Lung conditions
Diabetes	Diabetes	Alzheimer's disease
Vision Limitation	Lung conditions	Diabetes

[a,b] Freedman et al. (2007a), based on National Health Interview Survey.
[c] Center for Disease Control. National Vital Statistics System, National Center for Health Statistics. 10 Leading causes of death by age group, United States—2004.

COMORBIDITY, MULTIMORBIDITY, AND SELF-CARE

In later life, most adults do not have a single chronic condition. The term comorbidity, sometimes also called multimorbidity, is the presence of two or more health conditions in the same individual. The experience of having multiple conditions can lead to a long list of unfavorable outcomes, including mortality, poor functioning, and increased use of health care (see Gijsen et al., 2001, for a review of consequences). There are several common approaches to measuring comorbidity (John et al., 2003) including counts of conditions, weighted indices that take disease severity into account, examination of the proportion of the population with a condition who have a second condition, and analysis of measures of association and whether patterns and levels are greater than what would be found owing to chance (if conditions were independent).

In the United States, 35% of adults between ages 65 and 79 and more than 70% of adults ages 80 and older have more than one chronic condition (Fried, Ferrucci, Darer, Williamson, & Anderson, 2004b). Per capita annual medical expenditures double with each additional condition up to three, and persons with four or more chronic conditions on average have more than 12 times the medical expenditures of someone with one condition (Wolff, Starfield, & Anderson, 2002). Because of out-of-pocket medical expenses associated with treatments for chronic disease, comorbidity leads to significant wealth depletion in later life, especially for unmarried older adults (Kim & Lee, 2006).

We know very little about specific patterns of multimorbidity in the older population. Recent data from Sweden suggest that in older persons with multimorbidity, there exists co-occurrence of specific types of diseases beyond chance (Marengoni, Rizzuto, Wang, Winblad, & Fratiglioni, 2009). That is, there seem to be a higher probability than just due to chance of reporting clusters of circulatory conditions, clusters of cardiopulmonary conditions, and both mental health and musculoskeletal conditions.

Today, older individuals who have multiple conditions are expected to participate in the management of their conditions. An older adult with hypertension may be encouraged to have his or her pressure checked between visits to the physician, perhaps with a home monitor or at a local drug store. If he or she also has diabetes, that person will need to check his or her blood sugars, potentially several times a day, and follow a diet to help keep his or her glucose stable. If the person has another common condition, congestive heart failure, he or she may also be asked to follow a low-salt diet and weigh him- or herself daily. We know very little about how well patients manage these tasks in the face of multiple conditions. It is likely that family members—spouses and other people living with the patient or even children who live nearby—may play an important supportive role, but little research to date has focused on this topic.

What is known is that, because of shifts that took place many years ago in the educational system and in policies that provided education to soldiers returning from the Second World War, the older population today is better educated than it was just a few decades ago. This means that they may have more skills with which to manage their conditions. The concept of *health literacy*—the degree to which individuals have the capacity to obtain, process, and understand basic health information and services needed to make appropriate health decisions (CDC, *Healthy People 2010*, 2009)—has gained attention in recent years. People who have limited health literacy may have difficulty with a variety of self-care tasks, including finding providers and services, filling out forms, accurately sharing a medical history, taking medications according to directions, and following other instructions from providers for managing health conditions. Health literacy is different from literacy in that it encompasses skills that are needed to make treatment and self-care decisions. An individual who is literate (can read) but has a low health literacy might have difficulty finding and evaluating the credibility of health information, assessing risks and benefits of health care decisions, calculating the amount of a prescription to take, or understanding test results.

Health literacy may be measured in three domains: the ability to search, comprehend, and use information from a continuous text source ("prose"); the ability to search, comprehend, and use information from a noncontinuous text source like a bus schedule ("document"); and the ability to identify and perform calculations by using numbers found in printed materials ("quantitative"). According to the Federal Interagency Forum on Aging-Related Statistics, the health literacy of older adults in each of these areas is improving. In 2003, only 23%, 27%, and 34% of older adults had below basic prose, document, and quantitative health literacy skills, respectively (see Figure 4.2), whereas the figures in 1992 were 33%, 38%, and 49%, respectively.

Nevertheless, health literacy in later life remains a significant challenge. In 2003, 60%–71% of people age 65 and over had below basic or basic health literacy skills, depending on the measure. It is not surprising

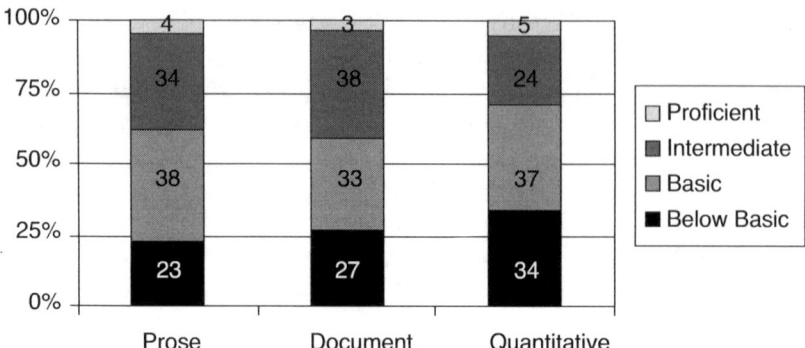

Figure 4.2 Percentage of people age 65 and over who demonstrate proficient, intermediate, basic, and below basic health literacy: 2003.

Source: From *Older Americans 2008: Key Indicators of Well-Being*, by Federal Interagency Forum on Aging-Related Statistics, March 2008. Washington, DC: U.S. Government Printing Office.

that limited health literacy increases with age, and is more common among minority populations, those with fewer economic resources, fewer years of education, and cultural or language barriers.

THE STATE OF HEALTH PROMOTION AND CHRONIC DISEASE PREVENTION FOR OLDER ADULTS

The idea of primary prevention in late life still strikes some people as strange. We have been unable to identify any comprehensive treatment of the subject. Even the field of "preventive" or "interventional geriatrics," which is further along, is still relatively new. In fact, efforts toward this end are underway in a number of fields, from neuroscience to occupational therapy, and continued progress toward primary prevention in late life is reported nearly weekly. Still, no comprehensive account is available.

In this section, we review current recommendations for older adults made by the U.S. Preventive Services Task Force (USPSTF). At this point, the Task Force does not provide separate guidelines for adults aged 65 and older but rather offers "adult health" guidelines. Indeed, there are so few recommendations that apply to older adults that they can be summarized in a single table. Here, we review the source and nature of these recommendations and how research was used in the process.

The U.S. Preventive Services Task Force

First convened by the U.S. Public Health Service in 1984, and now sponsored by the Agency for Healthcare Research and Quality, the USPSTF is the leading independent panel of private-sector experts in prevention and primary care in the United States. The panel's job is to conduct rigorous, impartial assessments of the scientific evidence for clinical preventive services. The range of services is unusually broad and covers screening, counseling, and preventive medications and procedures. The USPSTF's recommendations are considered the "gold standard" for clinical preventive services.

Initially published in 1989 as the Guide to Clinical Preventive Services, the USPSTF has made periodic updates (e.g., 1996). The current guide (2008) is available on the Web at http://www.ahrq.gov/clinic/pocketgd08/. The process by which these recommendations are made involves several steps: reviewing the existing evidence base, estimating the magnitude of the benefits and harms for each preventive service, reaching a consensus about the net benefit for each preventive service, and issuing a recommendation. The recommendation is made in the form of a grade from A to I, whereby A means strongly recommended, B means recommended, C means there is no recommendation for or against, D is a recommendation against, and I indicates insufficient evidence on which to base a recommendation. Of the 40 or so screen recommendations relevant to older adults, nearly half involved insufficient evidence. The remaining recommendations (5 strongly recommended, 8 recommended, and 10 interventions which are explicitly recommended *against* as of the 2008 report) are shown in Table 4.3.

Use of Evidence in Setting Recommendations

It would not be unusual for a student to wonder, at this point, just how does the task force decide that a particular preventive service should receive a "D" grade? To understand how research is used to determine a recommendation, one needs to have an appreciation for the concepts of reliability, validity, power, and diagnostic utility of screening. We turn to each of these concepts now.

Reliability is the extent to which a measurement instrument yields consistent results when repeated multiple times. Think of getting on a scale several times in a row: does the scale always read the same value? If so that scale is reliable. Another analogy that is helpful when thinking

Table 4.3

RECOMMENDATIONS, U.S. PREVENTIVE SERVICES TASK FORCE, 2008

STRONGLY RECOMMENDED (A)

1. Clinicians discuss aspirin chemoprevention with adults who are at increased risk for coronary heart disease
2. Clinicians screen adults aged 18 and older for high blood pressure
3. Clinicians routinely screen men aged 35 years and older and women aged 45 years and older for lipid disorders and treat abnormal lipids in people who are at increased risk of coronary heart disease
4. Clinicians screen men and women 50 years of age or older for colorectal cancer
5. Clinicians screen all adults for tobacco use and provide tobacco cessation interventions for those who use tobacco products

RECOMMENDED (B)

1. One-time screening for abdominal aortic aneurysm (AAA) by ultrasonography in men aged 65 to 75 who have ever smoked
2. Screening mammography, with or without clinical breast examination (CBE), every 1–2 years for women aged 40 and older
3. Screening adults for depression in clinical practices that have systems in place to ensure accurate diagnosis, effective treatment, and follow-up
4. Screening for type 2 diabetes in adults with hypertension or hyperlipidemia
5. Intensive behavioral dietary counseling for adult patients with hyperlipidemia and other known risk factors for cardiovascular and diet-related chronic disease
6. Clinicians screen all adult patients for obesity and offer intensive counseling and behavioral interventions to promote sustained weight loss for obese adults
7. Women age 65 and older and women age 60–64 who are at increased risk of osteoporotic fracture be screened routinely for osteoporosis
8. Women whose family history is associated with an increased risk for deleterious mutations in *BRCA1* or *BRCA2* genes be referred for genetic counseling and evaluation for BRCA testing

RECOMMENDED AGAINST (D)

1. Routine use of tamoxifen or raloxifene for the primary prevention of breast cancer in women at low or average risk for breast cancer
2. Routinely screening women older than age 65 for cervical cancer if they have had adequate recent screening with normal Pap smears and are not otherwise at high risk for cervical cancer

(Continued)

Table 4.3

RECOMMENDATIONS, U.S. PREVENTIVE SERVICES TASK FORCE, 2008 (*Continued*)

3. Routine use of combined estrogen and progestin for the prevention of chronic conditions in postmenopausal women
4. Routine screening for ovarian cancer
5. Screening for pancreatic cancer in asymptomatic adults
6. Routine screening for bladder cancer in adults
7. Routine screening for peripheral arterial disease (PAD)
8. Routine screening for testicular cancer in asymptomatic adolescent and adult males
9. Use of beta-carotene supplements, either alone or in combination, for the prevention of cancer or cardiovascular disease
10. Routine use of aspirin and nonsteroidal anti-inflammatory drugs (NSAIDs) to prevent colorectal cancer in individuals at average risk for colorectal cancer

about reliability is playing a game of darts. Hitting the same spot on the board over and over would mean you have reliable aim. Reliability is relatively easy to demonstrate or refute and, in general, takes the form of assessing how closely aligned (or correlated) are multiple measures of the same phenomenon.

Validity is a much harder concept to demonstrate. Validity is the extent to which a measure accurately reflects the concept that it is intended to measure. Think of the scale described above. It gives you the same value every time you get on, but is that scale showing you 5 pounds lighter than you are? If so, the scale may be reliable, but it is not valid. Invoking the dart board image, you may be hitting the same spot over and over again with the darts, but are you hitting the bull's eye (which in this case represents what you truly wish to measure)? If you are hitting the bull's eye, you have a valid and reliable measurement tool. Note a scale can be reliable but not valid (a scale that always shows you weigh 5 pounds less than you do), but a valid scale must always be reliable.

There are different types of validity that become important in assessing the validity of a research study. Internal validity is the extent to which conclusions can be drawn from the study sample about relationships among variables measured in the study. For a study to have internal validity its measures must be both valid and reliable. In addition, the study must be designed in such a way that one can compare individuals who received a preventive service with those who did not, and such comparisons must be valid over time—that is, the groups must be comparable before the service and nothing else but direct consequences of receiving the service should be different between the two groups after the services are given. Groups typically are made to be comparable through the process of randomly selecting who receives the treatment, but even randomized trials can have threats to internal validity if follow-up differs between the treatment and control groups.

Even if a study has excellent internal validity, there still may be threats to drawing conclusions beyond the study sample. External validity refers to whether such conclusions can be drawn more generally and depends on whether the sample was drawn probabilistically or if it relied on volunteers who did not look like people who would actually use the service in the real world. External validity also depends on whether all groups of interest are represented. A study of 40–59-year-olds, for instance, does not necessarily have external generalizability to older adults. Likewise, studies of men may not generalize to women, and studies that exclude minorities may not apply to groups that have not been represented.

A related concept that is important for the task force to set its recommendations is the notion of *power*. The power of a trial is the probability you will detect a meaningful difference, or effect, if one really exists. The larger the sample size, the more power a trial will have. Another way to define power is in terms of probabilities—in this case, the probability of NOT making an error in which you say there is no effect when there actually is one. This is the probability of not making a type II error, or falsely rejecting the null. By convention, most studies are designed to have a power of at least .80 or higher to detect clinically meaningful differences, so that type II errors will be minimized.

Finally, we turn to the *diagnostic utility of screening*. One of the best treatments diagnostic utility we have found was by T.-W. Loong in the *British Medical Journal* (2003). Here, we provide a brief summary, but we urge the reader to review the visual aids in Loong (2003). Imagine a hypothetical population in which 25% of the population has a disease. Twenty-five percent is the disease prevalence. Now imagine you have a screening test and you screen the entire population and find that 20% test positive for the disease. The *sensitivity* of your screening test is calculated as follows: among those with the disease, what percent test positive? The sensitivity tells you an important piece of information—were you able to identify when someone had the disease that they actually have it. Subtracting the sensitivity from 100% yields the false-negative rate—the extent to which you say someone does not have the disease when they actually do. Sensitivity and false-negative rates are only one way to evaluate your instrument. You also need to know the *specificity* of your screening test: among those without the disease, what percent test negative? The specificity tells you whether your test goes too far and identifies people as having the disease when they really do not have it. In fact, 100% minus specificity gives you the false-positive rate. Both sensitivity and specificity are considered to be "disease-denominator" measures—in the first case, people with the disease are in the denominator, and in the latter, people without the disease are in the denominator. The advantage of disease-denominator measures is that they are not sensitive to the prevalence of the disease. So you can use sensitivity and specificity with rare and common conditions alike.

There are two additional ways to evaluate your screening test. You can look among those who test positive and ask, what percentage truly have the disease? This is called *positive predictive value*. You can also look among those who test negative and ask, what percentage truly do NOT have the disease? Not surprisingly, this is called *negative predictive value*. Together these are referred to as "test-denominator" measures. Unlike disease-denominator measures, positive and negative predictive value change depending on the prevalence of the disease. For example, the rarer the disease, the lower the positive predictive value will be.

Now that we have covered all the basic concepts, we can turn to the question of under what circumstances does the USPSTF assign a "D" recommendation (recommend against)? A "D Grade" is given if:

- The condition has a low prevalence and the screen misses people with the condition, that is, has a low sensitivity or a high rate of false negatives.
- There is limited evidence that early treatment improves outcomes. Even if a screening tool has excellent sensitivity and specificity, if intervening early does not improve health outcomes, a preventive service may receive a "D" rating.
- There is harm that comes from a false positive (100% minus specificity). A range of harms may be considered from actual risks associated with the procedure to the experience of unnecessary anxiety.

Case Study of Breast Cancer Screening

Let's take a look at a specific example of how a recommendation is set. Currently the USPSTF recommends: screening mammography, with or without clinical breast examination (CBE), every 1–2 years for women aged 40 and older. The rationale for the recommendation follows:

> Rationale: The USPSTF found fair evidence that mammography screening every 12–33 months significantly reduces mortality from breast cancer. Evidence is strongest for women aged 50–69, the age group generally included in screening trials. For women aged 40–49, the evidence that screening mammography reduces mortality from breast cancer is weaker, and the absolute benefit of mammography is smaller, than it is for older women. Most, but not all, studies indicate a mortality benefit for women undergoing mammography at ages 40–49, but the delay in observed benefit in women younger than 50 makes it difficult to determine the incremental benefit of beginning screening at age 40 rather than at age 50.
>
> The absolute benefit is smaller because the incidence of breast cancer is lower among women in their 40s than it is among older women. The USPSTF concluded that the evidence is also generalizable to women aged 70 and older (who face a higher absolute risk for breast cancer) if their life expectancy is not compromised by comorbid disease. The absolute probability of benefits of regular mammography increase along a continuum with age, whereas the likelihood of harms from screening (false-positive results and unnecessary anxiety, biopsies, and cost) diminish from ages 40–70. The balance of benefits and potential harms, therefore, grows more favorable as women age. The precise age at which the potential benefits of mammography justify the possible harms is a subjective choice. The USPSTF did not find sufficient evidence to specify the optimal screening interval for women aged 40–49. (USPSTF, 2002)

In a report prepared for the task force and subsequent peer-reviewed article, Humphrey and colleagues (2002a, 2002b) searched the Controlled Trials Registry, medical literature databases, and reference lists of articles found to compile a list of randomized, controlled trials of screening with death from breast cancer as the outcome. The authors abstracted information about the patient population, the study design, issues of study quality, data analysis, and findings at each reported length of follow-up. They then rated each study in terms of internal validity, with good meaning all criteria were met and the study's findings were likely to be correct; fair meaning there were important but not major flaws so that the study was possibly valid; and poor indicating there were

Chapter 4 Chronic Disease in Older Adults   **121**

major flaws with the results likely to be invalid. Seven criteria were used for rating the studies:

1. The intervention was clearly defined
2. All important outcomes were measured
3. Data were appropriately analyzed according to how participants were initially assigned (also called "intention to treat" analysis)
4. The treatment and control groups that were initially assembled were demonstrated to be comparable, for example, through randomization, by showing equal distribution of confounders and similar mortality rates prior to the intervention
5. The treatment and control groups were equally maintained over time, through, for example, high adherence, low crossover from one group to another, and low contamination of information from one group to another
6. Low, nondifferential loss to follow-up across treatment and control groups
7. Valid and reliable measures applied equally in treatment and control groups

Humphrey and colleagues identified eight trials, seven of which were rated as "fair." The reasons for fair ratings varied. For instance, the Health Insurance Plan Study took place from 1963 to 1966, so its findings, although valid for that time period, are not necessarily relevant to the equipment in use today. Four Swedish trials all had issues with randomization and some had issues with measuring the outcome (death from breast cancer). Two Swedish (Malmo) trials were perhaps the best designed, one focusing on women ages 45–69 and the other on women ages 70–74, but still were deemed only "fair." The sensitivity and specificity of the trials rated as fair are summarized in Table 4.4.

Overall, the studies suggested that 77%–95% of cases with breast cancer are correctly identified as having cancer with 1-year screening. The rate is lower for women in their forties and lower for 2-year screening intervals. In terms of specificity, 94%–97% of cases without breast cancer are correctly identified as not having cancer. In other words, 3%–6% of those who did not have breast cancer are incorrectly screened positively (false-positive rate). The test-denominator measures (not shown), suggested that the positive predictive value ranged from 2% to 22%. That is, 2%–22% of cases with positive ("abnormal") results were found to have cancer upon further evaluation, and 12%–78% of cases

Table 4.4

SENSITIVITY AND SPECIFICITY OF STUDIES EVALUATING BREAST CANCER MAMMOGRAPHY FOR WOMEN IN THEIR 40s

	SENSITIVITY		
STUDY (AGES)	1-YEAR INTERVALS	2-YEAR INTERVALS	SPECIFICITY
Health Insurance Plan of Greater New York (HIP) (40–64)	NR	NR	—
Malmo, Sweden (45–69 / 70–74)	.92 / .81	—	.97
Swedish 2-County (40–74)	.95	.86	.96
Stockholm, Sweden (40–64)	.86	.68	.95
Canadian National Breast Screening Study-1 (40–49)	.77	.56	.94
Canadian National Breast Screening Study-2 (50–59)	.88	.56	—

From "Screening for Breast Cancer," by L. L. Humphrey, B. K. S. Chan, S. Detlefsen, & M. Helfand, 2002a, *Systematic Evidence Review No. 15*. Prepared by the Oregon Health & Science University (Practice Center under Contract No. 290-97-0018). Rockville, MD: Agency for Healthcare Research and Quality.

with positive ("abnormal") results were found to have cancer on biopsy. The positive predictive value increased with age.

What about effects on mortality? Four Swedish trials compared two to six rounds of mammography with usual care among 50–74-year-olds. They found a 9%–32% reduction in risk for death from breast cancer, but this result was significant in only one of the four trials. When the results were combined across studies (in a "meta-analysis"), the relative risk of dying for those who screened compared with those who did not was 0.84 (95% confidence interval 0.77–0.91), a statistically significant reduction. Of seven trials including 40–49-year-old women, five showed a benefit, but only one had sufficient power to show statistically significant results and only after many years (11–19) of follow-up. Combining the results in a meta-analysis resulted in a relative risk of mortality from breast cancer of 0.85 (95% confidence interval 0.73–0.99) after 14 years. The benefit appears to increase with longer follow-up.

Although the USPSTF is the leading panel evaluating preventive services in the United States, it is worth noting that not all scientists agree. Another view of the breast cancer trials that appeared in the *Lancet* (see Gotzsche & Olsen, 2000; Olsen & Gotzsche, 2001; and related commentaries) is instructive in this regard. The authors reviewed the same body of evidence and found that the practice of assigning breast cancer diagnoses was not blinded to researchers involved in the studies. So they chose to focus on deaths from all causes rather than deaths from breast cancer. They also focused exclusively on the Malmo and Canadian (CNBSS) studies, and chose to exclude the remaining trials as not having adequate validity. When only the Malmo and CNBSS studies were considered, the effect of screening on all causes of mortality was zero. Moreover, the incidence of mastectomies and lumpectomies was 30%–40% higher in screening groups compared with groups of every study done after 1970. The authors concluded that 40 unnecessary surgeries were conducted for every 10,000 women screened and that mammographic screening for breast cancer was unjustified.

The ensuing debate depicted the state of evidence-based medicine in crisis (Goodman, 2002). Others have suggested that there are flaws, albeit minor, in all of the trials, but nevertheless six show significant breast cancer mortality reduction for women who underwent screening (Jackson, 2002). Moreover, they argue that if a new trial were to be undertaken, systematically denying access to screening (the "control" group) today would be unethical, and the contamination between groups unacceptably large, making the conduct of such a trial an inevitable failure. We are as a nation, "stuck" with the "fair" evidence that we have. Perhaps the moral of this story is that we need well designed clinical trials *before* recommendations for preventive services are made. This may also help explain why it is so important that the USPSTF have and maintain a rating of "I" (insufficient evidence).

Older Adults and the Influenza Vaccine

Research suggests great benefit in a number of clinical preventive services but perhaps none greater than influenza vaccination. In a comparison of older adults who were vaccinated compared with those who were not over two flu seasons, Nichol et al. (2003) showed great reductions not just in hospitalization for pneumonia, but also hospitalization for stroke and cardiac disease. The reduction in risk and the number needed to treat to gain this benefit are shown in Figure 4.3.

Older adults who were vaccinated faced a much lower risk of mortality as well. This analysis is complicated by lack of a randomized,

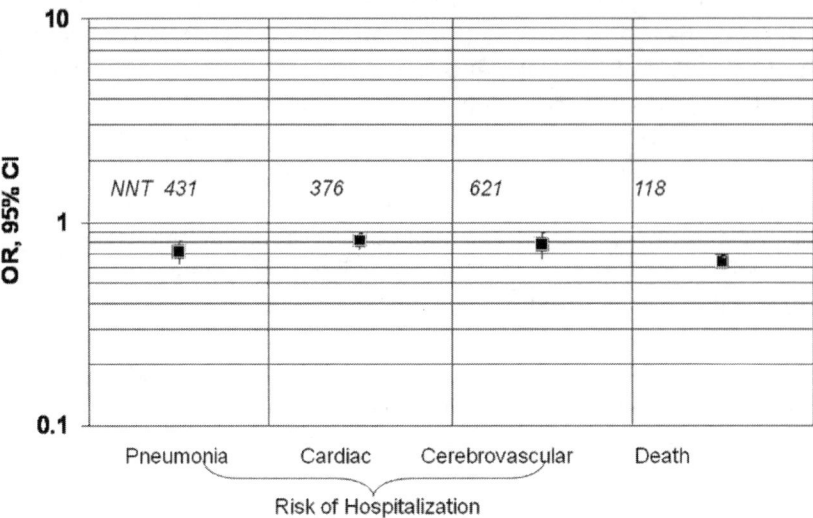

Figure 4.3 Generalized benefit on influenza vaccination.
Source: Nichol (2003).

controlled design (it would be unethical today not to vaccinate older people and people with chronic disease), and the investigators recognized that people who accept vaccination are different from those who do not. Vaccine acceptors are likely to be more proactive in health behaviors, but in this case were older and likely to have more chronic conditions as well. Nichol et al. (2003) and colleagues adjusted for differences between the group and made a strong case for the benefits of vaccination. More recently, Nichol and colleagues (2007) found, among older adults in the community, that influenza vaccination was associated with significant reductions in the risk of pneumonia- or influenza-related hospitalizations and mortality over 10 seasons. They concluded that vaccine delivery to older adults should be improved.

Results such as these suggest that the yearly prevalence of flu vaccination among older adults—which ranges from 40% to 60%—needs attention. Recognizing the need to increase vaccination among the older population, the Vote and Vax project makes vaccination clinics available to older adults at polling places. In November 2008, the program delivered 21,434 influenza vaccinations at 331 locations in 42 states and the District of Columbia. The effort is unique in its targeting of older adults at polling places and its recognition that older adults are most likely to vote.

Notwithstanding this program's success, it is useful to ask, do the nation's current efforts go far enough? Would it be possible, for instance, to have standing orders for older adults, in which nurses or other health personnel are able to vaccinate whenever someone comes to an appointment and is not up to date on vaccination? Is an even more proactive approach possible, one that is modeled, for example, after the U.S. experience with folate supplementation in bread? Folate is now added to all bread in the United States because of its clear benefit in preventing neural tube defects and spina bifida. It would be an interesting exercise to explore the effects of making flu vaccine similarly available. What might the effects on health and functioning of older adults be from such a program, and how might health effects differ in both the short and long term and at the individual and population levels? We offer some further insights into how to evaluate and compare different types of intervention in Chapter 5. Here, we take up the more fundamental issue of how criteria for setting up public health programs differ from the kinds of preventive services guidelines we have just reviewed.

Criteria for a Public Health Program

The preventive services guidelines are made based on whether there is sufficient evidence that individuals will benefit. But what if we are setting up a public health program? Recall from Chapter 1 that clinical geriatrics and public health differ in important ways. Clinical geriatrics stresses medical management of chronic disease and rehabilitation in the face of disabilities related to these conditions. Wallace (2005) explains that unlike clinical geriatrics, public health and aging places emphasis on prevention, proactive measures to preserve and promote health, rather than on a reactive treatment of disease. Moreover, public health focuses on the population rather than individual, and its programs and policies therefore address the community as a whole. How then might the criteria for such public health programs differ from clinical guidelines?

New York State's Department of Health offers some insight into the issue. They have outlined a set of principles to help guide adoption of public health screening efforts in that state. The Web site (http://www.health.state.ny.us/diseases/chronic/discreen.htm) suggests that the following criteria must be met for a condition to be a target of screening programs:

- Life-threatening diseases and those known to have serious and irreversible consequences if not treated early
- Conditions for which treatment at earlier stages is more effective than treatment begun after the development of symptoms
- Conditions for which screening tools have adequate sensitivity and specificity
- Conditions for which screening is low cost, easy to administer, safe, imposes minimal discomfort on administration, and is acceptable to both patients and practitioners
- Conditions that are high enough in prevalence for the program to be cost-effective
- Conditions for which appropriate follow-up care is available

Note that the public health concerns extend beyond those identified by the USPSTF to include administrative concerns related to cost and cost-effectiveness, ease of administration, and the availability of follow-up care.

MEDICARE AND FINANCING OF PREVENTIVE CARE IN AN AGING SOCIETY

In Chapter 3, we introduced the aging and public health systems in the United States, and described critical areas of commonality between the Center for Disease Control's public health apparatus and the Administration of Aging's area agencies on aging. A main focus of these agencies is prevention of chronic disease and disability, whether through exercise or fall prevention programs, immunization efforts, chronic disease management techniques, or other health promotion efforts. Yet most medical care for older adults in the United States is not financed or provided through the CDC or AoA, but through the Medicare program operated by the Centers for Medicare & Medicaid Services (CMS). Here, we review the Medicare program, providing an historic perspective of its development, ways in which its focus has been shifting toward preventive efforts, and issues the program will face in light of the aging of the population.

Medicare's Basic Benefit Structure

In 2008, Medicare provided health care coverage to 45 million people (CMS, 2009). Eligibility for this program is determined by another federal program: Social Security. Medicare covers 38 million people ages 65 and older with Social Security old-age benefits. In addition, the program serves about 7–8 million people under age 65 who receive Social Security disability benefits (most after a 24-month waiting period). Another 100,000 or so persons with end-stage renal disease also receive Medicare. In 2007, benefits amounted to $462 billion, making Medicare the largest public health program in the United States.

Signed into law by President Johnson in 1965, Medicare's original goal of was to provide "mainstream acute health care—hospital, physician, and related services—to persons ages 65 and older" (Moon, 2006). President Johnson (Public Papers, 1965) described the program as follows:

> During your working years, the people of America—you—will contribute through the social security program a small amount each payday for hospital insurance protection. For example, the average worker in 1966 will contribute about $1.50 per month. The employer will contribute a similar amount. And this will provide the funds to pay up to 90 days of hospital care for each illness, plus diagnostic care, and up to 100 home health visits after you are 65. And beginning in 1967, you will also be covered for up to 100 days of care in a skilled nursing home after a period of hospital care.
>
> And under a separate plan, when you are 65—that the Congress originated itself, in its own good judgment—you may be covered for medical and surgical fees whether you are in or out of the hospital. You will pay $3 per month after you are 65 and your Government will contribute an equal amount.

Over the past four decades, Medicare has been amended numerous times, but the basic benefit structure has remained largely intact. Medicare *Part A* (Hospital Insurance) covers inpatient care in hospital stays, skilled (short-term) nursing home stays, and some hospice and home care services for beneficiaries meeting certain requirements. Part A is financed through payroll taxes, and therefore most beneficiaries do not pay a premium for this benefit. Persons ages 65 and older who did not work or did not pay enough Medicare taxes while they worked may purchase Part A (premiums were up to $423 per month in 2008).

Medicare *Part B* (Medical Insurance) covers doctors' services and outpatient care as well as therapists and some home care when these services and supplies are medically necessary. Through the years, some preventive services designed to maintain beneficiaries' health and keep certain illnesses from getting worse have been added to Medicare Part B (see below). Most people pay a monthly premium for Part B. Starting in January 2007, the amount of the premium became tied to income.

In 2008, for example, a beneficiary earning less than $82,000 per year ($164,000 if married) paid $96.40 per month whereas a beneficiary earning more than $205,000 per year ($410,000 if married) paid $238.40 per month. In addition, beneficiaries are responsible for a deductible (the first $135 in 2008) and coinsurance (a percentage of every claim, with the percentage depending on the type of service).

Together Parts A and B are sometimes referred to as "original" Medicare (in contrast to Part C, described below). Beneficiaries who choose original Medicare may also choose to purchase supplemental coverage. These supplemental policies are designed to fill the gaps in Part A and Part B coverage. The majority of Medicare beneficiaries in original Medicare have some sort of supplemental coverage. In 2006, approximately 43% received supplemental coverage from an employer; approximately 22% purchased a Medigap policy from insurance companies, which must conform to specific standards set by CMS; and another 20% (so-called dual eligibles) were also covered by the Medicaid program (Gold, 2008). Economists and policy makers have long argued that older adults who have such supplemental policies use more medical care services because they are not required to pay out-of-pocket Medicare's cost-sharing requirements, although the extent to which reduction in Medigap policies would save Medicare dollars has been subject to debate (Lemieux, Chovan, & Heath, 2008).

Beneficiaries have been able to choose to receive services through managed care organizations since 1976. Beginning in 1997, however, the Medicare + Choice program (now known as *Part C*, Medicare Advantage) was enacted. This program initially allowed beneficiaries to receive combined benefits from Parts A and B through Health Maintenance Organizations (HMOs). In more recent years the types of plans available through Medicare Advantage have expanded. Today, most beneficiaries have a choice among at least two of the following: HMOs; local and regional Preferred Provider Organizations (PPOs), in which enrollees have lower out-of-pocket costs if they use network-based providers; Private Fee-for-Service Plans, which do not have restrictions on providers that a beneficiary can use; Medical Savings Accounts, which allow beneficiaries to deposit funds into a checking account to cover medical costs; and Special Need Plans, designed primarily for beneficiaries eligible for both Medicare and Medicaid, those in institutions, and those with serious or chronic disabling conditions.

The percentage of beneficiaries choosing to enroll in Medicare Advantage options increased from less than 10% in 1995 to approximately

19% in 2008 (Congressional Budget Office [CBO], 2007a; Gold, 2008) and is projected to increase substantially in the coming decades (CMS, 2009). Approximately 60% of Medicare Advantage enrollees are still enrolled in HMOs, which may include all the preventive services covered by Medicare described above, plus prescription drugs, and additional benefits such as vision, dental, and hearing services, physical examinations, and health/wellness education.

Growing Emphasis on Prevention

When the Medicare program was established in 1965, preventive services were not covered. Through the years, Medicare has increased the number of preventive services that are made available to beneficiaries. Specifically, since 1980, the Medicare program has been amended several times to add coverage for certain preventive services. During the 1980s, coverage for pneumococcal (1981) and hepatitis B (1984) vaccination became covered. From 1990 to 2000, coverage was extended to influenza vaccination (1993); screening for vaginal (1990), cervical (1991), breast (1993), colon (1998), and prostate (2000) cancers; bone mass measurements (1998); and diabetes screening (1998). In 2002, glaucoma screening tests and medical nutrition therapy were added. More recently, we have witnessed the addition of a one-time "welcome to Medicare" physical examination, cardiovascular screening, diabetes self-management training, smoking and tobacco-use cessation counseling, abdominal aortic aneurysm screening, and health risk assessments. According to Nelson and colleagues (2002b), most states experienced increases in mammography and adult vaccinations during the 1990s.

Table 4.5 shows current rates of preventive service use among Medicare enrollees by various demographic and socioeconomic characteristics. Two points are noteworthy. First, only cardiovascular disease screening exceeds the 50% mark; all other preventive benefits are used at much lower rates. Second, minorities, especially African Americans, have lower rates of preventive service use than White beneficiaries.

Not shown in the table is Medicare's most recent benefit addition: the prescription drug coverage benefit known as Medicare Part D, which was added in January 2006. For beneficiaries in original Medicare, a separate drug plan may be purchased from private companies that provide coverage. Beneficiaries enrolled in Medicare Advantage often have a prescription drug benefit as part of their plan; if not, they may enroll in a free-standing prescription drug plan. Beneficiaries pay a

Table 4.5

RATES OF USE OF MEDICARE PREVENTIVE BENEFITS BY SEX, AGE, AND RACE/ETHNICITY, 2006

DEMOGRAPHIC	INFLUENZA IMMUNIZATION	PNEUMOCOCCAL VACCINATION	MAMMOGRAPHY	PAP TEST	PELVIC EXAMINATION	PROSTATE CANCER SCREENING	DIABETES SCREENING	CARDIOVASCULAR DISEASE SCREENING	BONE MASS MEASUREMENT	WELCOME TO MEDICARE VISIT
Male	41.1	5.7	N/A	N/A	N/A	19.7	9.4	54.6	2	5.3
Female	46.5	6.3	37.9	11	5.9	N/A	9.7	58.2	13.7	6.3
Under 65	20.3	3	24.9	13.3	5.6	8.8	8.6	37.8	4	0.6
65–74	44.3	7.1	48.9	15.1	8.5	24.6	9.6	62	10.3	34.5
75–84	54.3	6.3	39.1	8	4.7	22	10.1	63.2	10	0.6
85 and Over	49.7	6.7	40.3	10.5	6	23	9.8	61.1	9.7	31
Caucasian	47.2	6.3	39.4	11.3	6.3	21	9.4	57.5	9.1	6.9
African American	24.9	4.5	31.6	9.6	4.1	13.4	10.7	50.5	5.1	1.3
Hispanic	22.7	4.1	25.1	7.3	2.7	9.7	11.1	55.1	7.5	0.5
Asian/Pacific Islander	43.8	6.2	23.8	6.9	3.1	11.4	10.1	60.3	9.5	1.8
National Total	44.2	6	37.9	11	5.9	19.7	9.6	56.7	8.6	5.8

From Centers for Medicare & Medicaid Services. Retrieved from http://www.cms.hhs.gov/PreventionGenInfo/20_prevserv.asp#TopOfPage.

monthly premium for prescription drug coverage, which may vary with the type of coverage. Those with incomes less than 150% of the federal poverty limit are eligible for subsidies for the new Part D prescription drug program.

How does the prescription drug benefit work? Enrollees have expenses covered (often with a copayment amount that depends on the generic status of the medication) until they reach a prespecified covered amount. Beneficiaries then enter a period of noncoverage (called the "donut hole") until they spend a prespecified out-of-pocket amount. At that point, the beneficiary is responsible for a minimal copayment (in 2008, $2.25 for a generic, $5.60 for a brand-name drug, or 5% of the cost of the drug, whichever is greatest). Actual benefit designs vary widely and some have argued for simplification of the program through standardization (Hoadley, 2008).

Early evaluations of the prescription drug benefit program suggest that, despite the voluntary nature of the program and its complexity, approximately 90% of Medicare beneficiaries had a drug benefit in 2006 (Heiss, McFadden, & Winter, 2006). That is, of 43 million beneficiaries, approximately 39 million had prescription drug coverage by June 2006, and 22 million of these had coverage through Medicare Part D (Kaiser Family Foundation, 2006). It is noteworthy that the program did not result in "adverse selection" in which those needing more prescriptions sign up and "healthy" beneficiaries refused coverage. Nevertheless, sizeable numbers of older adults—4.4 million in 2006—remain without coverage (Kaiser Family Foundation, 2006).

Medicare's Fiscal Health and Disability and Disease Prevention

The annual report of the Medicare trustees projects the fiscal health of the Medicare trust funds. According to the 2009 report (CMS, 2009, p. 3), the HI trust fund (Part A) is not adequately financed over the next 10 years and will be exhausted in 2017. This is not the first time the Medicare trustees have found the short-range financial status of the HI trust fund to be inadequate. The short-term outlook for the HI fund has been considered unsatisfactory since 2003; however, the outlook for this fund deteriorated substantially as a result of the economic downturn in late 2008/2009.

Parts B and D, the report explains, are adequately financed over the next 10 years, in part, because premium and general revenue income for these programs reset each year to match expected costs. However, Part B solvency could be jeopardized if Congress continues to override physician fee reductions that have been built into projections (as they have from 2003 through 2009) while maintaining a "hold harmless" provision that restricts premium increases for most beneficiaries. Without these reductions, Part B will increase at a rate of approximately 8%–9% per year. The trustees also project that expenditures for Part D will increase at a rate of approximately 11% through 2018. Both programs are projected to grow much faster than the U.S. economy.

Can a shift toward preventive services help defray the future costs of Medicare? It is too early to tell for sure, but early evaluation of the prescription drug benefit suggests perhaps not. It appears that prescription drug use *increased* for seniors newly insured under Part D. Some argue that Part D coverage will reduce medical problems and hospitalization costs enough to offset a significant portion of its cost. However, reduced adherence to therapies by consumers who hit the gap may adversely affect health outcomes. A study by Raebel and colleagues (2008) suggests that medication adherence declines after beneficiaries reach the gap, but how this influences other medical care utilization remains unclear.

Notably, the trustees' projections do not take into account shifts in the health and functioning of the older population. Some researchers have asked, if late-life disability rates continue to decline (say, as the result of more spending on preventive care), could Medicare spending slow? Projections by researchers at the RAND Corporation provide some insight into this question. Using a microsimulation model, Goldman and colleagues (2005) project that total health care expenditures for Medicare beneficiaries will more than double between 2000 and 2030, growing 3% per year from $300 to $621 billion (in 1999 constant dollars). Further technological breakthroughs will greatly increase spending beyond these levels. Varying assumptions about future declines in the prevalence of late-life disability, however, do not appear to have a large effect on projected health care spending.

Why is growth in health care spending so robust in the face of assumptions about disability declines? One study of lifetime expenditures provides some clues. Lubitz and colleagues (2003) found that an individual reaching age 70 is likely to spend approximately $140,000 (in 1998 dollars) over his or her remaining lifetime, whether that individual reaches age 70 with functioning intact, with some limitations, or with severe disability. Based on this analysis, Lubitz and colleagues conclude, "Health promotion efforts aimed at persons under age 65 may improve the health and longevity of the elderly without increasing health expenditures" (p. 1048). Because cumulative spending for older adults over their remaining lifetimes is largely invariant to health status, it also follows that disability prevention efforts may improve the health and longevity of older adults without *decreasing* such expenditures.

Where, then, might cost savings emerge? Some have argued that the highly variable practice patterns observed across the United States—and the apparent lack of association between intensity of care and outcomes—suggests that there is much excess waste in the current chronic care system (Wennberg, Fisher, Skinner, & Bronner, 2007). The authors propose that savings—and improved care—could emerge by transitioning to a system of prospectively managed, cost-effective, and coordinated care, one in which medical providers are paid for their performance (so-called P4P) based on measurable cost-effectiveness outcomes. Such a system would require extensive investments in creating the research base to support evidence-based medicine, as well as investment in the technological infrastructure of the medical care system. Others have argued that investing in prevention and wellness programs could result in substantial cost savings; however, this will undoubtedly depend on careful choices about the types of prevention, the groups targeted, and the costs of such measures (Russell, 2009). A recent article in the *New England Journal of Medicine* underscores this point with a demonstration that the distribution of cost-effectiveness ratios is very similar for preventive measures and treatments (Cohen, Neumann, & Weinstein, 2008).

PROMOTING CHRONIC DISEASE MANAGEMENT IN LATER LIFE

Of the $1.9 trillion spent on personal health care in the United States in 2007, Medicare accounted for 22%, or $409 billion (Medicare Payment Advisory Commission [MedPAC], 2009). On average, Medicare spending per beneficiary is about $7,500, but the roughly 10% of Medicare beneficiaries who describe themselves as being in poor health incur approximately one-fifth (20%) of Medicare expenditures (MedPAC, 2009). In 2005, for example, per capita expenditures were $4,286 for those with excellent health, $8,346 for those with good or fair health, and $15,705 for those with poor health. An effective means of identifying this group at highest risk for medical care would be an important addition to the armamentarium of public health. As Boult and Pacala (1999) argue, "this dense concentration of morbidity and use of health-related services is unfortunate for those afflicted, but it offers hope for effectively focusing resources where they will do the most good."

Who is the high-risk senior? In ambulatory and hospitalized patients, one way to identify the high-risk elder is to identify factors associated with hospitalization (and repeated hospitalization). An effective tool for identifying the high-risk elder is the P_{ra}, the Probability of Repeated Admissions (Pacala, Boult, Reed, & Aliberti, 1997). The eight items of the P_{ra} reliably identify people with high likelihood of repeated hospital admissions. The items include self-rated health, hospital stays over the prior 12 months, number of physician visits in the prior 12 months, diabetes, heart disease (coronary heart disease, angina, myocardial infarction), gender, presence of a person "who would take care of you for a few days, if necessary," and age. Thus, a male with coronary artery disease, angina pectoris, diabetes in the past year, and a self-rating of only "fair" health faces a high risk for hospitalization. He meets five of the eight P_{ra} risk factors, and Pacala and colleagues have developed regression equation weights for combining the factors into a single-risk index. We could also add additional risk factors. If this person also has a medication regimen of five or more prescriptions and a medical condition that requires regular injections or catheter care, he would obviously be at even higher risk. The P_{ra} is useful for its identification of eight simple indicators that reliably identify high-risk elders.

Covinsky and colleagues (2006; Lee, Lindquist, Segal, & Covinsky, 2006) have developed risk indices for mortality and decline in competency in the ADLs. The goal in this effort was to develop very simple indices that do not depend on laboratory biomarkers or extensive assessments, which could thus be useful for a clinical management or interpretation of new conditions in older adults. Mortality over 4 years was significantly associated with a series of these independent risk factors, which included age, male gender, disease status (diabetes, lung disease, heart failure), low body mass index (<25), current smoking, and functional status (difficulty with bathing, walking several blocks, and pushing or pulling heavy objects). Each of the factors was weighted as 1 or 2 points (except age, which ranged from 1 to 7) and the presence of the risk factors was summed, yielding a composite score ranging from 0 to 23. Among older adults with scores of 0–5 on this index (the lowest quartile of risk), 4% died over 4 years. Among older adults in the higher quartile risk categories, mortality was 15%, 42%, and 64%, respectively.

A similar approach with respect to decline in ADLs yielded nine risk factors: age older than 80 years, diabetes, difficulty walking several blocks, difficulty bathing or dressing, needing help with personal finances, difficulty lifting 10 lbs, unable to name the vice president, falling in the past year, and low body mass index. A simple count of these risk factors was highly related to onset of need for help in ADLs. For example, less than 1% of people in this large sample without any risk factors developed ADL dependency over 2 years. In people with five or more risk factors, by contrast, incidence was 40%.

Once the high-risk elder is identified, how should this person's medical care be managed to maximize effective treatment and minimize disability? Three areas of progress in this area, offering major benefit to older people, include geriatric evaluation and management, self-management of chronic disease, and reduction in polypharmacy.

Geriatric Evaluation and Management

The core of geriatric evaluation and management (GEM) is comprehensive geriatric assessment. This assessment includes a medical, psychological, and functional assessment that is integrated to develop an overall plan for treatment and follow-up (Beswick et al., 2008; Boult & Pacala, 1999; Fletcher et al., 2004; Gravelle et al., 2007; Rubenstein, Stuck, Siu, & Wieland, 1991; Stuck, Egger, Hammer, Minder, & Beck, 2002). Interdisciplinary teams meet to establish a comprehensive care plan for each patient that takes into account the full picture of this person's medical risks, ongoing preserved abilities, personal resources, and preferences for care. GEM works best when the team making the care plan is also involved in its implementation; otherwise, recommendations from comprehensive geriatric assessment may go unfulfilled (Stuck, Siu, Wieland, & Rubenstein, 1993).

A meta-analysis of controlled clinical trials involving GEM showed that effects were stronger in inpatient than outpatient settings (Stuck et al., 1993). A number of randomized trials in inpatient settings have shown benefits for GEM in a variety of areas, such as improvement in diagnostic accuracy, reduction in disability risk, improvement in mental health, and reduction in nursing home admission and mortality. Elders in the treatment arms of these trials were more likely to report satisfaction with medical care, and their family caregivers also reported lower stress. Finally, some of the trials reported decreases in hospital and emergency department services. Although the interventions usually involve greater use of home care and other long-term care services, these expenses are balanced and, in some cases, offset by lower hospitalization costs.

However, GEM results must be interpreted cautiously, that is, in light of the particular program elements involved and specific outcomes (and time frame) assessed. In early randomized clinical trials assessing GEM in inpatients, one showed no benefit in mortality risk, disability, or health status over 12 months (Reuben et al., 1995). The 1-year mortality rate in the two arms of the study was approximately 25%, typical of the mortality risk in older people discharged from hospitals. A second study showed no benefit in survival, but significant reductions in disability risk and admission to long-term care facilities (Landefeld, Palmer, Kresevic, Fortinsky, & Kowal, 1995). However, the two studies are not truly comparable. The second study examined only the change from hospital admission to discharge, whereas the former study involved a full year of follow-up.

Improvements in discharge status, as shown in this second GEM program, should translate into longer term benefits. If they do not, as shown in the first trial, it may be because selection criteria in these trials do not always identify people likely to benefit (i.e., they may be too ill or, conversely, too healthy to show benefit), or because the trials take place in settings where control group participants already receive services and assessment protocols typical of GEM.

Table 4.6 shows key elements in the GEM program that successfully improved outcomes at hospital discharge. The program illustrates well how hospital care can be modified to promote appropriate discharge planning from the point of admission by use of the many resources required for such a focus. The hospital environment was remodeled to focus on readying the patient for the return home, the patient-centered care protocol stressed skills and interventions that patients would need to bring with them when they returned home, and the barrier between the hospital and home care was broken down through active involvement of case management teams.

GEM has also been applied outside the inpatient and ambulatory care setting. In a randomized, controlled trial of annual in-home GEM, Stuck and colleagues showed that a program of home visits by geriatric nurses, who consulted with geriatricians, reduced disability risk (12% vs. 22% in ADL) and nursing home admission (4% vs. 10%) over 3 years (Stuck et al., 1995). These benefits came with the additional cost of significantly more visits to physicians, but the total incremental cost of the program was very favorable, with a cost of approximately $6,000 for each

Table 4.6

INPATIENT GERIATRIC EVALUATION AND MANAGEMENT PROTOCOL

KEY ELEMENT	FEATURES
Prepared environment	Make hospital ward approximate adapted natural living conditions: carpeting, handrails, uncluttered hallways, large clocks, calendars; elevated toilet seats, door levers
Patient-centered care	Daily nursing assessment Nursing interventions to improve self-care, continence, nutrition, mobility, sleep, skin integrity, mood, cognition Daily multidisciplinary assessment
Planning for discharge	Emphasis on return to home Early involvement of case manager/social worker to develop appropriate discharge plan
Medical care review	Daily review of medications Protocols to minimize iatrogenesis

From "A Randomized Trial of Care in a Hospital Medical Unit Especially Designed to Improve Functional Outcomes of Acutely Ill Older Patients," by C. S. Landefeld, R. M. Palmer, D. M. Kresevic, R. H. Fortinsky, & J. Kowal, 1995. *New England Journal of Medicine, 332*, 1338–1344.

additional well (disability-free) year. Other in-home intervention studies have shown benefit with different program elements (i.e., preventive home visits without comprehensive geriatric assessment, one-shot comprehensive assessment with follow-up, telemedicine contact); thus, it is unfortunately not clear which element of the program was most responsible for the beneficial effect.

A less extensive application of GEM principles is visible in geriatric case management. In this approach, a specially trained case manager arranges social- and health-related services and coordinates these services across long-term care settings. Results from this approach to GEM, on the whole, have been favorable. One randomized assessment of geriatric case management to increase access to primary care did not show a benefit in hospitalization or quality of life (Weinberger, Oddone, & Henderson, 1996). This was a study of veterans with a variety of conditions. Studies involving other elderly patient groups, such as patients with congestive heart failure, have shown benefit (Rich et al., 1995).

The benefits of geriatric assessment in the case of older people with chronic disease are becoming clearer now that a number of randomized trials have been completed. It is sometimes difficult to compare results of such trials because of differences in patient populations, bundling of intervention elements, duration of follow-up, and outcomes. Still, Berwick and colleagues (2008) conducted perhaps the best research synthesis to date. Their meta-analysis suggests that significant benefit of these interventions can be realized in chronic disease populations, as shown in Figure 4.4.

Figure 4.4 shows that community-based care after hospital discharge was associated with significantly lower risk of nursing home admission and repeat hospitalization. Similar results were obtained for interventions involving general geriatric assessment, fall prevention programs, group education and counseling, and a composite of all such interventions. Combining results across interventions showed benefit for all care transition outcomes (nursing home admission, hospital admission, falling, and declines in physical function), but no reduction in mortality. Aggregation across these randomized trials involved outcomes from nearly 40,000 people in the intervention and control arms and nearly 90 randomized clinical trials.

It is noteworthy that this meta-analysis did not find the expected dose-response relationship, given these findings. That is, interventions with more intensive services, more involvement of health professionals, longer duration, or more clinical specialties involved did not offer greater

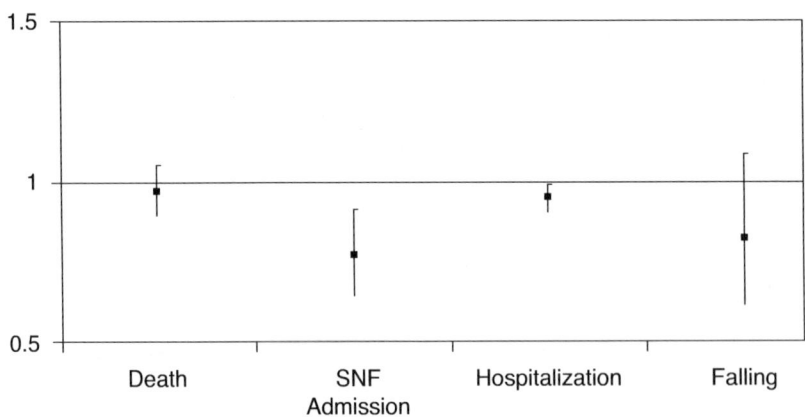

Figure 4.4 Meta-analysis: Community-based care after hospitalization. SNF, skilled nursing facility. Odds ratios and confidence intervals shown.

Source: After Berwick, et al., (2008).

benefit than less intensive forms of intervention. Thus, even short, less intensive home- and community-based services may offer great benefits to seniors.

Making Patients and Families Partners in Medical Care

Chronic disease is highly prevalent among older people, as we have seen. People aged 60 and older have a mean of over two chronic conditions, and these conditions account for the vast majority of health care expenditures (Hoffman, Rice, & Sung, 1996; Rothenberg & Koplan, 1990). Clinical and personal experience suggest that people differ in their capacity to manage the disability and symptoms typical of chronic disease. Some adapt well and maintain relatively active lifestyles, whereas others are less able to do so. Given these differences, it would be valuable to know what is involved in the successful management of chronic disease. Second, assuming these tasks can be identified, it would be valuable to know whether such skills can be taught. Finally, it would also be valuable to know whether disease management in this sense is associated with important health outcomes, such as physician utilization or hospitalization.

Recent research has examined the elements of effective chronic disease self-management. Lorig and colleagues (1999) identified 12 common features of successful disease self-management. These allow people to adapt to states of limited health and minimize the effects of disease on function. They include "recognizing and acting on symptoms, using medication correctly, managing emergencies, maintaining nutrition and diet, maintaining adequate exercise, giving up smoking, using stress reduction techniques, interacting effectively with health providers, using community resources, adapting to work, managing relations with significant others, and managing psychological responses to illness" (Lorig et al., 1999). These elements have been incorporated into a program of patient education, the Chronic Disease Self-Management Program (CDSMP), which has been used to teach patients with a variety of chronic conditions to manage symptoms well, to communicate effectively with health professionals, and to develop realistic appraisals of the health risks they face. Principles of this program include use of peer patient educators, mobilization of small groups of patients who develop joint problem-solving strategies, and a stress on self-efficacy, that is, development of weekly action plans with realistic goals and expectations of success. CDSMP is now considered an evidence-based model of self-management and may soon be tested in a Medicare demonstration effort.

A randomized trial of this model involving different chronic disease groups showed encouraging results for a variety of outcomes. One hundred eight CDSMP groups were convened for the 664 participants in the self-management treatment arm. Outcomes for these patients were compared with the experience of a waiting-list control group ($n = 476$) over 6-months of follow-up. Participants were drawn from people with a diagnosis of chronic lung disease, heart disease, stroke, or arthritis. People in the treatment arm completed a mean of 5.5 of 7 program sessions, showing effective delivery of the intervention, an important consideration in behavioral interventions of this type.

The trial showed significant benefit for CDSMP on a variety of outcomes, including health behaviors (self-reports of exercise, symptom management, effective communication with physicians), health status (self-rated health, disability, fatigue, and distress over health), and health service use (physician visits, hospitalization). These benefits were maintained over 2 years (Lorig et al., 2001) and were replicated when the control was offered the intervention. Comparing the CDSMP group with other samples assessed with a common measure of disability (HAQ, the Health Assessment Questionnaire) showed that CDSMP participants were more or less stable in disability scores, where other samples, matched for age and health status, declined.

These are impressive findings, and as a result CDSMP has been embraced by large HMOs, such as Kaiser Permanente, and by the National Health Service's (UK) Expert Patient program (AHRQ, 2002). Still, some caution is in order. Lorig and colleagues (1999) do not report participation rates in their initial randomization (i.e., how many patients randomly assigned to the intervention declined to participate). They do report that only 72% of controls agreed to enter the intervention when offered the chance to do so after the end of the initial 6-month trial. This suggests that the intervention group may have been enriched with more highly motivated participants, that is, people able to benefit from the program, or more motivated to self-manage their disease in any case. These selection effects are difficult to assess in behavioral trials.

CDSMP can also be faulted for ignoring a number of other factors that may be central to effective self-management. One is the availability of objective ways to monitor a chronic disease condition, such as urine or blood tests to identify hypoglycemia, as in diabetics. Access to these indicators allows patients to monitor and adjust medications or behaviors (Tattersall, 2002). Another factor is fostering effective partnerships between patients and health professionals. The "copy letter," in which physicians send patients a copy of their recommendations and the results of jointly planned care plans, is one way to build such partnerships. Finally, more needs to be done from the physician side, especially giving patients approval, or permission, to take a more active role in their care. Tattersall (2002) suggests that "many doctors and other healthcare professionals feel uncomfortable with the idea of empowering their patients."

In the case of some medical conditions, such as arthritis and diabetes, self-management has recently become the focus of randomized clinical trials that seek to determine whether patients trained in appropriate exercise, control of fatigue, adequate nutrition, stress reduction, and effective medication management manage symptoms more effectively. A large trial of an arthritis intervention showed benefit in patient mental health but not pain or physical function (Buszewicz et al., 2006). A smaller trial showed benefit for physical function (Heuts et al., 2005). Efforts to promote self-management and train "expert patients" have become widely adapted in the U.K. National Health Service as a promising way of reducing morbidity in chronic disease (www.expertpatients.nhs.uk). One interactive Internet-based self-management program to develop expert patients reported reductions in most symptoms and in health services utilization as well (Lorig et al., 2008). However, this effort did not involve a control group or a randomized design and should be interpreted in that light. More generally, a Cochrane Collaboration review of self-management education by peer leaders examined 17 randomized trials involving nearly 7,500 patients with chronic disease (Foster, Taylor, Eldridge, Ramsay, & Griffiths, 2007). The review found that lay-led self-management education promoted short-term reductions in pain, disability, fatigue, and depression, but it did not alter health care utilization.

Albert and colleagues explored self-management in osteoarthritis with reference to CDSMP guidelines for optimal self-management in a large biracial sample of Medicare beneficiaries (Albert, Musa, Kwoh, & Silverman, 2008). Lorig and colleagues recommend exercise, management of activity, and use of hot compresses on affected joints to manage pain and stiffness in osteoarthritis (Lorig et al., 2000). To operationalize this approach, the study considered optimal self-management to include at least two of the three behaviors. Only 20% practiced optimal self-management by this definition. Both White and African Americans who practiced optimal self-management reported significantly less pain than suboptimal self-managers, but other outcomes were not related to self-management competency.

Apart from promotion of effective self-management of chronic disease, it is also worth asking how older people actually manage chronic conditions. In fact, for the most disabled and oldest patients, management usually involves a patient-physician-family triad, rather than the traditional patient-physician dyad. Little is know about self-management behaviors in the home, or outside of contact with physicians or other health professionals. Up to one third of older people are accompanied by other family members in their physician consults (Silliman et al., 1996). Presumably, the patient's family plays an even larger role in management decisions beyond physician contact. This would be an important topic for future research on self-care.

Avoiding Inappropriate Medication Use and Managing Polypharmacy

Inappropriate medication use is a common problem in older people. One community-based study of people aged 75 and older found that 14% were using at least one inappropriate drug (Stuck et al., 1994), and a second study found a higher prevalence of 23.5% over a 1-year period (Willcox, Himmselstein, & Woolhandler, 1994). Forty percent of nursing home residents have been reported to receive one or more inappropriate drugs (Beers et al., 1992). "Inappropriate medications" in these studies are defined as drugs that should generally be avoided by older people, as specified in expert consensus panels. The drugs have all been shown to be ineffective or have been replaced by safer alternatives. For example, long-acting benzodiazepines (sedative-hypnotic agents) have been replaced by short-acting benzodiazepines with better side-effect profiles. The same is true for a number of antidepressant agents, antihypertensives, nonsteroidal anti-inflammatory agents, oral hypoglycemic agents, analgesics, dementia therapies, platelet inhibitors, muscle relaxants, and gastrointestinal antispasmodic agents (Stuck et al., 1994).

In these efforts to identify inappropriate medication use, the authors obtained valuable information on the prevalence of medication use in older people in general. In the sample of community-resident people aged 75 and older, medication use was fairly high. People were taking an average of 2.4 prescription and 2.4 nonprescription medications. A very small proportion, less than 5%, managed to avoid all medications, and about one third were taking six or more medications. The 14% of the sample taking at least one inappropriate drug were more likely to be older, on an antidepressant, and taking many medications (Stuck et al., 1994).

Chapter 4 Chronic Disease in Older Adults 143

More recent prevalence surveys continue to show that at least one potentially inappropriate medication is prescribed for approximately 20% of elderly patients living in the community each year (Fialová et al., 2005; Hanlon et al., 2001). Although overuse (polypharmacy) and underuse are likely to account for a larger amount of avoidable morbidity in the elderly, studies have focused on potentially inappropriate medications because modifying prescribing behavior may be easier than addressing polypharmacy or underuse. In addition, the consequences of inappropriate medication use may be severe. In an analysis of pharmacy and medical claims from a large employee retiree database, we have shown that use of medications on "do not prescribe" lists is associated with elevated risk of hospitalization in analyses that control for sociodemographic status, medical status, and total use of medications (Albert, Colombi, & Hanlon, in press).

A distinction should be drawn between inappropriate and excessive use of medications on the one hand, and polypharmacy on the other (Stuck, 2001). Inappropriate or excessive medication use involves use of medications in which the harm exceeds the benefit, as described above. Polypharmacy, by contrast, is simply use of many medications, all potentially appropriate. It is a problem, however, because of the greater risk of adverse events associated with a greater number of medications, which is complicated further by interactions between medications (drug-drug interactions) and between medications and nonindicated medical conditions (drug-disease interactions). Also, the greater the number of medications, the less likely compliance, and, hence, the greater the risk that people will not take the medications they should be taking.

One operational definition of polypharmacy is regular use of four or more prescription medications. By this definition, approximately 50% of the oldest old meet criteria for polypharmacy. A challenge to geriatric care is to determine which medications are inappropriate, because it is possible for diseases to be poorly managed and symptoms undertreated even with an excessive number of medications. The following tests can be used to determine the appropriateness of medications: Is there an indication for the drug and is the drug effective for the condition? Is the dosage correct (taking into account changes in renal clearance and other features of pharmacokinetics and pharmacodynamics associated with aging)? Are there drug-drug or drug-disease interactions? Are directions for administering the drug reasonable for the patients, that is, is the patient likely to be able to take the drug according to directions and for as long as indicated? Does the drug duplicate an existing drug? Can the drug be replaced with something less expensive? (Stuck, 2001).

In pursuit of proper polypharmacy, physicians may have to take patients off medications as part of a comprehensive examination of medication profiles. It is much easier to add a medication than to remove one, but good management of patients may also require taking patients off drugs. Evidence suggests that physicians, like patients themselves, are reluctant to remove medications that have been prescribed for a long time. For example, in-home evaluations of medicine cabinets show a great number of expired and obsolete medications, stored just in case (Rubenstein et al., 1991). Likewise, with the passage of time, patients are likely to accumulate medications, with a comprehensive assessment of medications undertaken by physicians only when adverse events or a medical event requires it.

The rational management of polypharmacy is a major challenge of public health and aging. Some success in this effort will likely come from new partnerships between physicians and pharmacists (Weinberger et al., 2002), and from greater consumer awareness, and perhaps increased regulatory pressure.

SUMMARY

Prevalence and Incidence. Prevalence refers to the number of persons who have a particular disease among the population at a given point in time, whereas incidence refers to the number of new cases of a disease that occur within a specific time frame in a population that is at risk for developing the disease.

Prevalent vs. Debilitating vs. High-Mortality Conditions. If the public health goal is to prevent the onset of or to detect chronic conditions early in the process (primary and secondary prevention), highly prevalent conditions such as hypertension, heart disease, and arthritis make excellent targets. If the goal is to maximize life expectancy, targeting high-mortality conditions such as heart disease, cancer, and strokes is appropriate. However, if the aim is to maximize functioning, then conditions such as mental distress, strokes, and vision and hearing limitations, all of which can be highly debilitating, must be considered.

Managing Comorbidity and Multimorbidity. The experience of having multiple conditions can lead to a long list of unfavorable outcomes, including mortality, poor functioning, and increased use of health care.

Today, older adults are increasingly responsible for managing their chronic conditions. Although health literacy has increased over the past decade, 60%–71% of people age 65 and over had below basic or basic health literacy skills, and may have difficulty finding and evaluating the credibility of health information, assessing risks and benefits of health care decisions, calculating the amount of a prescription to take, or understanding test results.

U.S. Preventive Services Task Force. The USPSTF's recommendations are considered the "gold standard" for clinical preventive services. The USPSTF recommendation is made in the form of a grade from A to I, whereby A means strongly recommended, B means recommended, C means there is no recommendation for or against, D is a recommendation against, and I indicates insufficient evidence on which to base a recommendation. Of the 40 or so screen recommendations relevant to older adults, nearly half involved insufficient evidence (I). The remaining recommendations include 5 A's, 8 B's, and 10 D's. In setting recommendations the USPSTF considers issues of reliability, internal and external validity, diagnostic utility (including sensitivity, specificity, and positive and negative predictive values), and the power of a study design. The panel also considers which negative consequences might occur as the result of screening. Despite agreement that USPSTF is the "gold standard" for preventive services recommendations, there have been disagreements in the literature as to how to correctly interpret the evidence base.

Public Health Screening Program Criteria. Criteria for public health screening programs go beyond those identified by the USPSTF to include administrative concerns related to cost and cost-effectiveness, ease of administration, and the availability of follow-up care.

Prevention and Medicare. When the Medicare program was established in 1965, preventive services were not covered. Through the years, Medicare has increased the number of preventive services that are made available to beneficiaries. Specifically, since 1980, the Medicare program has been amended several times to add coverage for certain preventive services. In 2006 a prescription drug benefit was added. It is unclear whether these preventive efforts will result in cost savings in terms of the lower prevalence of chronic conditions. Projections suggest that even if disability prevalence were reduced, costs to the Medicare program would not be affected, because average lifetime costs would not be altered. Medicare is not adequately financed to meet its obligations over the next 10 years

Managing High-Risk Elders. A small share of "high-risk" elders are responsible for a disproportionately high share of medical care expenditures. Such high-risk elders are subject to repeated hospitalizations and can be identified with an eight-item scale called the Probability of Repeated Admissions (P_{ra}). Items include self-rated health, hospital stays over the prior 12 months, number of physician visits in the prior 12 months, diabetes, heart disease (coronary heart disease, angina, myocardial infarction), gender, presence of a person "who would take care of you for a few days, if necessary," and age. Once the high-risk elder is identified, this person's medical care should be managed to maximize effective treatment and minimize disability. Three areas of progress in this area, offering major benefit to older people, include geriatric evaluation and management, self-management of chronic disease, and reduction in polypharmacy.

5 Disability and Functioning

Disability and functioning are central outcomes for public health and aging. The prevalence of chronic disease increases with older ages, as does the development of senescent changes that lead to frailty. As such, older people are at risk for dropping below the thresholds of physical, cognitive, affective, and sensory functioning required for safe, independent, and efficient completion of everyday self-maintenance and domestic-related tasks and for participation in social and community life. Self-maintenance tasks include, the basic "activities of daily living": bathing, dressing, grooming, feeding oneself, and getting to and using the toilet. Domestic-related activities include getting groceries, preparing meals, cleaning clothes, and performing everyday household chores. Participation restrictions refers to reduced involvement for reasons related to functioning in major life activities such as working, volunteering, or caring for others, or in social or community activities, such as participating in organized activities or attending religious events.

As we will see, the term "disability" is not used consistently by those conducting research on aging or by those working in public health. In this chapter, we use disability as a broad term that encompasses reductions in physical, cognitive, affective, and sensory functioning, difficulty with self-maintenance and domestic-related tasks, and restrictions in the ability to participate in productive, social, and community life. When compensatory mechanisms (such as environmental modification, use of assistive technology, or other behavior adaptations) are unavailable or no longer suffice for completion of tasks that have become difficult, older adults may need the assistance of other people to manage their daily lives. Individuals who adopt such compensatory strategies, even if they do not report having difficulty with daily activities, are also included under the disability umbrella to the extent that they are at increased risk for developing limitations.

Public health and aging professionals benefit from the perspectives of many fields as they attempt to understand the intersection between disability and aging. Demographers have focused largely on the population-level trends in disability, their causes, and identifying high-impact opportunities for intervention. Epidemiology has been concerned with identifying risk factors for the onset of activity limitations and functional decline, and more recently with understanding trajectories that individuals follow from onset through end of life. Clinical geriatrics emphasizes prevention of the loss of capacity and, in the face of such loss, the deceleration or mitigation of the effects of such losses on the progression of basic activity limitations—difficulty and dependence in bathing, dressing, eating, toileting, and basic mobility. The rehabilitation and professional therapy fields (occupational, physical, and speech) have focused on regaining and maintaining antecedent skills and making changes to the environment that translate into participation in a much broader range of activities.

The field of public health and aging draws on each of these perspectives but yet maintains a unique focus on implementing programs to create the conditions under which older adults can maintain and maximize physical function well into late life. To some extent, each of these fields speaks a slightly different language, so we begin this chapter with a review of the language and measurement of disability.

THE LANGUAGE OF DISABILITY

Well-trained graduate students know that before formulating a research hypothesis, whether for their thesis, dissertation, or graduate course in Public Health and Aging, they should first review and synthesize the relevant literature on their topic. Now imagine you are interested in designing a public health intervention to prevent the onset of disability among older adults through physical activity. A Medline search of studies using key words "exercise," "prevent," and "disability" with limitation fields set to find only clinical or randomized trials and age group 65 and older, yields 10 articles. After eliminating the five that do not actually examine disability or functioning as an end point in a trial, the remaining five studies define and operationalize disability (or functioning) in at least four different ways: (a) impairments in physical capacity related to mobility including strength, gait, and functional reach; (b) speed of performance of daily tasks and/or walking; (c) self-reports of difficulty with self-maintenance; and (d) self-reports of difficulty or the need for personal assistance with self-maintenance or mobility.

Such a finding—that the term disability is used at least a half a dozen different ways—is not atypical in the study of disability and aging. In some studies, the term may mean having impaired physical functioning; in others, it may mean reporting difficulty with daily activities, needing help with such activities, or receiving help. Policy discussions around public health goals for disability have been hampered by such a lack of a universally accepted and understood terminology. Not only have researchers used the term to connote a variety of concepts about undertaking activities important in daily life, but federal policies also use an equally wide range of definitions. A search of the United States Code found 67 acts or programs that define disability in at least 14 different ways (CESSI, 2003). Whether discussing the size of the population with late-life disabilities or interventions to minimize avoidable dependency, diminished quality of life, and lost productivity of older individuals and family members, the clarity surrounding such conceptual distinctions is critically important.

Recognizing the absence of universally accepted and understood terms and concepts as a major barrier to consolidating knowledge about disability and developing interventions to maximize functioning, the Institute of Medicine's Committee on the Future of Disability in America recommended in its 2007 report the adoption and refinement of the World Health Organization's International Classification of Functioning, Disability and Health (ICF) as the language for disability monitoring and research.

The International Classification of Functioning, Disability and Health (ICF)

The ICF language is presented in Table 5.1. The framework starts with the concept of *health conditions*, which encompasses disease, disorders, injuries, and trauma. Examples of health conditions include cataracts, chronic obstructive pulmonary disease (COPD), or congestive heart failure (CHF). *Impairments* may occur to either body functions (for example, impaired vision, reduced lung function, or reduced cardiac function) or body structures (loss of a lens or narrowing of a heart valve). *Activity limitations* are difficulties an individual may have in executing activities related to learning, communicating, mobility, self-care, or domestic life. *Participation restrictions* are problems an individual may experience in involvement in life situations such as school, work, or community life.

Disability and functioning are used as umbrella terms, rightly reflecting the myriad of uses that currently exist in the research, public health, and policy spheres. In fact, in the pictorial representation of the ICF, the terms do not appear at all (Figure 5.1).

What do appear are the terms "environmental factors" and "personal factors," and these clearly influence and are influenced by all other functioning domains. Environment is defined broadly in the ICF to include products and technologies, the physical environment and human-made changes to it, and attitudes, as well as services, systems, and policies. Personal factors are contextual factors related to the individual, such as age, gender, social status, and life experiences.

Table 5.1

MAJOR CONCEPTS IN THE INTERNATIONAL CLASSIFICATION OF FUNCTIONING DISABILITY AND HEALTH

Health condition: includes disease, disorder, injury, or trauma

Impairment in body function or structure: problems in body function or structures, including physical, mental, and sensory

Activity limitation: difficulties in executing activities related to learning, communicating, mobility, self-care, or domestic life

Participation restriction: problems in involvement in life situations such as school, work, or community life

Disability: umbrella term for impairments, activity limitations, and participation

Functioning: umbrella term for body functions and structures, activities, and participation

Adapted from *The Future of Disability in America* (p. 38, Box 2-1), by Institute of Medicine, 2007, Washington, DC: National Academies Press.

Embedded in the various documents that accompany the classification system, including the introductory guide (World Health Organization [WHO], 2002), is another important distinction between the *capacity* to carry out activities and the actual *performance* of those activities. The former relates to an individual's ability to function without aids or help from another person, whereas performance concerns itself with whether, how often, and with what supports an individual actually carries out particular activities.

Thus, the revised WHO model blends both social and medical models of disability. Disability is not an attribute of the individual, but rather a feature of person-environment relationships (WHO, 2001). In contrast, definitions that frame disability as exclusively caused by a health condition—with treatment of that condition the only focus—are symbiotic with the medicalized model of disability.

The ICF language, which has broad acceptance worldwide, offers several advantages for public health and aging. First, components can be expressed in both "positive and negative terms" (WHO, 2001, p. 10; e.g., functioning and disability), thus changing the dialogue from disability prevention to maximizing functioning. Second, it introduces the notion of participation in activities beyond those necessary for self-care

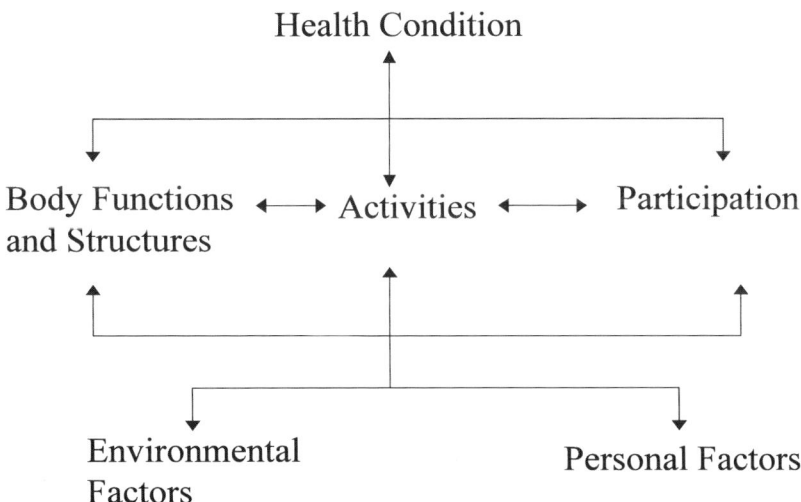

Figure 5.1 International Classification of Functioning, Disability and Health (ICF).

Source: From *International Classification of Functioning, Disability and Health*, by World Health Organization (p. 18), 2001, Geneva, Switzerland: Author.

(so-called ADLs) and domestic life (so-called IADLs). Gerontology and to some extent public health and aging has been almost singularly focused on these outcomes for many years. The ICF facilitates research and policy around additional activities and life situations that may be valued at different points in the life course. Third, in the ICF there is an explicit role for environmental factors of central interest to public health, including services, systems, and policies in filling the gap between capacity and performance.

Despite these advantages, the Institute of Medicine (2007) also pointed out several directions for refining and improving the ICF to better serve research and public policy purposes. The ICF does not currently offer crisp distinctions between activity and participation, an omission that researchers are working to rectify (Jette, Haley, & Kooyoomjian, 2003; Jette, Tao, & Haley, 2007). Current measures available in most surveys and studies of later life have measures that were developed in line with the Nagi disablement model (described below) and, therefore, do not map precisely into the ICF, making it difficult to use with many existing data resources. Nor does the ICF language link directly to quality-of-life measures and paradigms (see Chapter 8 for discussion of quality of life).

Finally, and perhaps most important in the public health and aging context, the ICF is not inherently a dynamic model. Like the International Classification of Diseases (ICD-10), the ICF is inherently a classification system that offers standardized internationally accepted language. For understanding dynamic relationships among factors predicting changes and maintenance of functioning, however, elements of the Nagi model of disablement (described below) remain useful to consider.

The Nagi Model of Disablement

The Nagi disablement model (Verbrugge & Jette, 1994) differs from the WHO approach in asserting a strict four-part temporal and causal sequence shown in Figure 5.2.

In the Nagi model, *pathology* (e.g., sarcopenia) first leads to *impairment* (e.g., lower extremity weakness evident in manual muscle testing). When lower extremity weakness crosses some threshold, *functional limitation* becomes evident, measurable perhaps in gait speeds below age- and gender-appropriate norms. When gait speed in turn drops below the minimum speed required to cross at a signaled intersection, a person is

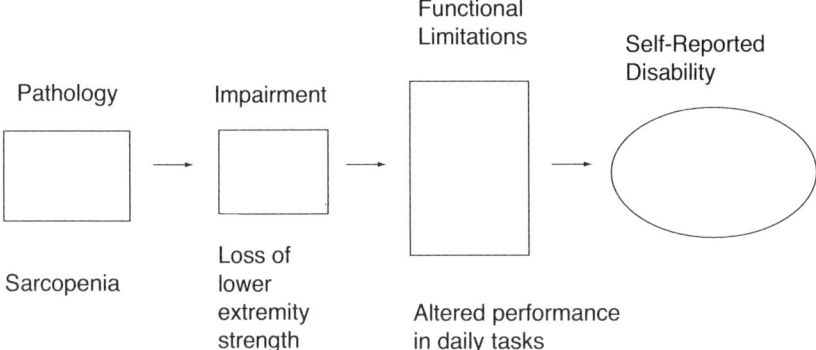

Figure 5.2 Nagi Disablement Model.

likely to report difficulty or a need for help crossing the street, that is, *disability*.

Note that in this framework, unlike in the ICF approach, the term disability more narrowly encompasses only: (a) *self-reported* difficulty or need for assistance, (b) a *need* rather than use or receipt of assistance, and (c) difficulty or need due to impairment, that is, a problem with one's *health*. The first condition construes disability is a matter of subjective evaluation. The second condition, the stress on need rather than on use, is important because it gives due recognition to unmet need (Allen & Mor, 1998). Only some of the elders with a need for assistance receive such assistance, so that restricting disability to the group actually receiving assistance would severely underestimate disability. Indeed, difficulty and dependence define important distinctions (Gill & Kurland, 2003), with the former more prevalent among older adults than the latter. Finally, the third condition requires that self-reports of disability be due to health conditions rather than solely to an environmental restriction, personal motivation, or other nonhealth sources of task restriction. This distinction may be hard to maintain in some cases, because environmental restrictions can also be considered legitimate targets for public health interventions and disease may affect motivation (as in the case of depression).

What of the older adult who uses personal assistance or equipment to complete ADL tasks? Ambiguity exists in the Nagi model, as specified above, as to whether this person would be considered to have a disability. In their elaboration of the model Verbrugge and Jette (1994) have made the additional important distinction between underlying difficulty—the level of difficulty without help or special equipment—and residual difficulty—that is, with whatever assistance is generally used. (The former is similar to the notion of capacity in the ICF.) Agree and Freedman (2003) refer more generally to behavioral compensations for impairments, such as using personal care, update of devices, or altering the demands of the environment, as accommodations. Individuals who make such compensations to complete daily tasks and carry out social roles would be considered to have underlying disability but, depending on the effectiveness the compensation, perhaps not residual disability.

The Nagi model has been used as a framework to identify early signals for the development of disability later in life. One advantage of the Nagi model for such work is the solid tradition of measurement behind it (Guralnik & Ferrucci, 2009). Even in people who do not report mobility problems, for example, weakness in lower extremity strength predicts future mortality and onset of limitations in daily activities (Guralnik et al., 1995). Likewise, people who do not report difficulty in ADL but report they have changed the way they perform these tasks have an increased risk for incident mobility limitations (Fried et al., 1996, 2000). More recently, the Nagi model has been used as the basis for identifying older adults at risk for interventions designed to deter the onset of activity limitations (Pahor et al., 2006).

Yet the Nagi model also has some important limitations. Because the environment is not an explicit domain in the model, for example, the emphasis to date in the literature has been on individually focused rather than population-level levers to reduce activity limitations. Indeed, many public health interventions that might reduce residual difficulty in a population—for example, changing the timing of traffic lights or extending health insurance to cover assistive technologies or motorized wheelchairs that may be used to enhance participation—have been overlooked. The ICF, in contrast, makes clear that environmental factors influence all aspects of functioning.

The Nagi model also makes disability an outcome and uses a fairly narrow definition of disability. This approach has been criticized for neglecting other components of daily life, such as non-ADL activity and general participation in social life, which can be preserved even with severe ADL limitations, and which may be more important to personal identity and self-worth than independence in ADL. Studies focusing, for example, on the ill effects of social isolation (both objective and subjective) among frail older adults (Simonsick, Kasper, & Phillips, 1998) and the beneficial effects of social engagement, in particular, volunteerism (e.g., Fried et al., 2004) might benefit from the more inclusive language that ICF has to offer.

Which approach is superior? The question sets up a false choice and is inappropriate because the ICF is not meant to describe disablement, but rather to inspire more extensive integration of environmental and personal factors into the management of impairing conditions. While the disablement model suggests clinical strategies, the ICF language offers a broader, common framework and language for taking action (Jette, 2009). As the authors state, if "disability is not an attribute of the individual, but rather a complex collection of conditions, many of which are created by the social environment," then "the management of [disability] requires social action, and it is the collective responsibility of society at large to make the environmental modifications necessary for the full participation of people with disabilities in all areas of social life" (WHO, 2001, p. 20). Efforts to bring the ICF language into studies of aging with a dynamic context are in progress (see for example, Freedman, 2009).

THE MEASUREMENT OF DISABILITY

Centrality of the Activities of Daily Living in Measuring Late-Life Disability

Activity limitations have long been a central focus of studies of late-life disability. Indeed, avoiding difficulty and need for help with the tasks of everyday life has been a focal point of chronic disease research. Chronic disease can also cause symptoms or changes in physical, social, affective, and cognitive capacity, an increased risk of hospitalization and death, a need for regular medications and physician visits to monitor indicators of disease progression or therapy, changes in behaviors such as dependency on people or equipment in daily self-maintenance activities, depression and anxiety, and changes in self-image and sense of control. All of these outcomes are appropriate targets for public health inquiry, but activity limitations are central because of their implications for each of these alternative outcomes.

Chronic disease, as described in Chapter 4, may cause difficulty or make it impossible for people to learn, go to school, work, play sports, travel, participate in conversation, drive, or complete the basic tasks required for independent living, such as eating, bathing, dressing, grooming, using the toilet, or moving between a bed and a chair. In short, chronic disease may lead to activity limitations or participation restrictions. The former are often operationalized in later life as the "activities of daily living" (Katz et al., 1963) or "personal self-maintenance activities" (Lawton & Brody, 1969), which over time have picked up the prefix of "basic" or "physical" ADL (hence, BADL and PADL) to distinguish them from more complex, household (or "domestic") tasks usually considered IADLs.

In public health and aging, there has been an almost exclusive focus on the activities of daily living. The reasons for this focus are numerous. Perhaps the most salient reason is that, traditionally in public health ADL competencies were typically considered the primary sphere of activity in old age, on a par with attending school for children and working or running a household for adults (Sullivan, 1966). Whereas older adults do not work or attend school at rates anywhere near those of younger people, an increasing proportion do; and we may want to rethink this rationale for the focus on ADL. (Indeed, the early Sullivan [1966] classification also considered housework the primary sphere of activity for adult women under age 65.)

Second, *ADLs are the basic and universal competencies of adulthood.* The loss of basic ADL competencies—the ability to toilet or bathe oneself—is a severe threat, not just to social participation and safety, but also to adulthood as we understand it, and hence self-worth. (However, note that there is some variability by culture in the degree to which this sort of independence is considered central to adulthood [Albert & Cattell, 1994]). Loss of ADL competency, then, represents a major milestone in the progression of chronic disease. From a public health perspective, providing the services to care for individuals who do not have the basic competencies in place is an enormous intergenerational obligation, one that is projected to grow in the United States as the population ages.

A third reason is *the universality of ADLs: all people need to accomplish ADL tasks; and people perform these tasks on all or most days.* Thus, all older people can be asked whether they have difficulty bathing or dressing or using the toilet. The tasks are not gender-specific, optional, or subject to variation in lifestyle. This is not the case with other competencies, such as the IADLs. The IADLs are household competencies, which typically include managing finances, going shopping, doing housework, doing laundry, using the telephone, and taking medications. The need, desire, and training to perform IADL tasks varies by gender, education, health status, lifestyle, and culture. The same applies to the so-called advanced ADL, such as using a microwave oven, programming a VCR, or using a computer, and to any of the more general lists of activities that have been proposed as indicators of adult competencies.

A fourth reason for the focus on ADLs relates to their measurement properties; that is, the tasks are hierarchical in nature. *ADLs differ in task complexity, and hence in motor and cognitive demand, and as a result appear to be gained and lost in a generally consistent (but not necessarily fixed) order.* Early on, Katz et al. (1963) suggested that the order in which ADL tasks are acquired in childhood development (first, feeding and transfer; later, toileting and dressing; last, bathing) is the reverse of the order in which they are lost in chronic disease (so that the first lost is bathing, the most complex of the tasks), as well as the order in which they are regained in recovery from stroke or brain injury (so that the last competency reacquired is again bathing). For this reason, Katz considered the ADL a measure of "primary sociobiologic function." His early research showed that the disability status of almost all elders in a skilled care setting adhered to this rough hierarchy of preservation and loss of task ability, which formed a Guttman scale. That is, people who were unable to do just one task from this set of tasks almost always had lost the ability to bathe. Likewise, people who could not dress themselves independently were also very likely to have trouble bathing independently. People who could perform only one task independently from the set of ADLs were likely to have retained the ability to feed themselves. In fact, a simulation study has shown that a number of alternative patterns, mostly relating to the order of the most primitive of the ADL tasks, form equally good hierarchical scales (Lazirides, Rudberg, Furner, & Cassel, 1994). However, it is well to remember that Katz and his colleagues (who developed the measure in the late 1950s and early 1960s) did not have access to sophisticated modeling software and that their clinical judgment regarding the scalability of the items was essentially accurate.

It is worth mentioning, as well, that a number of changes in task items have been introduced since Katz first proposed the measure. The original Katz items included bathing, dressing, toileting ("going to the toilet room for bowel and urine elimination; cleaning self after elimination, and arranging clothes"), transferring, continence (ability to control urination and bowel movements), and feeding. These items were initially developed as observations made by clinicians in institutional settings. Over the years these measures have made their way onto national surveys and studies in which older adults, typically in a community setting, are asked to self-report their level of difficulty or need for help or use of help with daily activities. Current measures of ADL competency generally include only one toileting item, and have added indoor mobility and expanded dressing in some cases to include personal grooming. Also, the original Katz scale items had very detailed descriptors for categories of ability. Each item was assessed on a three-point scale, and the scale values were quite detailed. For example, the middle scale point for dressing was "gets clothes and gets dressed without assistance except for assistance in tying shoes." Current versions of the measure typically use a single underlying measure for all ADL tasks: either level of difficulty (none, some, a lot, unable) or need for help (none, sometimes, all the time).

A last point involves the source of information about ADLs. While the ADL items have been selected to minimize "does not apply" or "don't know" responses (since the tasks are both basic and universal), cognitive impairment prevents a small proportion of the young-old (approximately 6% of people under age 75) and a much larger proportion of the old-old (about 20% of people aged 75 and older and perhaps 50% of people residing in nursing homes) from answering the questions. For information about the ADL status of these respondents, researchers and clinicians must rely on proxy reports, that is, information from family or service providers. But for people able to report on ADL status, it is their judgment that defines disability. As in the case of quality-of-life measures (see Chapter 8), this seems appropriate: who other than the person at hand is better able to report on the degree of difficulty he or she faces in performing daily tasks (Gill & Feinstein, 1994)? In fact, studies comparing patient and proxy reports of patient ADL status show moderate levels of agreement, and if patient factors affect accuracy (i.e., denial, loss of insight, wish for a more intense level of services), so do proxy factors (i.e., degree of contact with patient, mental health, perceived burden as caregiver) (Magaziner, Simonsick, Kashner, & Hebel, 1988).

Still, even with these limitations, the ADL hierarchy is highly robust. For example, the Venn diagram shown in Figure 5.3 demonstrates that in a sample of more than 2,000 elders *none* had difficulty with feeding or toileting without also having difficulty in bathing, grooming, or dressing.

Functional Status: WHICAP

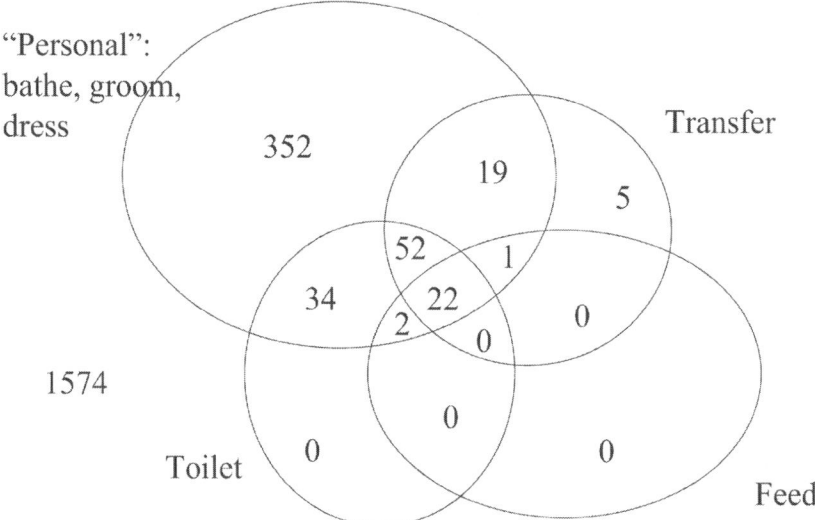

Figure 5.3 Functional status: Washington Heights-Inwood Columbia Aging Project.

Difficulties in Measuring Activity Limitations Among Older Adults

The centrality of BADLs and IADLs as measures of disability is clear, but measuring these most basic tasks is not simple. Kovar and Lawton (1994) describe many issues to be considered in assessing self-reports. These include:

1. Decisions about which activities should be assessed ("the number of possible IADL tasks seems almost limitless");
2. Ceiling effects ("the ADL/IADL scales do best at identifying the most-disabled minority");
3. Problems with the standardization of question formats to control for interpretation of environmental effects ("estimates of functioning reflect an unknown mix of personal disability and contextual constraint");
4. Effect of emphasizing different components in question formats ("dependence" vs. "difficulty" vs. "limitation") or combining them (Gill, Robison, & Tinetti, 1998);

5. Effect of proxy reporting (proxy respondents are more likely to report limitations than self-respondents, but they may be the only source of information for people with severe impairment);
6. Relevance of cultural differences ("socially or culturally assigned roles are obvious conditioners of IADL task performance and, conceivably, capability");
7. Cognitive factors in interpreting questions ("help from another person" can mean ongoing help, occasional help, or indirect help, that is, purchasing an assistive device).

An additional challenge relates to the variation across questions in whether underlying or residual difficulty is being assessed (Freedman, 2000). That is, sometimes questions explicitly ask, "without help or special equipment, do you have difficulty," whereas others ask simply, "do you have difficulty ____." The former are problematic in that respondents may not consider their assistive devices "special" and those who use equipment all the time may be answering about a hypothetical situation; the latter are problematic in their ambiguity, particularly for people who may not always carry out a task the same way every time (e.g., use their cane only some of the time).

These measurement challenges may be responsible for the different prevalence estimates of ADL limitations evident in national surveys. In their now classic study, Wiener, Hanley, Clark, and Van Nostrand (1990) identified substantial variation among the major national probability surveys of disability in the 1980s in the number of ADLs queried, whether "disability" in an ADL required a specified period of duration, and whether distinctions were made between need for assistance and receipt of personal assistance, use of special equipment, and standby help. The prevalence of receiving help with any ADL ranges from 5.0% (Supplement on Aging, 1984) to 7.8% (National Long Term Care Surveys, 1982 and 1984). Given the common definition of "receives help from another person," these differences are impressive. This variability applies to disability in all the ADLs, both those with relatively high prevalence, such as bathing (4.6%–6.3%), and those with low prevalence, such as eating (0.7%–2.5%).

Rodgers and Miller (1997) conducted a similar exercise, analyzing the prevalence of reporting any difficulty and receiving help with six ADLs in the Asset and Health Dynamics of the Oldest Old Study (now the oldest cohorts in the Health and Retirement Study). At the end of their interviews, respondents to the survey were randomly assigned additional ADL questions from existing health and aging surveys. Thus, unlike the comparisons in Weiner et al. (1990), estimates from Rodgers and Miller are generated from the same study sample. A summary of their findings is presented in Table 5.2.

Note the differences in prevalence for the same respondents in the same survey are even greater for different measures of difficulty than they are for measure of help. The difference between the estimate from the Asset and Health Dynamics of the Oldest Old (AHEAD) Study and the National Long Term Care Survey (NLTCS) is especially striking: one survey yields a prevalence of approximately 24% and the other survey yields closer to 11%. Such a large discrepancy is potentially of major public health significance. One only needs to consider the costs of providing support in the community for 24% of the population versus 11%

Table 5.2

PREVALENCE OF ACTIVITY LIMITATIONS AMONG ASSET AND HEALTH DYNAMICS OF THE OLDEST OLD COHORT, NHIS SUPPLEMENT ON AGING, AND NATIONAL LONG TERM CARE SURVEY (AGES 70 AND OLDER AND LIVING IN THE COMMUNITY)

	RECEIVES HELP		HAS DIFFICULTY/ UNDERLYING DIFFICULTY		HAS DIFFICULTY/ PROBLEM	
	AHEAD	SOA	AHEAD	SOA	AHEAD	NLTCS
Waking	3.2	3.9	17.2	24.3**	19.3	6.7**
Dressing	3.8	2.7	8.9	5.0**	10.0	4.6**
Bathing	3.9	3.1	8.0	6.3*	7.9	5.8**
Eating	2.6	0.8**	3.9	2.1**	2.7	1.0**
Transferring	1.3	1.8	6.5	6.9	7.8	3.5**
Using Toilet	0.6	0.6	1.9	3.4**	2.4	1.6*
Any	9.1	6.7+	26.7	24.1+	24.4	10.8+
N (Module)			N = 845 (3)		N = 915 (4)	

* $p < .05$, ** $p < .01$ difference from AHEAD; +, statistical test not reported.
From "A Comparative Analysis of ADL Questions in Surveys of Older People," by W. Rodgers and B. Miller, 1997, *The Journals of Gerontology. Series B, Psychological Sciences and Social Sciences, 52*, Tables 5, 8, 13, and 15.

of the population to begin to appreciate how meaningful these estimates are. And, although significance tests were not reported for this particular contrast, given that all the other contrasts between the AHEAD and NLTCS approach to asking ADL items—including some much smaller differences—reach statistical significance, it is highly likely that this difference also reached statistical significance.

Measuring Capacity: Performance-Based Tests

Elicitation of capacity to perform activities—in Nagi's model, functional limitations—usually involves self-reports of difficulty or need for assistance in a global sense; for example, "By yourself, that is, without help from another person or special equipment, how much difficulty do you have climbing stairs?" As explained previously, these types of questions pose problems of interpretation (Is the handrail or my cane special equipment?) and may even require some individuals to consider a hypothetical situation (Would I have difficulty climbing if I did not use the railing or my cane?).

Fortunately, a growing arsenal of tools is available to the field of public health and aging to measure capacity with performance-based assessments. Physical performance measures involve an individual performing a movement or task according to a standardized protocol and a trained observer rating the performance by use of objective, predetermined criteria. Batteries have been developed to measure the basic components of functioning (strength, balance, coordination, flexibility, endurance) as well as physical movements (e.g., walking speed) and goal-oriented functions (e.g., ADLs and IADLs). For example, the Short Physical Performance Battery (SPPB; Guralnik et al., 1994), assesses the time it takes respondents to walk 4 m and stand up repeatedly from a chair, and asks participants to hold progressively more complicated stances. Quartiles established within each of the three tests are then used to establish a "physical performance" score with a range of 0 (poorest performance on all three measures) to 12 (top quartiles of performance on all three measures). Such tests have been administered by interviewers in the home environment in population-based studies such as the Established Populations for Epidemiologic Study of the Elderly (EPESE) and the Women's Health and Aging Study (WHAS), and are now incorporated into the designs of population-based studies such as the large, national studies, the Health and Retirement Study and the English Longitudinal Study of Ageing (ELSA). Evaluations of the SPPB suggest that it is a strong predictor of incident activity limitations (Guralnik, Fried, Simonsick, Kasper, & Lafferty,1995b; Guralnik et al., 2000) and is particularly useful for detecting change within individuals (Guralnik et al., 1999; Onder et al., 2002).

Other tools from the occupational therapy field may also be useful, because they tap the antecedent skills necessary to perform a range of activities. In the Assessment of Motor and Process Skills (AMPS) test mentioned earlier, occupational therapists obtain *performance-based ratings of specific motor and cognitive skills* used in completing two tasks from a pre-specified list of 54 IADL/BADL tasks (Fisher, 2006a, 2006b). An occupational therapist, having undergone a 5-day training program in the AMPS, makes the ratings. Each of the motor and cognitive or "process" skills, drawn from extensive experience in occupational therapy with a variety of patient populations, is rated on a 4-point scale (competent, questionable, ineffective, deficit). The skills (and domains) are shown in Table 5.3.

An important advantage of the AMPS is its use of a many-faceted Rasch measurement model. The Rasch model has been used to (a) calibrate difficulty levels for the 54 tasks, (b) establish difficulty levels for ratings of each skill item, and (c) combine these skill ratings and task difficulty ratings to establish a single score for respondents on separate motor and cognitive/process skill dimensions. The equating of AMPS

Table 5.3

ASSESSMENT OF MOTOR AND PROCESS SKILLS

AMPS Motor Skills:

Posture: stabilizes, aligns, positions.

Mobility: walks, reaches, bends.

Coordination: coordinates, manipulates, flows.

Strength and Effort: moves, transports, lifts, calibrates, grips.

Energy: endures.

AMPS Cognitive/Process Skills:

Energy: paces, attends.

Using Knowledge: chooses, uses, handles, heeds, inquires.

Temporal Organization: initiates, continues, sequences, terminates.

Space and Objects: searches/locates, gathers, organizes, restores, navigates.

Adaptation: notices/responds, accommodates, adjusts, benefits.

tasks, linked by common skill items, makes it possible to compare the ability of respondents who perform *different* sets of tasks.

An advantage of this approach is its explicit focus on the skill elements elders use *to get tasks done,* as observed in home settings by using prespecified but ecologically valid tasks. In this way it differs from existing IADL or BADL performance tests (e.g., Karagiozis, Gray, Sacco, Shapiro, & Kawas, 1998; Lowenstein et al., 1992; Muharin, DeBettignies, & Pirozzolo, 1991; Myers et al., 1996), which are limited to only a few tasks, require subjects to perform tasks they may not do in normal activity, and do not yield measures of ability or skill that are involved in all IADL/BADL tasks.

Measuring the Environment

The emergence of the ICF highlights the need to improve measures of the environments in which older adults conduct their daily activities. Indeed, the expansion of measures of assistive technology and the physical environment would allow analysts to more fully understand the reasons for population-level changes in disability prevalence, and could further understanding at the individual level of the accommodation process and interventions to enhance independence and participation.

Keysor (2006) summarizes three general approaches to environmental measurement. The first approach involves assessment of an individual's perceptions of how the environment influences his or her participation. For example, the CHIEF (Whiteneck et al., 2004) is a 24-item self-report instrument that asks how often various barriers in the environment have been a problem in the past 12 months (and, if so, whether it has been a big problem or a small problem). The CHIEF focuses on barriers related to attitudes and support, services and assistance, physical and architectural features, policies, work, and school. A second approach is to literally observe study subjects and characterize avoidance and/or encounters with various features in the physical environment. Shumway-Cook and colleagues (2003), for example, used this approach to assess eight dimensions of the physical environment that may influence mobility: temporal, physical load, terrain, postural transitions, distance, density, attentional demands, and ambient conditions. A third approach is to ask research participants to characterize the presence or absence of various features in the environment (rather than perceptions about their roles as barriers). Keysor, Jette, and Haley's (2005) 36-item Home and Community Environment Instrument and the Pilot

Study of Aging and Technology (PSAT) instrument (Freedman, Agree, & Cornman, 2005) are examples of the latter strategy.

Such measures are beginning to make their way into clinical studies and national surveys. An example of the latter, the items from the PSAT were incorporated into an experimental module in the Health and Retirement Study in 2006, to assess the existence, acquisition, and use of assistive home features and devices by adults ages 52 and older (Freedman & Agree, 2008). Findings suggest that assistive home features are common: 78% of this age group have one or more features, 37% have added them, and 53% used them in the past 30 days. Of particular concern for public health and aging, one in four near-elderly and older adults were found to be at risk for a home modification, that is, had a mobility limitation and an unmodified barrier at the entry to their home, inside their home, or in the bathroom (either shower/bath area or toilet area). Adults receiving Medicare through the Disability Insurance program were identified as having elevated chances of being at risk for a home modification, suggesting a possible programmatic opportunity for reaching such a population.

TRENDS IN DISABILITY PREVALENCE AND ACTIVE LIFE EXPECTANCY

A central question for demographers interested in population aging is, "what are the implications for lengthening life for the health of the older population?" Simply put, the question is, are these additional years spent in good health and function or in a state of dependence?

Trends in Prevalence

Early studies on this question suggested that longer life implied worsening health, as measured by increases in self-reported activity limitations and chronic disease. Some researchers have questioned whether these increases were due to changing social forces during the period that made reports of disability more acceptable. The evidence for the 1980s and early 1990s was much more mixed, with Manton and colleagues first noting large declines in activity limitations (Manton, Corder, & Stallard, 1993) and Crimmins and colleagues concluding that there was no clear ongoing trend (Crimmins, Saito, & Reynolds, 1997b). A review of these inconsistencies by the Committee on National Statistics of the National

Research Council (Freedman & Soldo, 1994), concluded that there had been modest declines in the proportion of older people with limitations in IADLs, but inconsistencies across surveys in trends in ADLs.

In the 15 years since that workshop more than a dozen studies have focused on late-life disability trends. A review by Freedman, Martin, and Schoeni (2002b) highlighted methodological considerations in the comparison of trends in prevalence across surveys and reported findings for a range of outcomes, including physical, cognitive, and sensory limitations, as well as ADL and IADL limitations. Of the 16 studies identified, the authors analyzed 8 unique surveys: for the purposes of trend analysis, 2 were rated as good, 4 were rated as fair, 1 was rated as poor, and 1 was rated as mixed (fair or poor, depending on the outcome). Studies rated fair or good consistently showed substantial declines in IADL limitations. For example, evidence from the National Health Interview Survey (NHIS) suggests that between 1982 and 2004 there was a 6% decline in the population ages 70 years and older needing help with only routine care (but not personal care) activities, such as shopping, preparing meals, and managing money, sometimes called IADLs. Subsequent analysis of data from the NLTCS suggested that declines in limitations in three IADL activities—managing money, shopping for groceries, and doing laundry—were notably large from 1984 to 1999; however, among those reporting a limitation in ADL or an IADL, the severity of disability increased over time (Spillman, 2004).

At the time that the review was published, disagreement remained about whether there had been a decline in the proportion of older Americans having difficulty with self-care activities, such as bathing, dressing, toileting, and walking around inside, sometimes called ADLs. The answer was sorted out by a technical working group that analyzed five national surveys conducted from the early 1980s through 2001 (Freedman et al., 2004). The 12-person panel prepared estimates by use of identical methodologies and investigated sources of the inconsistencies among the population age 70 years and older. They found that during the middle and late 1990s consistent declines on the order of 1%–2.5% per year for two commonly used measures in the disability literature: difficulty with daily activities and help with daily activities. Mixed evidence was found for a third measure: use of help or equipment with daily activities. In comparing findings across surveys, the panel found that the time period, definition of disability, treatment of the institutional population, and standardization of results by age were important considerations.

More recently, the NLTCS suggested that declines continued from 1999 to 2004 (Manton, Gu, & Lamb, 2006), but other surveys, such as the Medicare Current Beneficiary Survey (Federal Interagency Forum on Aging-Related Statistics, 2008), suggested a possible leveling off of "any limitation." Disagreement also exists about trends among the generations approaching late life (see Martin et al., 2009; Seeman, Merkin, Crimmins, & Karlamangla, in press; Soldo, Mitchell, Tfaily, & McCabe, 2007; Weir, 2007) and some have warned that trends in obesity and other potentially disabling conditions among working-age adults could offset future improvements in late-life functioning (Bhattacharya, Choudhry, & Lakdawalla, 2006; Sturm, Ringel, & Andreyeva, 2004). Hence, reconciling disparate findings remains an important focus among demographers.

Trends in Active Life Expectancy

Prevalence measures are helpful policy and planning tools but do not yield information on whether increasing years of life are active. Measures of active life expectancy are needed to ask whether, on average, older adults spend more of their lives living free from limitations. Active life expectancy is a summary measure that combines information on age-specific mortality with age-specific activity limitations. Some researchers use cross-sectional activity limitation information ("Sullivan method") and others have drawn on transition probabilities in making these calculations, but in either case the concept is similar: how many years on average could an individual be expected to live without activity limitations if age-specific rates of such limitations and mortality held over a hypothetical cohort's lifetime. Comparisons of active life expectancy estimates over time are subject to many of the same threats to validity as are prevalence trends.

What have the studies shown? Several studies of the 1970s suggested that increases in active life expectancy were being accompanied by an increase in the number of years lived with a limitation, but this trend appeared to reverse during the 1980s and more recently. Three studies using different measures, methods, and dates (Cai & Lubitz, 2007; Crimmins et al., 1997b; Manton et al., 2006) suggest surprisingly similar results: all three show an increase in the expected number of years of active life and in the percentage of life expectancy expected to be spent without activity limitations. A fourth study (Crimmins, Hayward, Hagedorn, Saito, & Brouard, 2009) suggests stable levels of active life expectancy between the 1980s and 1990s that are the result of several underlying processes: declines in the onset of limitations, increases in the chances of recovery, and reductions in mortality among those living with an activity limitation at age 70.

Disparities in Trends and Causes

Adopting a public health focus, we may ask, have all groups benefited equally from these trends or are some groups being left behind? Although the evidence is thin, and with few exceptions, statistical tests have not been performed to determine whether these differences are due to chance, the answer appears to be no, at least when the population is sliced by major racial and socioeconomic groups. In one of the few studies including such tests, Schoeni, Martin, Andreski, and Freedman (2005), found persistent gaps in activity limitations between Blacks and other groups and widening gaps between socioeconomic groups from 1982 to 2002. Educational disparities in both the prevalence of activity limitations and in the extent of expansion in active life are also evident. For instance, older adults with less than a high school education as a group have experienced increases in the prevalence of basic activity limitations, while other groups have experienced declines (Schoeni et al., 2005). Similarly, a study by Crimmins and colleagues found a compression of morbidity—that is, an increase in the percentage of life expectancy to be lived in an active state—for highly educated groups but an expansion of morbidity for less educated groups (Crimmins & Saito, 2001).

In searching for ways to promote further declines in late-life disability prevalence, we might ask, what are the causes of trends to date and are those forces expected to continue as the Baby Boom generations reach late life? Four distinct realms of explanation have been explored to date: demographic and socioeconomic shifts; changes in chronic disease and related treatments; trends in underlying physical, cognitive, and sensory functioning; and environmental changes, in particular, growth in the use of assistive devices.

Research to date suggests that the decline is likely the result of a combination of factors and not any single underlying trend (Schoeni, Freedman, & Martin, 2008). For example, the improvement has been attributed in part to the greater educational attainment of older adults today compared with cohorts who were in late life in the mid-1980s. Yet such changes account for only a portion—and not all—of the decline in limitations. One analysis suggests that impending increases in education levels will continue to contribute to improvements in late-life functioning, albeit at a reduced rate (Freedman & Martin, 1999).

Other evidence also suggests that the extent to which some chronic conditions are expressed in terms of disability may have been ameliorated in recent decades. In particular, arthritis, vision-related conditions such as cataracts, and cardiovascular diseases appear to be less debilitating even as the prevalence of these and related conditions has increased in the older population (Schoeni et al., 2008). It could be that earlier diagnosis and better management of such conditions has led to lower reported rates of disabilities. Evidence supporting this possibility is lacking, however.

A third area of focus has been on trends in underlying physical, cognitive, and sensory functioning. Self-reported measures of capacity (using Nagi's functional limitations—difficulty with body movements such as reaching, bending, and lifting) have shown consistently large declines (Freedman, Martin, & Schoeni, 2002b), but no study of trends in performance measures has been conducted to date because of data limitations. Evidence regarding trends in cognitive function among the elderly population is not as well developed, although there may be some positive movement in that regard (Langa et al., 2008). Vision impairments appear to be less debilitating than they were 10 years ago, possibly because of the increases in cataract surgery over the past decade (Schoeni et al., 2008).

A final avenue of inquiry has focused on the role of assistive technology in disability trends. Well-known shifts have been occurring in the forms of assistance available to help people cope with disability in later life, and the use of technology without personal care has increased markedly among those reporting reduced functional capacity (Freedman, Agree, Martin, & Cornman, 2006a). Some researchers have also attributed declines in IADL disabilities to the increased availability of modern conveniences, such as no longer having to go to the store to shop or to the bank to manage money, and having microwave ovens to facilitate cooking (Spillman, 2004). Moreover, many more seniors are living in supportive living environments that provide assistance with these tasks, such as continuing-care retirement communities, assisted living facilities, and other retirement communities. The role of these pervasive technologies and specialized living environments has not been quantified.

THE EPIDEMIOLOGY OF DISABILITY: RISK FACTORS FOR FUNCTIONAL DECLINE

Prospective cohort studies have proven very productive in helping to identify factors that increase the risk of developing an activity limitation in later life. In these studies, a group of people without difficulty in daily activities at baseline is monitored during some defined interval. Onset of disability is recorded, typically at 1- or 2-year intervals, sometimes more frequently. We are thus able to identify incident (new) cases and go back to baseline assessments to see how these people differ from people who never reached the end point of interest. Typically, we examine a series of baseline risk factors and calculate the risk associated with a factor, independent of other risk factors that make up a person's profile. Features associated with the disability outcome are "risk factors"; features that reduce likelihood of incidence are called "protective factors." We often calculate these risks by use of logistic regression models, or proportional hazards models if we wish to incorporate a time dimension into analyses (i.e., time to onset rather than simply onset).

In a comprehensive review, Stuck and colleagues (1999) summarized findings across a large number of such studies, with a focus on potentially modifiable risk factors for functional loss. Findings varied somewhat between studies, according to the demographic composition of the cohort, the length of follow-up, how attrition was handled, how risk factors were categorized, and how competing risks (for death and disability) were handled. Nevertheless, the review identified some consistent findings across studies. Consistent predictors of functional loss included, for example, cognitive, vision, and lower body impairments; depression; comorbidity; high/low body mass index; few social contacts; low physical activity; and smoking as consistent predictors of functional loss. Stuck also identified several areas that required further investigation, including the role of biological factors (earlier in the disablement pathway) and the environment.

Since Stuck's review, progress has been made on both fronts. On the biological front, potential biomarkers for disability have been identified. For example, serum albumin level (g/liter) is a risk factor for both incident activity limitations and mortality. Within the EPESE cohort, serum albumin concentration and activity limitations were strongly related at baseline. Moreover, at follow-up, greater serum albumin concentration was associated with a greater risk of mortality within categories of baseline functioning. A new set of biomarkers for function is currently under investigation, including C-reactive protein, interleukin-6 (IL-6), and other cytokines.

In addition, strides have been made in understanding the relationship among inflammation, frailty, and loss of physical capacity that precedes limitations and frank limitations. Chronic inflammation, visible in elevations in IL-6, fibrinogin, C-reactive protein, and tumor necrosis factor-alpha, and decreases in serum albumin, are associated with loss of lean muscle mass (shrinking), low energy, decreased appetite, and the other symptoms of frailty. For instance, in the Women's Health and Aging Study, high levels of IL-6 and C-reactive protein were shown to predict incident difficulty with daily activities independent of other risk factors (Ferrucci et al., 1999). The mechanism for this effect is the catabolic effect of IL-6 on muscle, which leads to sarcopenia and, hence, loss of muscle strength in the lower extremities. This, in turn, leads to limitations in mobility and ultimately ADLs. Examination of changes in knee extensor strength and walking speed suggest that IL-6 affects muscle mass, and that this effect is responsible for the increased risk of disability. That is, the effect of IL-6 on risk of disability was attenuated when changes in muscle mass were introduced into regression equations. This attenuation in risk suggests that "change in muscle strength is intrinsic to the causal pathway leading from high IL-6 to the development of new disability" (Ferrucci et al., 2002). This is an indirect demonstration of the causal mechanism, but it is consistent with other research showing an association between high levels of IL-6 and lower muscle mass and strength (Visser et al., 2002a), as well as lower muscle mass and poorer lower extremity function (Visser et al., 2002b). A stronger demonstration would show an increased risk of disability among people whose IL-6 serum levels have increased (or a lower risk of disability in a group whose IL-6 levels have declined, perhaps as a result of a therapeutic intervention). This growing body of work suggests that intervention strategies that might prevent IL-6 and other cytokines from affecting muscle may be ready for investigation.

With respect to environmental influences, the role of neighborhoods in facilitating or impeding late-life function has been a recent focus (e.g., Balfour & Kaplan, 2002; Clarke & George, 2005; Freedman, Grafova, Schoeni, & Rogowski, 2008; Schootman et al., 2006). Balfour and Kaplan (2002), for example, found that functional loss among persons 55 and older in Alameda County, California, was related to self-reported problems with neighborhoods, including excessive noise, inadequate lighting at night, heavy traffic, and limited public transportation. Clarke and George (2005) found that among adults age 65 and older living in North Carolina, greater independence in IADLs (e.g., shopping, managing money, household chores) was reported among those living in environments with more land-use diversity, and that among those with functional limitations, housing density was inversely related to self-care disability. Schootman and colleagues (2006) found that among middle-aged African Americans around St. Louis, Missouri, adults living in areas with 4–5 versus 0–1 fair/poor conditions were more than 3 times as likely to develop a lower body limitation. And, Freedman et al. (2008) have found by using tract- and county-level data linked to the nationally representative Health and Retirement Study that neighborhood economic advantage is associated with a reduced risk of lower body limitations for both men and women, and that high connectivity of the built environment is associated with reduced risk of limitations in instrumental activities for men.

While of interest to public health, such studies stop short of providing communities with the information they need to create environments that support functioning and well-being of older adults. Fortunately, progress has been made on this front through the Visiting Nurse Service of New York's AdvantAge Initiative (Feldman, Oberlink, Simantov, & Gursen, 2004). Based on the premise that communities matter in the daily lives of older adults, AdvantAge began by exploring what makes a neighborhood "elder friendly." By talking with people in four communities, they identified four domains of the elder-friendly community: (a) addressing basic needs, (b) optimizing physical health and well being, (c) maximizing independence for older adults who are frail or have disabilities, and (d) promoting social and civic engagement. They then developed a 33-item instrument for communities to rate their elder-friendliness (Feldman & Oberlink, 2003). In addition, they surveyed older adults in 10 communities to understand older adults' perceptions of the 33 indicators. Information was reported back to communities in chart book form. National survey results (Feldman et al., 2004) based on 1,500 older adults made norms available to communities so that they had a basis of comparison for each indicator. The national survey underscored the disparate experience of two groups of older adults—the vibrant, successfully aging seniors dubbed the "fortunate majority" and a smaller group referred to as the "frail fraction." The latter are living in ill health, with inadequate resources, and in nonsupportive and sometimes dangerous communities.

In an equally important companion project, the AdvantAge initiative identified and profiled best practices to promote health and independence among older adults. The resulting report highlighted several key "ingredients" to the success of community-based programs (Feldman & Oberlink, 2003). These ingredients are so fundamental to successful community-based interventions—whether related to elder friendliness or any other public health and aging topic—that we provide a summary here:

1. Broad stakeholder support throughout the planning, implementation, and life of the program
2. Knowledge of the community and how to tailor programs to that community
3. Leadership—both in terms of lead agency and lead person
4. The "right" lead agency and person
5. Building and sustaining relationships with all those involved in the effort
6. Marketing with tailored messages
7. Flexibility to change and grow with community needs

The information provided to participating AdvantAge Initiative communities has been used to help give a voice to the older adults of the community, as well as to identify barriers and solutions to promoting elder friendliness.

A CLINICAL PERSPECTIVE: IDENTIFYING DISABLEMENT PATHWAYS

For prevention of disability progression and frailty in older adults, a good target is the older adult with reduced capacity to carry out the building blocks of activities—those with mobility limitations, upper and lower body limitations, sensory limitations, and mild cognitive impairments. In ICF-language, by focusing on capacity in the domains upon which activities are built, it is possible to identify persons at risk for activity limitations and participation restrictions. (Put in terms of the Nagi formulation, it is important to measure *functional limitation* antecedent to *disability*.) The aim is to identify factors associated with reports of disability among individuals who demonstrate a range of limitation in the abilities or skills needed to undertake daily activities. Such "skill elements"—for example, sequencing steps in a task, organizing a workspace, or maintaining bodily alignment—have been well-examined in occupational therapy research and have been defined, with clear scoring criteria, as in AMPS (Fisher, 2006a, 2006b).

The Link Between Capacity and Performance

What is the relationship between the motor and cognitive skills used in performing daily activities (functional limitation) and IADL/BADL limitations? A first investigation in this area involved the relationship between leg strength and gait speed. Buchner et al. (1996) found that the relationship between leg strength, measured in an exercise machine test, and gait speed was nonlinear. In such a nonlinear relationship (or flattened S-shaped curve), three regions are defined, as shown hypothetically in Figure 5.4. The figure relates gait speed, a measure of mobility capacity, to difficulty or needing help in bathing, a measure of activity limitation. However, this type of nonlinear relationship between capacity and activity limitations has been established for other indicators, including balance and gait speed, and between gait speed and IADL/BADL measures (Jette, Assmann, Rooks, Harris, & Crawford, 1998).

When mobility speed is extremely low, people are essentially unable to walk or stand, and disability in bathing is complete. The curve is flat (region A), indicating that until gait speed exceeds a certain minimum (despite some minor improvements), limitation in bathing will not change. In other words, there is a threshold of leg strength or gait speed required for bathing. Once this threshold is crossed, gait speed and independence in bathing are directly related, as shown in region B, so that each additional unit of leg strength or gait speed is associated with a proportional gain in independence or efficiency (or ease) in bathing. Once leg strength or gait speed exceeds a certain level again, a second threshold is crossed, defining the beginning of region C. At this point, additional gait speed or leg strength does not translate into greater bathing efficiency. Given the biomechanical and ergonomic properties of the task, individuals are already performing as efficiently as possible and any additional leg strength contributes to physiological reserve but does not affect the speed or efficiency of bathing. Above this threshold, increments in strength or skill are not associated with reduction in disability but only with increased reserve (Buchner et al., 1996; Sonn, Frandin, & Grimby, 1995).

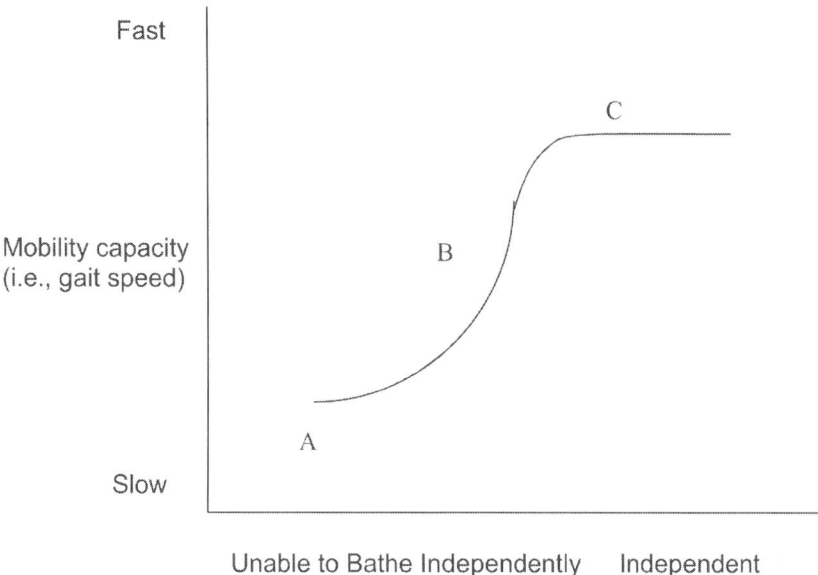

Figure 5.4 Hypothetical relationship between mobility capacity and bathing disability.

Identification of these thresholds may be clinically important, because these indicate the point on a continuum of ability, physical or cognitive, when capacity has implications for limitations. The thresholds also help set goals for intervention and rehabilitation. For example, a clinical trial seeking to prevent or reduce activity limitations by improving strength would not show benefit if targeted to individuals in region C of the curve. These individuals are already beyond the threshold where improvements in strength will affect performance of daily tasks. Similarly, only with large improvement in capacity could we expect to see reduction in limitations in region A. By contrast, people along region B of the curve might be the best target for such a trial. In this group, even small changes in underlying capacity can be expected to translate into increases in independence and efficiency.

Buchner et al. (1997) have shown the relevance of these considerations in a clinical trial of exercise to reduce the incidence of falls. The trial was part of the FICSIT initiative, "Frailty and Injuries: Cooperative Studies of Intervention Techniques." The study recruited elders with extensive functional limitation; all were unable to do an eight-step tandem gait test without errors, and all were below the 50th percentile in knee extensor strength based on norms for weight and height. A program of endurance and strength training led to increases in isokinetic strength and aerobic capacity, but no improvements in gait speed or balance. This lack of consistent benefit (reduction in measures of impairment, no benefit in measures of functional limitation) already suggests that selection criteria for the study were too stringent. People recruited for the study were likely near or within region A of the curve shown in Figure 5.4, so that improvement in underlying capacity might not lead to reduction in limitations. Indeed, in this study 1-year fall rates in the intervention group were 42%, better than the control group rate of 60%, but no different than the risk of falls typical of older people living in the community (Tinetti, Speechley, & Ginter, 1988). Buchner concludes that "the eligibility criteria selected a sample on the verge of substantial decline, and exercise prevented this decline." A more efficient design would have selected a less impaired sample.

The nonlinear relationship between underlying capacity and activity limitations also appears to hold for cognitive capacity. Figure 5.5 is a scatterplot of limitations (reported by caregivers) by number of errors by care recipient on a cognitive screening measure, derived from a sample of caregivers to elders with a diagnosis of Alzheimer's disease. Scores ranged from 24 (best score: independent all the time in 12 tasks) to 0 (worst score: dependent all the time in all 12 tasks assessed). Elders completed a 15-item cognitive screening test, which included items from a series of brief cognitive status tests (CARE-Diagnostic Screen; Gurland et al., 1995). These items assess a person's orientation, short-term memory, attention, and language ability. The scatterplot stratifies by number of comorbid conditions to better isolate the effect of cognitive capacity on dependence in daily activities.

The least-squares regression lines shown in Figure 5.5 were derived using a curvilinear regression model. The R^2 for the model in subjects without other comorbid conditions (thick line, $n = 78$) increased from 0.41 to 0.52 with introduction of a quadratic term, suggesting that the nonlinear curvilinear model offers a better fit. By contrast, in the two groups with other concurrent disease, linear models provided an adequate fit. Subjects with cognitive impairment in the absence of other comorbid disease are not likely to have reported limitations until they made five or more errors on the cognitive screen. This relationship should be compared with that of subjects with cognitive deficit and one or two or more comorbid conditions. They report greater dependency at every

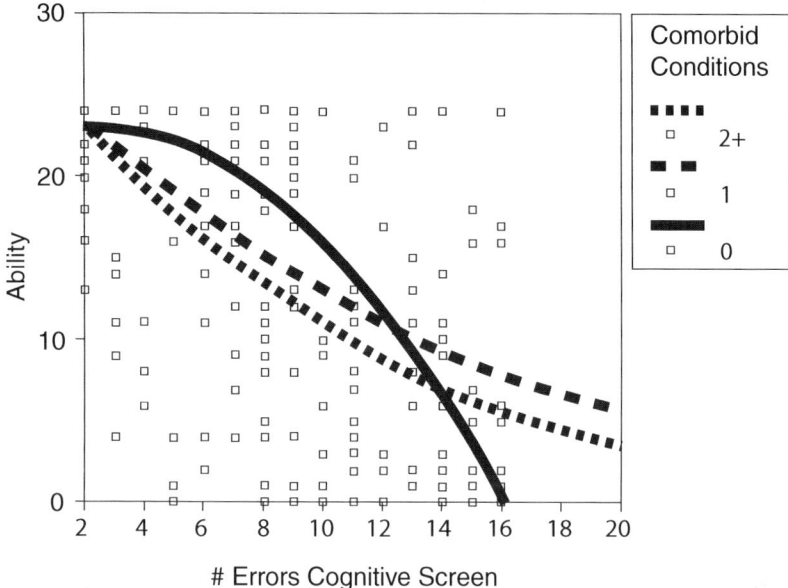

Figure 5.5 Relationship between disability and cognitive status.

level of cognitive ability. We conclude that the relationship between cognitive impairment and activity limitations may follow that demonstrated for physical indicators and disability.

The Role of Accommodations

Both the ICF language and the Nagi disablement model support questions about the compensatory processes and environmental modifications that prevent reduced capacity from resulting in activity limitations or participation restrictions. Four major types of accommodations exist: change in how the activity is performed (e.g., frequency, duration, or positioning), uptake of assistive technology, changes to the environment to support performing the activity, and reliance on help from another person. Although much attention has focused on the latter, in particular, caregiving to older adults, these other types of accommodations that may facilitate independent performance of activities have only recently come into focus.

Perhaps the most common—yet least studied—accommodation is simply altering the frequency of a task or changing the way a task is performed (Weiss, Hoenig, & Fried, 2007). This is the first and most basic adaptation. If a shoulder range-of-motion limitation makes it difficult for someone to wash his or her hair, the first response probably will be a reduction in the frequency of hair washing or a change in bathing routine, such as washing hair only when someone is available to help. These are effective modifications for mild-to-moderately severe functional limitation. With progression of functional limitation, completing ADL tasks may become impossible without further modifications, either alteration of the physical environment (washing hair in the sink rather than shower, use of a grab bar or bath stool, use of walk-in shower stall), or recourse to personal assistance (regular help getting into the tub, balance support, and personal assistance with the application of shampoo).

More subtle forms of behavioral adaptation involve drawing on other faculties to compensate for reduced capacity in another area. For example, older persons with severe balance deficit (impairment) who still perform well in daily tasks, such as vacuuming or cooking, have presumably relied more on other faculties to prevent the balance disorder from disabling them in these daily tasks. We know very little about these processes, although efforts from kinesiology and neuroscience are underway to specify this effect. A simpler example is seen in the elder with mild cognitive impairment who uses other brain regions, visualized in functional magnetic resonance imaging, to perform better than expected in certain memory tasks. This elder probably uses mnemonics or other strategies to perform the memory task and, hence, draws on other relatively spared domains of brain function. Such subtle changes may suggest that a person's capacities might be increased through recruitment of remaining, relatively spared abilities. This process is less well explored than any of the other behavioral accommodations described here, but may be at least as important. It suggests far more extensive use of rehabilitative technologies to teach older people (and, indeed, anyone facing reductions in capacity) how to reorganize the way they do tasks by drawing on other remaining abilities.

One challenge for defining the population with activity limitations, already mentioned, is that people who have made successful adaptations of this sort may not report difficulty with the task. After all, they are successfully performing the task and have, to a great extent, overcome the change in capacity that might have otherwise caused this difficulty. Behavioral changes that individuals make to compensate for changes in underlying capacity may then be an important clue for clinicians to look for in predicting who will develop limitations—or who might benefit from an intervention to prevent this process from unfolding. For example, people reporting no difficulty with ADL, but who also say they have reduced the frequency of these ADL tasks, have lower grip strength, gait speed, dexterity, and balance scores, and a higher risk of developing ADL limitations (Fried et al., 1996).

Also widespread is the use of assistive technologies and environmental modifications. Cornman and colleagues (2005) have found, for example, that estimates of assistive device use across several national surveys range from 14% to 18% for the population of adults aged 65 and older, and range from 39% to 44% for the 85 and older population. Devices are used most often for mobility and bathing, and less often for toileting and transferring. However, questions about such devices are often restricted to individuals who report difficulty with daily activities and, therefore, omit a potentially sizeable group—those who use assistive devices but report no difficulty with daily activities. If this group is included the prevalence of both device use—and of those at risk for developing limitations because of reductions in capacity—are significantly higher.

The fact that assistive technology may in many cases bridge the gap between capacity and the environment is not surprising. Using the 1994–1995 Disability Supplement to the NHIS, for example, Verbrugge and Sevak (2002) show that equipment only or equipment with personal assistance is more likely to reduce difficulty than personal assistance alone. To explain this result, they point out "First, equipment is designed for the task, can be modified to suit the individual, and is generally on hand when needed. . . . Second, equipment maintains an individual's self-sufficiency. This can foster pride and keen perception of task improvements." This is an important result and suggests the need for further development of assistive devices. However, it is also worth recognizing the limits of equipment use in the case of cognitive disability, a major source of disability in late life (see Chapter 6).

An Example of Accommodations: Bathing

We can tie these insights on disability and efforts to mitigate the effects of reduced capacity with a closer look at a particular activity. A good candidate is bathing. As we have seen, it is the most prevalent ADL limitation and one that lends itself to a variety of accommodations and the use of compensatory processes.

In a study of nearly 200 older adults, all aged 70 and older, with mild to moderate activity limitations (reported difficulty in one to three domains of upper extremity, lower extremity, IADL, and ADL function, but not all four), 9.5% reported they had difficulty with bathing (Albert, Bear-Lehman, Burkhardt, Merete-Roa, & Noboa-Lemonier, 2006). These self-reports were quite stable. In the whole sample, less than 2% changed their self-report between a telephone interview and an in-home assessment. Respondents reported a variety of sources for their difficulty bathing, including fear of falling and concern about balance, pain, weakness, swollen legs (edema), and shortness of breath. People who reported difficulty bathing were more likely to report they had changed the frequency of bathing and the way they bathed. For example, of those reporting difficulty bathing, 87.5% said they had changed the way they bathe during the past 12 months. In people who did not report difficulty bathing, only 24.8% reported a change in the way they bathe. Thus, reports of difficulty and attempts to modify environments to mitigate difficulty go hand in hand.

If we look only at people who said they had no difficulty bathing, we find further evidence that environmental modification is a response to changes in underlying capacity. People who reported they had changed the way they bathe showed lower grip strength, slower gait speed, and less efficient performance on the AMPS assessment (the occupational therapy assessment described above) than people who reported no change. We find this pattern even when we restrict the sample further to people who report they have not changed the frequency with which they bathe. People who have changed the way they bathe score more poorly on the measures. Thus, changes in behavior, indicated by changes in frequency and mode of performing the ADL, are clearly related to degree of capacity.

In the same sample, we also investigated one facet of compensation in the face of reduced capacity. We established the poorest balance group by examining the distribution of scores on a series of progressively more difficult static stances. Those in the lowest tertile (or third) showed a great range of motor performance in the AMPS assessment. In fact, nearly half scored above the cutting score on the motor dimension, indicating an ability to live independently despite poor balance. Of those with poor balance but good motor performance, 13.3% reported difficulty bathing. By contrast, nearly 40% of people with poor balance and poor motor performance reported difficulty bathing. Thus, some elders in the poor balance group were able to draw on other abilities to achieve reasonable motor performance despite balance deficit. These elders were also less likely to report bathing difficulties. We need to know more about this process.

PUBLIC HEALTH INTERVENTIONS TO MAXIMIZE LATE-LIFE FUNCTIONING

To this point we have considered disability and aging from three vantage points. The demography literature teaches us that, although activity limitations may be declining, not all groups have benefited equally, and continued declines in prevalence will be important to achieve as the large Baby Boom cohorts begin to retire this decade. Epidemiology has pointed to a list of important risk factors—from biological, to medical, to social and behavioral to environmental—that increase individuals' chances of developing activity limitations. Clinicians have added important insights about how accommodations and compensatory strategies may be individualized to bridge gaps between an individual's capacity to perform activities and their desire to perform both essential and valued activities. The public health and aging professional's interest cross cuts these disciplines as it seeks to establish public programs to ensure maximization of functioning among older adults. Here, we illustrate this sprawling literature by reviewing one especially important and promising avenue—fall prevention programs, and follow this with a discussion of how to compare the likely effects of interventions at the population level.

Preventing Falls

Falling is a common event among older people. Approximately 30% of people aged 65 and older residing in communities and 40% of people aged 80 and older fall each year (Tinetti et al., 1988). According to the Web-based Injury Statistics Query and Reporting System, available at http://www.cdc.gov/injury/wisqars/index.html and shown here in Table 5.4, in 2006, nearly 17,000 people aged 65 years or older died because of falls, up from 10,000 in 1999.

The number of reported injuries because of falls in this population exceeded 1.8 million. Approximately one in four older people who fall experience either a severe injury (e.g., fracture, trauma to the head, serious lacerations, joint dislocation) or limitation. Among those who sustain hip fractures, recuperation from depressive symptoms, cognitive loss,

Table 5.4

FALL-RELATED DEATHS AND INJURIES, 2001–2006, 65+ AND 85+ POPULATION

YEAR	# DEATHS	CRUDE DEATH RATE	# INJURIES	CRUDE INJURY RATE	POPULATION
65 and Older Population:					
2001	11746	33.25	1,642,533	4649.12515	35,329,945
2002	12961	36.42	1,640,080	4608.48203	35,588,294
2003	13820	38.44	1,822,590	5069.980707	35,948,651
2004	15028	41.4	1,851,602	5101.258967	36,296,965
2005	15917	43.32	1,802,172	4904.367212	36,746,273
2006	16747	44.95	1,840,564	4940.703674	37,253,065
85 and Older Population:					
2001	5366	121.47	504,704	11425.32486	4,417,415
2002	6020	132.41	503,708	11079.13089	4,546,457
2003	6436	136.5	554,978	11770.56146	4,714,967
2004	6993	144.26	555,070	11450.80042	4,847,434
2005	7561	149.57	545,958	10800.07957	5,055,128
2006	8052	152.33	573,804	10855.21849	5,285,976

From Web-based Injury Statistics Query and Reporting System (WISQARSTM).

and upper-body limitations generally occurs within a few months; however, lower body functioning takes on average a year or so to regain pre-fall status (Magaziner et al., 2000). Some older adults who fall also curtail activities because of a fear of falling again. As a result, individuals who experience falls have two or three times the relative risk of developing activity limitations as those who do not fall.

There are many known risk factors for falling. Tinetti et al. (1998), for example, found in a cohort of community-dwelling adults age 70 and older that sedative use, cognitive impairment, functional limitation in the lower extremities, poor reflexes, abnormalities of balance and gait, and foot problems were all risk factors for falling. An important finding from this study was the important role of environmental and ergonomic factors in falls. While 77% of the falls occurred at home, in a familiar environment, 44% of the falls involved modifiable home hazards. In these falls, people tripped over objects or slipped on stairs. Also, most falls involved particular kinds of activities, mainly those that displaced a person's center of gravity. These activities included getting up or sitting down, bending over or reaching, or stepping up or down. These particular environmental and ergonomic factors, along with medical risk factors identified in this effort, suggest a number of interventions to reduce the risk of falling.

Over the past two decades, a series of randomized clinical trials have shown that the risk for falls can be reduced. In a review of 40 such fall prevention trials, the most effective interventions were multifactorial falls risk assessments with management programs (Chang et al., 2004). Exercise programs alone were also effective in reducing the risk of falling, but not as effective as multifactor approaches. For example, one of the early, yet most notable, intervention studies linked reduction in the risk of falling to modification of particular risk factors. In the trial conducted by Tinetti and colleagues (1994), the Yale FICSIT trial, 35% of the intervention group fell, compared with 47% of controls, over a 1-year period. In this trial, one inclusion criterion was use of four prescription medications, a risk factor for falling, and a target of this multifactorial intervention. As part of the intervention, medication use for people in the intervention group was evaluated and adjusted, as needed. Sixty-three percent of the intervention group continued to take four or more medications, compared with 86% of controls. The trial also showed that many other risk factors for falling were modifiable, including balance impairment, difficulty with toilet transfer, and gait impairment. Each was modified through a combination of behavioral training, exercise program, or environmental change. The prevalence of impairments in the intervention group declined relative to controls; and this reduction appears to have been responsible for the reduction of falls.

A reanalysis of the data (Tinetti, McAvay, & Claus, 1996) showed that improvements in balance and reduction in blood pressure (to lower fall risk associated with orthostatic hypotension) were associated with lower rates of falling. Also, the reanalysis showed that fall risk declined in both treatment and control groups according to degree of reduction in a composite measure of fall risk. In the treatment group, the average number of risk factors declined by about one (of seven different risks), but this degree of risk factor reduction was enough to reduce falls by approximately 35% (Buchner, 1999). Together, these findings suggest that altering or eliminating specific risk factors for falls can reduce fall risk.

In other developed countries these types of tailored programs have been packaged with community-focused interventions, with reasonable success (McClure et al., 2005). Specific interventions varied but generally involved a combination of community-wide education, reduction in risks in homes and communities, training of health care personnel, and/or visits to the homes of high-risk individuals. A review of five prospective community trials with matched control communities suggested that, despite methodological limitations, fall-related fractures potentially could be reduced by 6%–33%.

In the United States, public health efforts to prevent falls have greatly expanded since the FICSIT trials. The AoA, for example, has been providing grants to states to mobilize the aging, public health, and nonprofit networks at the state and local level (see Chapter 3). Four evidence-based fall prevention programs have been included in these grants in more than a dozen states: Matter of Balance, Stepping On, Tai Chi, and Step by Step. In partnership with AoA, the CDC has funded evaluations of these fall prevention packages, and has also independently funded projects to translate this research into practice and to disseminate findings to communities. With respect to the latter, CDC has compiled a compendium of successful interventions for public health practitioners and community-based organizations, which covers exercise programs, home modification programs, and multifactor fall prevention programs (Stevens & Sogolo, 2008).

A companion guide for community-based organizations offers practical advice for planning, development, implementation, and evaluation of fall prevention programs (Stevens & Sogolo, 2008). In addition to providing essential program components (e.g., education, exercise, medication management, vision assessment, and home hazard identification), the guide also provides tips to communities on building and maintaining partnerships that will foster sustained prevention programs. Like the AdvantAge Initiative described earlier, critical ingredients for a successful and sustained fall prevention program involve community building, leadership and resources, and flexibility.

Comparing Potentially High-Impact Interventions

How does one go about comparing potentially high-impact interventions at the population level? That is, if one were to attempt to maximize the population's functioning, what approaches would be most effective? An interdisciplinary team recently tackled this question (Freedman et al., 2006) and identified critical information needed to compare the effects of interventions at the population level. Their framework drew on the notion of illness trajectories, that is, that individuals follow one of several prototypical experiences in terms of declines in function at the end of life, and that interventions might alter these trajectories or the demands placed on individuals by the environment. Their exercise started with the simple goal of reviewing the literature to identify the interventions with the greatest potential to reduce disability prevalence in the older population.

Their plan to compare interventions was complicated by several factors. First, most randomized studies evaluate interventions in terms of their influence on one or more proximate risk factors for disability, rather than on disability itself. Thus, to assess short-run effects, they considered three pieces of information—the prevalence of the risk factor of interest, the effect of the intervention on the targeted risk factor, and the relationship between the risk factor and the disablement process. Second, a variety of measures of functioning were found in the literature, and many studies evaluating interventions omitted measures of functioning altogether and instead focused on more proximate outcomes (e.g., leg strength or balance). Thus, the effects of interventions on the progression of activity limitations in many cases cannot be calculated precisely. Third, because interventions may influence not only disability, but also length of life, their short- and long-term effects may differ. Despite these complications, however, the investigators were able to assess the *relative* magnitude of effects on the prevalence of activity limitations by comparing interventions according to the following dimensions: the size and selectivity of the intervention's target population, the risk of disability associated with the risk factor addressed by the intervention, the effect of the intervention on the targeted risk factor, and the influence of the intervention on length of life and competing risks.

The team implemented this strategy for three potentially high-impact strategies: physical activity, depression screening and treatment, and fall prevention. Because of the large population at risk for falling, the demonstrated efficacy of multicomponent interventions in preventing falls, and the strong links between falls and activity limitations, they concluded that in the short run, multicomponent fall-prevention efforts would likely have a higher impact than either physical activity or depression screening and treatment. However, they stressed that "longer-term comparisons [could] not be made based on the current literature and may differ from short-run conclusions, since increases in longevity may temper the influences of these interventions on prevalence" (p. 493).

More generally, although there are a number of promising approaches to facilitating functioning in later life, there are real challenges to widespread implementation of high-impact interventions. Here, we outline five such challenges:

1. Disablement and functioning are complex processes with multiple risk factors at work. In general, multifactor interventions that are tailored to individual needs seem to work better than single interventions, but public health and aging programs are not always equipped to individualize services.
2. Ideally, public health and aging interventions need to be developed at multiple levels—not just aimed at the individual, but also at the families and communities in which people live. As we have seen, some examples of fall prevention interventions combine individual- and community-based approaches, but on the whole these have not been adopted in the United States.
3. Identifying the appropriate target population and window of time for targeting an intervention is critical to its success. The curvilinear relationship between underlying capacity and activity limitations complicates this targeting effort.
4. Attention throughout the process to the issue of sustainability and/or adherence is critical for long-term success.
5. Finally, the complex interactions between functioning and length of life complicate the equation. Interventions can influence both but will only reduce the prevalence of activity limitations and/or participation restrictions if the intervention lengthens active life at least as much as it lengthens life expectancy. These relationships are very difficult to predict and more research is needed to link interventions to disability and mortality outcomes.

SUMMARY

Language of Disability. The internationally accepted World Health Organization's International Classification of Functioning, Disability and Health (ICF) provides a useful language for disability research and public health interventions. Key terms include activity limitation, participation, the environment, and distinctions between capacity and performance. Unlike the Nagi model of disablement, the ICF language is not a dynamic model. To blend the benefits of the ICF language with those of the Nagi model is an important next step for disability and aging research.

Measuring Disability. Difficulty and need for help with activities of daily living have been central measures of interest in the study of public health and aging. New measures capturing the capacity to perform daily activities, the environment, and behavioral accommodations that individuals make to bridge the gap between capacity and the environment are gaining importance in the field.

Disability Trends. The prevalence of activity limitations declined during the 1980s and 1990s and active life expectancy increased. Declines were larger for instrumental activities of daily living than for the more severe activities of daily living, and more advantaged groups experienced larger declines. The reasons for these trends are complex and include shifts in socioeconomic status of the older population, in the distribution of underlying conditions and limitations in capacity that may be related to use of medical treatments, and in the uptake of assistive and other convenience technologies. In recent years this trend may have leveled off, and there are some signs that, in the future, this course may even reverse. Reconciling disparate findings remains an important focus among demographers.

Risk Factors for Functional Loss. Consistent predictors of functional loss included cognitive, vision, and lower body impairments; depression; comorbidity; high/low body mass index; few social contacts; low physical activity; and smoking as consistent predictors of functional loss. In addition, in recent years, our understanding of the biology of disability and the role of inflammation has increased. Studies of environmental factors, especially those focused on neighborhood characteristics that influence late-life disablement, suggest a role for the economic and built environments as well. These latter findings have not yet been translated into multilevel interventions.

Disablement Pathways. Clinicians have documented nonlinear relationships between measures of physical and cognitive capacity and activity limitations. Such findings indicate that there may be zones of opportunity for maintenance or improvement in functioning and other subgroups for whom intervention around underlying capacity may be less productive. Three distinct types of behavioral accommodations were also discussed in detail: changes in how the activity is performed (e.g., frequency, duration, or positioning), uptake of assistive technology, and changes to the environment to support performing the activity. The latter two are highly prevalent, but less is known about behavioral accommodations. One promising, but poorly understood, type of behavioral adaptation involves drawing on other faculties to compensate for reduced capacity in another area.

Public Health Interventions to Maximize Physical Functioning. Research to date is incomplete in guiding public health practitioners as to which interventions will maximize the functioning of the population in the long run. However, it appears that fall prevention efforts may be a useful place to start for short-term results. One especially promising avenue includes combining individually and community-focused efforts. The design and implementation of interventions to maximize physical functioning holds many challenges. Such challenges include the need to design multifactor, multilevel interventions that are targeted at the appropriate population, that are sustainable, and that lengthen active life expectancy at least as much as life expectancy.

6 Cognitive Function: Dementia

Alzheimer's disease and the other dementias are a major source of morbidity and disability in older people. The medical and supportive care needs of people who have dementia are a major challenge to families, medical care, and every component of long-term care services, not to mention to older people themselves, who perceive declining memory. More and more, they are given a diagnosis of "mild cognitive impairment," often without being told what the diagnosis means for risk of Alzheimer's (Albert, Dienstag, Tabert, Pelton, & Devanand, 2002a). Because the risk of dementia is highly related to age, with diagnosis of dementia occurring in the vast majority of people at the oldest ages, dementia is a central problem in geriatric care. The strong association between age and risk of dementia also makes the study of cognitive deficit and its consequences a key element in the epidemiology of aging.

The Alzheimer's Association reports a prevalence of 5.1 million Americans with Alzheimer's disease (AD) in 2009, with a projected increase to 7.7 million in 2030 (Alzheimer's Association, 2009). About 5%–10% of people aged 65 and older and between one-third and one-half those aged 85 and older meet criteria for the disease. Survival with the disease from the point of diagnosis averages about 8 years, but evidence suggests a very long latency, with progressive cognitive decline over a period of 20 or more years before people come to medical attention and receive the diagnosis. In fact, many older people in the community meet criteria for AD but have not received a diagnosis (Ross et al., 1997) and may not receive the diagnosis until quite late in the course of the disease (or may even die without ever receiving the diagnosis).

Families confronting the disease face the very difficult problem of deciding when driving should cease, when supervision is required for safety, when older people can no longer live alone, and when parents or spouses are no longer competent to handle money, take medications, or manage their lives independently. They will likely have to contend with the personality changes, psychiatric symptoms, and challenging behaviors typical of the more advanced stages of the disease. They may have to perform ADL care or manage supportive care staff hired to assist the elder, or more likely both sets of tasks, possibly at a distance. They may face the difficult decision to admit the Alzheimer's patient to a nursing home. Or, as is increasingly common, older people themselves may choose residences (such as assisted living or continuing care retirement communities) that can accommodate Alzheimer's or nursing-home levels of care, should they need such services.

A central question for public health with respect to Alzheimer's disease is to ask whether early diagnosis would make lives better for patients and families. A new array of technologies, including magnetic resonance imaging (MRI), that allows quantification of amyloid load and impaired hippocampal blood flow, now offer increasingly early detection. Does early detection do any good? Does it translate into better use of existing therapies, more effective planning for the future, and reduction in the excess morbidity associated with the disease, such as falls, depression, car accidents, weight loss and dehydration, or self-neglect? At this point, cognitive assessments, with notification of families and physicians, are not standard elements in primary care, and research is only now underway to determine whether such testing leads to changes in clinical management or family planning for long-term care needs.

The explosion of research in Alzheimer's and other dementing diseases makes this realm difficult to summarize. We address the following topics in this chapter: definitions of dementia, the question of normal memory decline and pathological changes, including the significance of awareness of declining cognitive ability and early effects of cognitive decline on daily activities; estimates of the incidence and prevalence of AD; risk factors for AD (genetic and environmental risk factors, as well as concurrent medical status predictors); and outcomes for people with dementia.

WHAT IS DEMENTIA?

DSM-IV (*Diagnostic and Statistical Manual of Mental Disorders*, 2000) has established criteria for a dementia diagnosis. A person meets criteria for dementia if he or she has:

- *Memory impairment*, defined as an impaired ability to learn new information or recall previously learned information; and
- One or more of the following additional impairments in cognition:
  - *Aphasia*, difficulty in language comprehension or production manifested in difficulty finding the right words, and marked by the presence of frequent word substitutions, breaking off in midsentence, and repetition;
  - *Apraxia*, difficulty performing movements in response to verbal commands despite intact motor function;
  - *Agnosia*, difficulty recognizing familiar faces, objects, and places despite intact sensory function; or
  - *Executive function deficits*, difficulty in planning or sequencing activity, or difficulty completing a task in the presence of interference from another task.

In addition, these cognitive deficits must be severe enough to cause significant impairment in social or occupational function and must represent a significant decline from a previous level of functioning.

For Alzheimer's disease to be diagnosed, the course of this general cognitive disorder must, in addition, be characterized by gradual onset and continuing, progressive decline. The defect in cognition should not be attributable to other central nervous system conditions that cause progressive deficits in memory and cognition, such as cerebrovascular disease, Parkinson's disease, Huntington's disease, subdural hematoma, normal-pressure hydrocephalus, or brain tumor. Nor should the cognitive disorder be caused by systemic conditions that are known to cause dementia, such as hypothyroidism, vitamin B12 or folic acid deficiency, niacin deficiency, hypercalcemia, neurosyphilis, or HIV infection. Substance-induced conditions should also be excluded. Finally, the cognitive deficits should not occur exclusively during the course of delirium, an acute and temporary confusional state. Delirium, unlike dementia, is usually the result of a general medical condition, a medication reaction, or substance use, and resolves with treatment.

The distinction between dementia and delirium is important. Delirium is characterized by fluctuating disturbances in cognition, mood, attention, arousal, and self-awareness. This clouding of consciousness and disorientation is acute, and will resolve with appropriate medical treatment. It is highly prevalent in some settings: 10%–30% of hospitalized medical patients, and up to 80% of terminally ill patients in the last weeks of life, have been reported to have episodes of delirium (Inouye et al., 1999). It is also common in nursing homes. Delirium can affect a patient with dementia, and, in these cases, distinguishing between the two may be difficult.

The Alzheimer's Disease and Related Disorders Association (ADRDA) (McKhann et al., 1984) has developed additional criteria for diagnosing dementia of the Alzheimer's type. A definitive AD diagnosis requires that clinical criteria for probable AD be met and, in addition, that histopathological evidence from biopsy or autopsy be available. "Probable AD" is defined by the criteria listed above, but a diagnosis of "possible AD" can also be made based on the dementia syndrome described above in "the presence of variations in the onset, presentation and clinical course" or in "the presence of a second systemic or brain disorder sufficient to cause the dementia but not considered to be the cause of the dementia." These are the criteria for diagnosis of the National Institute of Neurological Disorders and Stroke-Alzheimer's Disease and Related Disorders Association (NINCDS-ADRDA).

The "possible AD" distinction is important because dementia can also be a feature of other neurodegenerative diseases, such as Parkinson's or vascular disease, and can also accompany stroke or trauma. In other adults, these diseases or effects from disease can co-occur. In such cases, the diagnosis of AD may depend on which came first; for example, if dementia precedes Parkinson's disease, it is reasonable to call this person an incident case of AD, with a further complication from Parkinson's. In other cases, the temporal sequence is less clear and a diagnosis of "possible AD" may be warranted.

Lack of diagnostic specificity in the NINCDS-ADRDA criteria and the discovery of a series of biomarkers for Alzheimer's disease have led to a new set of proposed criteria. These biomarkers include imaging technologies (structural MRI to identify characteristic brain signatures), molecular neuroimaging (positron emission tomography [PET] scanning with use of new ligands to quantify amyloid), cerebrospinal fluid analyses (that identify amyloid and tau proteins), and familial genetic mutations that cause AD. The newly proposed diagnostic criteria for Alzheimer's disease include memory impairment along with a positive finding in one of the biomarkers (Dubois et al., 2007). The new criteria are designed to reflect the activity of drug therapies ("disease modifying agents") that affect these basic processes (such as amyloid clearance). Indeed, changes in the biomarkers are now viewed as indicators of successful therapy.

This shift to a biological rather than purely clinical phenotype is notable. Apart from the absence of clear definitions (for example, the amount of brain atrophy or combination of cerebrospinal fluid markers required for diagnosis), the newly proposed criteria shift attention from clinical problems, such as memory loss or IADL limitations, to the neurodegenerative process assumed to underlie Alzheimer's. This approach is reasonable if these are indeed the primary neurodegenerative processes and if therapies can successfully modify them. But without clear specification of the level of biomarker required for diagnosis, the new criteria introduce uncertainty in the meaning of the diagnosis and may allow a vast expansion of the prevalence of the disease based on the presence of risk factors alone.

A comparison with osteoporosis may be instructive. Based on norms available for people at much younger ages, we define osteoporosis as bone mineral densities less than a certain T score (bone mineral densities in the lowest 2.5% or 5% of a population distribution of 35-year-old women, for example). We consider women with this level of bone loss to have the disease and prescribe therapies, such as bisphosphonates, that help with bone remodeling and turnover and can be said to modify the disease. This is precisely what is missing in the revised criteria for Alzheimer's. We lack norms and distributions for the proposed biomarkers. Moreover, we cannot be sure that these biomarkers are the critical ones. Finally, we still have only equivocal evidence that current therapies modify these measures of underlying neurodegeneration.

MAKING AND RECEIVING THE DIAGNOSIS OF ALZHEIMER'S DISEASE

When an elder is brought to medical attention because of memory disorders or progressive inability to manage independently in a household, the treating physician is likely to assess cognitive status with the Folstein Mini-Mental State Examination (MMSE), a 30-point assessment of orientation, memory, attention, language, calculation, and visuospatial construction skills, typically used as a screening test. The MMSE is shown in Table 6.1. Current recommendations suggest that a score greater than 24 is considered normal, a score of 15–24 shows mild-to-moderate impairment, and a score less than 15 shows definite impairment. Nevertheless, the test is not a diagnostic tool and should be considered only a first-line glimpse at cognitive function.

Properties of the MMSE have been investigated intensively. Performance on the measure is related to age and education, apart from dementia status, suggesting that these influences must be considered when interpreting scores on the test. In one effort, the MMSE was administered to over 18,000 adult participants selected in a probability sample within census tracts and households (Crum, Anthony, Bassett, & Folstein, 1993). Median MMSE scores ranged from 29 in people 18–24 years of age, to 27 in people aged 70–74, and to 25 in people aged 80 and older. The median MMSE score was 29 in people with 9 or more years

Table 6.1

EXCERPT FROM MINI-MENTAL STATE EXAMINATION (MMSE)

Orientation to Time

"What is the date?"

Registration

"Listen carefully. I am going to say three words. You say them back to me after I stop. Ready? Here they are . . .

APPLE (pause), PENNY (pause), TABLE (pause). Now repeat those words back to me."

[Repeat up to 5 times, but score only the first trial.]

Naming

"What is this?" [Point to a pencil or pen]

Reading

"Please read this and do what it says." [Show examinee the words on the stimulus form]

CLOSE YOUR EYES

Reproduced by special permission of the Publisher, Psychological Assessment Resources, Inc., 16204 North Florida Avenue, Lutz, Florida 33549, from the Mini-Mental State Examination, by Marshal Folstein and Susan Folstein, Copyright 1975, 1998, 2001 by Mini Mental LLC, Inc. Further reproduction is prohibited without permission of PAR, Inc. The MMSE can be purchased from PAR, Inc. by calling 813-968-3003.

of school, 26 for people with 5–8 years, and 22 for people with 0–4 years. Because a score of less than 24 is often taken as an indicator of possible dementia, education obviously needs to be taken into account in interpreting performance. The need for caution in applying cutoff scores in the MMSE is even clearer when we examine older people with low education. For people with 0–4 years of school, the median MMSE score for people under age 65 ranges from 22 to 25, but it is 21–22 in people aged 70–79 and 19–20 in people aged 80 and older. Research suggests that literacy may be as important as years of school for MMSE performance (Albert & Teresi, 1999), and that quality of education should also be considered when interpreting education-referenced scores, especially among minorities (Manly, Jacobs, Touradji, Small, & Stern, 2002).

One way to grade the severity of dementia is through instruments such as the Clinical Dementia Rating, or CDR (Hughes, Berg, Danziger, Cohen, & Martin, 1982). The original scoring categories and criteria are shown in Table 6.2. The CDR involves six dimensions: three cognitive (memory, orientation, and judgment and problem-solving) and three functional (home and hobbies, community affairs, and self-care). The original system allows a diagnosis of normal, "questionable," "mild," "moderate," and "severe" dementia. The CDR has also been expanded to include a "profound" and "terminal" level of severity (Dooneief, Marder, Tang, & Stern, 1996).

Scoring of the CDR requires a semistructured interview with both the caregiver and patient. In particular, caregivers provide information that the clinician can use in his or her discussion with the patient to check a patient's level of insight on the extent of memory deficit. Washington University has prepared a series of training videotapes that illustrate effectively the variation in the severity of dementia. The tapes are good teaching tools not only for rating severity, but also for showing features of dementia, such as lack of insight, difficulty with verbal production and comprehension, retardation of motor activity, depression, and confabulation to mask memory difficulty. Students unfamiliar with dementia who view the tapes report how difficult, even excruciating, it is to see someone struggle with language and the simplest comprehension tasks.

Scoring of the CDR can take a number of forms. Clinicians can use it to formulate a global impression, or they can more formally assign severity according to the sum of box scores or some other algorithm for weighting dimensions in making an assignment.

The CDR score offers an important end point for studies of dementia progression or treatment efficacy. What proportion of patients with mild

Table 6.2

CLINICAL DEMENTIA RATING (CDR)

	IMPAIRMENT LEVEL AND CDR SCORE (0, 0.5, 1, 2, 3)				
	NONE 0	QUESTIONABLE 0.5	MILD 1	MODERATE 2	SEVERE 3
Memory	No memory loss or slight inconsistent forgetfulness	Consistent slight forgetfulness; partial recollection of events; "benign" forgetfulness	Moderate memory loss; more marked for recent events; defect interferes with everyday activities	Severe memory loss; only highly learned material retained; new material rapidly lost	Severe memory loss; only fragments remain
Orientation	Fully oriented	Fully oriented except for slight difficulty with time relationships	Moderate difficulty with time relationships; oriented for place at examination; may have geographic disorientation elsewhere	Severe difficulty with time relationships; usually disoriented to time, often to place	Oriented to person only
Judgment & Problem Solving	Solves everyday problems & handles business & financial affairs well; judgment good in relation to past performance	Slight impairment in solving problems, similarities, and differences	Moderate difficulty in handling problems, similarities, and differences; social judgment usually maintained	Severely impaired in handling problems, similarities, and differences; social judgment usually impaired	Unable to make judgments or solve problems

Community Affairs	Independent function at usual level in job, shopping, volunteer and social groups	Slight impairment in these activities	Unable to function independently at these activities although may still be engaged in some; appears normal to casual inspection	No pretense of independent function outside home; appears well enough to be taken to functions outside a family home	No pretense of independent function outside home; appears too ill to be taken to functions outside a family home
Home and Hobbies	Life at home, hobbies, and intellectual interests well maintained	Life at home, hobbies, and intellectual interests slightly impaired	Mild but definite impairment of function at home; more difficult chores abandoned; more complicated hobbies and interests abandoned	Only simple chores preserved; very restricted interests, poorly maintained	No significant function in home
Personal Care	Fully capable of self-care		Needs prompting	Requires assistance in dressing, hygiene, keeping of personal effects	Requires much help with personal care; frequent incontinence

From http://www.adrc.wustl.edu/adrc/cdrGrid.html.

dementia (CDR 1), for example, progress to moderate or more severe dementia (CDR 2+) over a defined interval? Natural history studies of incident cohorts provide information of this sort, which is important for assessing the efficacy of a therapy in delaying progression. The risk of progression from mild to more advanced dementia in an incident AD cohort is approximately 6%–10% per year (see below); thus, a reasonable goal for delay of disease progression would be a rate significantly lower than this.

Measures that tap cognition alone (as opposed to cognition and function, like the CDR) are also valuable tools. Neuropsychological assessment allows fairly fine differentiation of strengths and weaknesses in a variety of cognitive domains. Age- and education-based norms, in different languages, are now available for an increasingly wide range of tests (which now offer multiple forms, an advantage for longitudinal studies that must consider "practice effects"). With so many tests, scored in so many different ways, however, it is often difficult to decide how best to use the measures. Should tests be aggregated according to the cognitive domain they have been designed to assess (such as memory, visuospatial skill, language, or executive function), or according to data reduction techniques (such as factor analysis)? Assuming we combine tests, should we count the number of tests 1 or 2 standard deviations below norms to compute a "deficit score," or should we standardize scores and compute a sum of z scores? After we have computed a composite measure, should we be concerned with mean performance or variation in the test scores over time (Holtzer, Verghese, Wang, Hall, & Lipton, 2008)?

One factor-analytic study of neuropsychological test performance offers some reassurance for these questions. Mayeux and colleagues reported a stable and plausible factor structure for test performance in a sample of elders without dementia (Mayeux, Small, Tang, Tycko, & Stern, 2001). In this effort, three factors emerged:

Memory: Total recall, long-term recall, delayed recall, long-term storage, cued long-term recall, and total recall over six trials of the Selective Reminding Test (Buschke & Fuld, 1974);
Visuospatial/Cognitive Skill: Matching and recognition components of the Benton Visual Retention Test (Benton, 1955), Rosen Drawing Test (Rosen, 1981), and Identities and Oddities of the Mattis Dementia Rating Scale (Mattis, 1976);
Language: Boston Naming Test (Kaplan, Goodglass, & Weintraub, 1983), Controlled Oral Word Association Test (Benton, 1967), and WAIS-R Similarities (Wechsler, 1981).

In this study, composite scores for each factor were computed and used to examine decline in cognitive performance over follow-up in a community-dwelling cohort of elders without dementia drawn from Medicare enrollee files. The authors used the scores without reference to norms because the purpose of the study was not to establish impaired performance, but rather to track change in different cognitive domains.

Change in cognitive test scores may be an unreliable indicator of drug efficacy in clinical trials if these changes are small. The clinical significance of such small changes is not clear. For example, if participants in the active arm of a trial retain baseline scores and participants in the placebo group decline by a mean of 1.2 words on a 15-word memory test, is the difference meaningful? Can we say the therapy has blunted the memory decline typical of AD? Does this difference in short-term memory performance matter for daily performance of ADL or IADL tasks? Research to establish the clinical significance of such often subtle change is difficult. In the absence of such research, the gold standard for clinical trials is to insist on an additional favorable global impression of clinical change as a criterion (Leber, 1991; Schneider & Olin, 1996). Thus, the Food and Drug Administration (FDA) considers therapies efficacious only if they demonstrate improvement in cognitive performance along with a global impression of relative improvement. The latter establishes the clinical significance of otherwise small changes in performance.

COGNITIVE DECLINE WITH AGE: DISTINCT FROM ALZHEIMER'S DISEASE?

Earlier, in Chapter 1, we showed that people enter late life with different cognitive and health resources, along with differences in wealth and family support. Differences in the case of cognitive resources, or "cognitive reserve," are especially important. By age 65 or 70 any sample of older adults without dementia will show a wide range of performance on tests of memory and other cognitive domains. But older people scoring more poorly on measures of memory, for example, can be expected to reach the dementia end point, or "convert" to AD, sooner (adjusting for other differences) than older adults with better memory performance. This difference in cognitive resources at the beginning of old age means some people are closer to the threshold of detectable dementia even when they are not very old, as shown schematically in Figure 6.1.

The figure shows that we must consider the decline in memory performance typical of aging and also ask whether the pathological process of AD is something separate from this decline. Figure 6.1 shows two groups of older persons, one entering old age (for convenience, age 65) with high cognitive reserve (a score of 1.5 on a hypothetical cognitive score), the other entering old age with low reserve (cognitive score of 0.5). The two groups can have different trajectories according to whether memory changes in ways typical of "normal aging," or whether memory declines much more quickly as the result of a potentially distinct Alzheimer's pathological process. The figure also includes an "Alzheimer's threshold," a cognitive score (for convenience, set at zero) that is associated with disability and clinical diagnosis.

If we look only at the decline in memory associated with normal memory (see below), we see that the high-reserve group does not reach the Alzheimer's threshold even as late as age 85. The low-threshold group, by contrast, crosses the dementia threshold shortly after age 75. Note that this difference would occur even if the slope of memory decline in the two groups were equivalent, shown by parallel or nearly parallel lines. If we look instead at the declines in memory associated with the pathological process, we see that the high-reserve group now crosses the Alzheimer's threshold at approximately age 80 and the low-reserve group crosses at age 75 or so. Again, the slope of decline in the two groups could be equivalent, represented by parallel lines, or we might hypothesize an important interaction, in which low reserve and the pathological process together result in a steeper slope of decline.

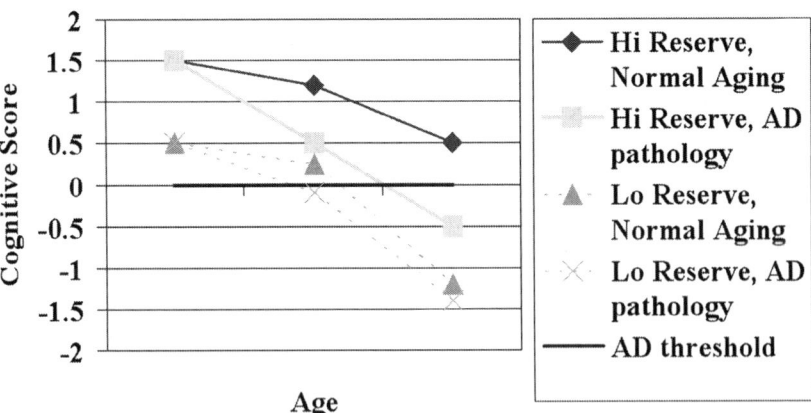

Figure 6.1 Schematic presentation of cognitive resources/reserve as risk factor for dementia.

Chapter 6 Cognitive Function: Dementia

The big question in this kind of inquiry is whether distinct slopes for normal and pathological memory change in aging exist at all. Within the high- or low-reserve groups, we will find variation in rates of change. Do the changes in memory at either end of this range represent different underlying brain processes, or is a single process enough to account for this variation? More simply, are the declines typical of Alzheimer's just one end of the continuum of changes typical of aging?

Research suggests that memory declines typical of Alzheimer's disease may be distinct from normal aging. Mayeux et al. (2001) first identified a cohort of nearly 600 older people who never met criteria for dementia over 7 years, who were evaluated, on average, every 20 months. The mean age of the cohort was 75.9 at baseline, and 14.2% had one or more *APOE*-e4 alleles. The *APOE* gene is the only gene identified so far for Alzheimer's risk in older adults (as opposed to *PS1, APP, SORL,* and other genes associated with familial disease and much younger onset). The increased risk of AD associated with the e4 allele has been confirmed repeatedly in large prospective cohort studies (Maestre et al., 1995). Mayeux and colleagues (2001) monitored their cohort to investigate the relationship between declines in cognitive performance and *APOE* status. Declines in cognitive domains in people without the e4 allele could plausibly identify normal age-related changes in cognition. People with the e4 allele, who have a higher risk of AD, could plausibly represent early AD and should show steeper declines in memory performance.

In this cohort, memory performance mostly declined over time; two-thirds had a negative slope on the composite memory measure described earlier. Older age and lower education were each associated with poorer memory scores at baseline and at follow-up assessments. Individuals with an *APOE*-e4 allele had steeper declines in memory performance, suggesting early changes typical of Alzheimer's disease. This steeper slope was evident only in people with low education, or low cognitive reserve, suggesting an interaction between low reserve and the Alzheimer's pathological process.

It is noteworthy that memory was the only cognitive domain that declined in this cohort of people who never met criteria for dementia. Visuospatial and language performance were stable across the 7 years of follow-up. Scores in the visuospatial and language domains were stable even in people with an *APOE*-e4 allele.

These findings suggest that memory decline typical of aging can be separated from the pathological aging typical of AD. They also suggest the sensitivity of the memory domain for identifying age-related changes and the risk of AD. In a second set of analyses, Mayeux et al. (2001)

also examined changes in the three domains in a separate group of 228 people who did not meet criteria for AD at baseline but progressed to AD over the follow-up period. These people showed significant declines with time in all three domains, showing a more generalized decline of cognition in people closer to the Alzheimer's threshold.

Mayeux's study is valuable for showing that memory decline is common in a group of older people who do not develop AD over a long period, but also more pronounced (steeper, in terms of Figure 6.1) in a group with an AD risk factor who are still, however, far from the AD threshold. These elders showed declines in memory only. It stands to reason, then, that areas of the brain involved in memory, such as the entorhinal cortex of the hippocampus, should be different in younger people and older people without AD. Differences in anatomy would not be expected, because the older people in this case do not have AD and would not be expected to show the pathological lesions (amyloid plaques, neuritic tangles) typical of the disease. However, differences in physiology might be expected, because poorer memory presumably must reflect differences in cellular processes. In fact, recent research suggests just such a difference, with older people selectively showing less MRI signal than younger people only in this region of the hippocampal formation (Small, Tsai, De La Paz, Mayeux, & Stern, 2002).

These kinds of differences have been confirmed in studies using Pittsburgh Compound B (PiB), an amyloid ligand, in PET imaging (Klunk et al., 2004). Amyloid deposition correlates with AD severity, presence of *APOE*-e4 alleles, and therapeutic activity. In addition, PiB studies have shown that seniors without AD or with mild cognitive impairment short of frank AD have more amyloids than elders who perform at normal levels on cognitive assessments (Aizenstein et al., 2008).

COGNITIVE DECLINE PRIOR TO FRANK DEMENTIA

Mild cognitive impairment (MCI) is typically defined by the following criteria: subjective complaints of memory problems and memory performance below age- and education-referenced norms, with normal performance in other cognitive domains and absence of impairment in the instrumental and basic activities of daily living (Peterson et al., 1997; Peterson, 2000). Another definition of mild cognitive impairment is "questionable dementia," which involves both mild deficits in cognitive status and mild deficits in functional status. This state is recognized in the 0.5 category of the CDR (Hughes et al., 1982). Still other alternative nosologies include "age-associated memory impairment," which involves poor memory performance relative to people under age 50 (Crook et al., 1986; Feher, Larrabee, Sudilovsky, & Crook, 1994) and "aging-associated cognitive decline," which involves defective performance in any cognitive domain, relative to age-matched elders (Levy, 1994; Richards, Touchon, Ledesert, & Ritchie, 1999). The different definitions all strive to establish an intermediate cognitive status: people with MCI do not meet criteria for dementia but show deficits in memory or other domains of cognition. These deficits are evident to elders and distressing enough to lead them and their families to seek medical attention. They may presage advancing Alzheimer's disease.

Even within the domain of "questionable dementia" it is possible to make distinctions based on prognosis. Morris and colleagues assigned MCI patients ascertained in a clinic setting into three groups: CDR 0.5 but likely demented, CDR 0.5 with likely progressive dementia ("incipient AD"), and CDR 0.5 with uncertain dementia (Morris et al., 2001). All three groups faced a high risk of developing Alzheimer's disease (CDR 1.0 or greater) over a 5-year follow-up period: 60.5% for the likely dementia group, 35.7% for the likely progressive dementia group, and 19.9% for the uncertain dementia group. These rates should be compared with a control group (CDR 0, no cognitive or functional impairment) over the same time period, in which the incidence of Alzheimer's disease was 6.8%. Given these results Morris and colleagues conclude, "individuals currently characterized as having MCI progress steadily to greater stages of dementia severity at rates dependent on the level of cognitive impairment at entry." People in the three groups who died and came to autopsy had neuropathogical evidence of AD, again suggesting that MCI, at least when defined by CDR 0.5 criteria, is a dementia prodrome rather than a benign variant of aging.

The situation is less clear for patients who do not meet CDR 0.5 criteria but whose cognitive performance is lower than expected. Ritchie and colleagues assessed mild cognitive impairment in a population-based, rather than a clinic-based, sample (Ritchie, Artero, & Touchon, 2001). Only 11.1% of patients progressed to dementia. Moreover, these people moved back and forth across the dementia threshold, changing diagnostic category at different assessments. With more restrictive definitions identifying greater cognitive impairment, 28.6% met the dementia end point over 3 years.

In general, studies suggest that dementia incidence in elders who report cognitive complaints and demonstrate mild deficits in cognitive assessment is much higher than that for elders as a whole, 18% over 3 years, compared with perhaps 3%–6% in the population of older adults as a whole (Ritchie et al., 2001). Consequently, mild cognitive impairment cannot be considered benign or a normal feature of healthy aging, and elders with mild cognitive impairment in this sense (i.e., complaints of memory impairment supported by neuropsychological performance >1 SD below age norms) are indeed at risk for developing Alzheimer's over a 3- to 5-year period.

Of course, the annual risk of transition to AD among people with mild cognitive impairment will depend heavily on the definition of MCI, and even limiting definitions to a single type of MCI shows substantial variation. The "isolated amnestic" variant, that is, memory performance below age- and education-adjusted norms without involvement of other cognitive domains, ranges from 3% to 12.5% in community-based samples (Manly et al., 2005). The annual risk of progression to Alzheimer's disease was 5% in a New York City sample (Manly et al., 2008). If we examine this risk among people who already demonstrate some kind of cognitive impairment, but one short of dementia, the annual risk of transition to AD is 10%–12% (Plassman et al., 2008).

Insight on Declining Cognitive Ability

Older adults with MCI describe their difficulties with memory in this way:

> I do feel the difference. I can't retrieve words easily. I lose words. It will take me a few minutes . . . and it takes me a while to retrieve it. Sometimes I can't, and that's disturbing. And to think of walking into a room and forgetting why you walked in is a killer. It's strange. Or getting a list in my head, and not writing it down . . . and then forgetting what I want to do. That kind of thing. I'm sure it happened before, but not as frequently as now. It's happening more.

The woman reporting these memory problems met criteria for MCI. She had a Global Deterioration Score (GDS) of 3, as indicated by a score below age- and education-adjusted norms on the Logical Memory II subscale of the Weschler Memory Scale; she did not meet criteria for dementia, as indicated by a Mini-Mental State Examination (MMSE) score greater than or equal to 24; and she did not report difficulty in daily occupational, self-care, home management, or community activities, as indicated by a Clinical Dementia Rating of 0.5.

Still, she was concerned that her memory problems might presage Alzheimer's disease. Mainly, she was concerned that she might be denying the extent of her problems, which she recognized as a feature of memory impairment and incipient Alzheimer's disease. She was also concerned that she was not pushing herself as hard as she might and that this circumscription of daily activities and interests might be the result of her memory deficit. Was she actually avoiding situations that would reveal her difficulty with memory?

Her assessment and the new label of "MCI" did not help. She reported great frustration with the clinical label: "They said there was some memory loss, that it might not mean anything, and that they would like to re-evaluate me in a couple of years to see if it's progressing. [But] the significance of it is what I'm interested in, and [that] they didn't tell me" (Albert et al., 2002).

Mild Cognitive Impairment and Disability

Aside from "questionable dementia," the other definitions of mild cognitive impairment, reviewed earlier, assume no impairments in instrumental (household management) or basic (personal self-maintenance) activities of daily living, but leave open the possibility of deficits in higher level functions, such as the ability to work, travel, participate in community affairs, or manage complex activities (such as driving to a new place, appearing in front of an audience, planning an event, participating in competitive games, or taking part in activities that involve some degree of risk from slow reaction times or poor judgment). As Ritchie et al. (2001) point out, "No guidelines have been given as to what constitutes activities of daily living restriction in MCI." Recent studies show that people with MCI who ultimately progress to Alzheimer's disease do show mild functional deficits (such as occasional need for help or need for cuing and supervision in activity) and reductions in physical activity before AD diagnosis (Friedland et al., 2001; Touchon & Ritchie, 1999).

Estimates of the proportion of seniors with cognitive impairment short of dementia vary, but are surprisingly high. The Aging, Memory, and Demographics Study (ADAMS) surveyed a national probability of Americans in 2002. It used a fairly liberal definition of "cognitive impairment without dementia." People were considered to fall into this category if (a) they did not meet criteria for dementia, and (b) participants or their proxies reported cognitive or functional impairment, *or* participants performed 1.5 *SD* below published norms for neuropsychological tests. By this standard, 22.2% of older people demonstrated cognitive impairment without dementia, of which 8.2% were considered to demonstrate prodromal AD.

Cognitive impairment short of dementia is clinically meaningful. In prior research, Albert and colleagues (1999) found that quite mild cognitive impairment is associated with less frequency and diversity of advanced functions, as indexed by the Pfeffer Functional Activities Questionnaire (Pfeffer, Kurosaki, Chance, & Filos, 1982). The Pfeffer scale records perceived difficulty with writing checks, assembling tax or business records, shopping alone, playing games of skill, making coffee or tea, preparing a balanced meal, keeping track of current events, paying attention and understanding while reading or watching a TV show, remembering to take medications and attend family occasions, and traveling out of the neighborhood. Close informants to people with "minimal cognitive impairment" reported that these elders had more difficulty in these tasks than a group with no cognitive impairment. In this study we considered someone to have mild cognitive impairment if they were not demented (score of 23 or greater on the MMSE), but had performance >1 SD below norms on one or more of a series of neuropsychological tests (recall of 2 of 3 objects at 5 minutes, delayed recall in the six-trial Selective Reminding Test (SRT), or a Wechsler Adult Intelligence Scale [WAIS] performance IQ score of >15 points below the WAIS verbal IQ score).

We have also shown that a discrepancy measure indicating lack of awareness of functional deficits (i.e., greater informant- than self-reported functional deficits) predicted risk of Alzheimer's disease more efficiently than self- or informant reports alone (Tabert et al., 2002). In these models, which controlled for sociodemographic differences and cognitive status, self-reports of functional status at baseline were not associated with the risk for diagnosis of Alzheimer's disease. By contrast, informant reports of deficits at baseline were a significant predictor of dementia over follow-up. A discrepancy of 1+ deficit in the Pfeffer scale, relative to those with no discrepancy, was associated with a fourfold increase in the risk of a future AD diagnosis. These findings support research by Tierney et al. (1996), who showed that informant- but not self-reported cognitive deficits (i.e., memory for lists, events, and names, finding one's way around home and neighborhood, and financial management) also predicted risk of AD.

Other research suggests that older adults meeting criteria for MCI performed worse than older adults performing within age- and education-based norms on tasks involving fine and complex motor skills (mainly tests of manual dexterity) (Kluger et al., 1997). These findings suggest a gradient of motor and cognitive performance in which people with MCI again fall between people with no cognitive impairment and people who meet criteria for Alzheimer's disease.

Finally, occupational therapist ratings of efficiency and safety in IADL tasks, such as cooking and cleaning, were lower in people with MCI compared with older adults without cognitive impairment. The therapists use the Assessment of Motor and Process Skills, a standardized measure of motor and process skills (Fisher, 2001), to rate older adults as they performed daily tasks. Therapists were blinded to the cognitive status of these seniors (Albert, Bear-Lehman, & Burkhardt, 2006).

The upshot of this research is that MCI affects high-level function, not basic self-care, that people with MCI are not fully aware of the extent of their functional impairment, and that families recognize functional deficits in people with MCI. Furthermore, functional deficit, as reported by families and *not* reported by elders, may be useful for identifying MCI patients with a high likelihood of rapid progression to Alzheimer's disease (Albert et al., 2002).

PREVALENCE AND INCIDENCE OF ALZHEIMER'S DISEASE

Surprisingly little information about the national prevalence and incidence of Alzheimer's disease has been available in the United States. Early estimates of the number of people with AD in this country ranged from 1.09 to 4.58 million (Brookmeyer, Gray, & Kawas, 1998). Such estimates were based on studies in four communities: Rochester, Baltimore, Framingham, and East Boston. Each study measured AD in a different way; for instance, the Rochester study included only cases coming to medical attention, whereas the East Boston study (which had higher rates) included both mild and moderate cases.

U.S. General Accounting Office (GAO) estimates from the 1990s fall in the middle of this range. In a synthesis of 18 prevalence surveys, the GAO estimated that 1.9 million people aged 65 and older were identified as meeting criteria for Alzheimer's disease in 1995. Prevalence rises to 2.1 million if we include possible or mixed cases, that is, cases marked by AD and some other source of dementia. If we restrict cases to moderate or more severe AD, the prevalence is 1.0 million with the narrow definition and 1.4 million if we include possible and mixed cases. All told, in the mid-1990s, 5.7% of Americans aged 65 and older had AD, with 3.3% meeting criteria for moderate or more severe AD (GAO, 1998).

In 2002 estimates became available from one of the first studies designed explicitly to produce national estimates of AD and other dementias. ADAMS, an add-on to the Health and Retirement Study, examined a nationally representative sample of people age 71 and older with cognitive assessments (Plassman et al., 2007). Of Americans over age 71, 13.9% met criteria for dementia, and 9.7% met criteria for AD. The absolute number of older adults with dementia was 3.4 million (with a 95% confidence interval [CI] of 2.8–4.0 million). The absolute number with AD was estimated to be 2.4 million (95% CI 1.8–2.9 million). Including people aged 60–70 yields a prevalence of 4.7 million Americans with dementia and 3.3 million with AD (Plassman et al., 2008). These prevalence estimates are considerably higher than the median reported for a recent synthesis of published studies, which suggested an AD prevalence of 2.5 million (Hirtz et al., 2007).

Table 6.3 reports the GAO prevalence by age and gender for the U.S population aged 65 and older in 1995. The table shows that prevalence doubles every 5 years, both for men and women, reaching approximately 40% for people aged 95 and older. The proportion with moderate or more severe AD in the oldest age group reaches approximately 25%. The prevalence of AD is higher in women than in men in every age group, with the gap widening at successively older ages. This gender disparity most likely reflects greater risk of AD for women, but this finding is controversial. Some prospective cohort studies have found a greater risk of AD for women (Launer et al., 1999); others have not (Tang et al., 2001). Results from ADAMS do not suggest differences by gender or race in the prevalence of AD. In addition, in ADAMS the prevalence of AD in people over age 80 was 18.1% and in people over 90, it was 29.7%.

If prevalence doubles every 5 years, then delaying the disease by 5 years would reduce prevalence by half. This is an important public health goal. With this delay, dementia-free life expectancy would increase, a greater number of older adults would live their last years without the need for costly supportive care, and older people at these late ages would die of other causes. Such a delay would obviously have a major impact on disability in late life and caregiving demands. In simulation studies using available data on population growth, Brookmeyer, Gray, and Kawas (1998) suggests that a delay of even 1 year in the incidence of the disease would result in nearly 800,000 fewer prevalent

Table 6.3

PREVALENCE OF ALZHEIMER'S DISEASE, UNITED STATES, 1995

	ALZHEIMER'S DISEASE			
	ALL		MODERATE+	
AGE	MEN	WOMEN	MEN	WOMEN
65–69	0.6	0.8	0.3	0.6
70–74	1.3	1.7	0.6	1.1
75–79	2.7	3.5	1.1	2.3
80–84	5.6	7.1	2.3	4.4
85–89	11.1	13.8	4.4	8.6
90–94	20.8	25.2	8.5	15.8
95+	35.6	41.5	15.8	27.4

Table entries are percentages meeting criteria for Alzheimer's disease, CDR 2+.
From "Alzheimer's Disease: Estimates of Prevalence in the U.S.," by GAO, 1998.
Retrieved from http://www.gao.gov/archive/1998/he98016.pdf.

cases over the next 50 years. A delay of 2 years would cut prevalence by 2 million cases.

A number of prospective cohort studies have examined the incidence of Alzheimer's disease. These studies are superior to retrospective studies that ask family proxies to date disease onset (i.e., "when did _____ first report memory problems or first go to the doctor because of difficulty with memory?" [Wolfson et al., 2001]). Retrospective studies do not allow formal diagnosis and are always subject to recall bias. Prospective studies begin with a dementia-free cohort and monitor the cohort over multiple assessments to track onset of disease.

However, prospective cohort studies of AD are complicated not just by differences in the definition of the disease, but also by different approaches to establishing the date of onset. Even with a regular schedule of follow-up assessments, it is not possible to establish the date when a person first met criteria for the disease. Further, most studies do not have long follow-up or closely spaced assessment intervals. The result has been imprecision in the true date of diagnosis, which affects calculation of person-years of dementia-free follow-up. In the face of this problem, the European Community Concerted Action on the Epidemiology and Prevention of Dementia Group (EURODEM) carried out a pooled analysis of AD incidence, which used a statistical adjustment: "To account for the fact that reliable data regarding when the dementia started is difficult to obtain, we used an iterative procedure that provides a best estimate for time of onset based on the patient's age and age-specific dementia rates" (Launer et al., 1999). A simpler approach, if multiple follow-up assessments are available, is to call the incidence date the date of the assessment when the respondent first met criteria for the diagnosis (Tang et al., 2001).

The incidence of AD is closely related to age. For people aged 65–74, the annual incidence ranges from <0.5% to 1.3%. For people aged 75–84, the range is 1.5%–4.0%, and for people aged 85 and older the range is 4.7%–7.9% per year (Launer et al., 1999; Tang et al., 2001). Thus, for someone aged 85 and older, the risk of meeting criteria for AD for the first time is approximately 5%–10% per year, a very high rate.

Even within age strata, the incidence of AD varies considerably among groups defined by race and ethnicity. In New York City, for example, incidence was considerably lower among Whites than among African Americans and Hispanics. African Americans and Hispanics were 2–3 times as likely to develop AD; thus, for example, the risk among Whites aged 75–84 was 2.6% per year and among African Americans and Hispanics it was 4.4% (Tang et al., 2001). This difference persisted even with adjustment for socioeconomic (education, literacy status, gender) and disease (hypertension, diabetes) factors. It also persisted when analyses were limited to people with the *APOE*-e3 allele (Tang et al., 1998) to control for the effects of this genetic risk factor (see below). Thus, minority status is among the most important risk factors for AD. Given the increasing number of older adults in the United States who belong to minority racial and ethnic goups, this disparity has great public health significance.

These rates for AD incidence apply to the entire population at risk in any given year. If we restrict risk estimates to the group of older people who report memory complaints or demonstrate mild cognitive impairment, annual AD incidence is, of course, much higher. The risk of AD in these older adults is between 10% and 25% per year, depending on ascertainment site (community versus clinic) and the stringency of the definition of mild impairment (Peterson et al., 2001).

How many older adults in the United States will have AD in the future? As the number of adults reaching old age increases, so will the number of Americans living with AD. Projections by Hebert suggest the number may reach 7 million in 2030. This estimate is based on incidence rates reported in several neighborhoods in Chicago. Projections based on Brookmeyer's study, which relies on rates from four community-based studies, put the figure closer to 5 million in 2030. To our knowledge, projections have not been undertaken that take into account both shifts in age and education level using national estimates of either prevalence or incidence.

RISK FACTORS FOR ALZHEIMER'S DISEASE

Genetic Risk Factors

The role of genetic factors in the development of AD is an active research area but at this point is still underdeveloped. Only approximately 7% of early-onset AD (younger than age 65) and less than 1% of late-onset AD has been linked to mutations on particular genes (Whalley & Deary, 2001; Whalley et al., 2000). Early-onset Alzheimer's disease has been linked to mutations on a number of genes (located on chromosomes 1, 14, and 21). Risk of late-onset AD is associated with the e4 allele of the *APOE* gene on chromosome 19. The mechanism for the APOE-AD relationship is not completely understood.

Although mutations for early-onset AD have been identified, their relevance for late-onset AD, which represents the vast majority of cases, is unclear. For public health purposes, attention is centered on *APOE*, the apolipoprotein E gene, which produces a plasma protein involved in the transport of cholesterol and other hydrophobic molecules (Farrer et al., 1995). Whereas some forms of apolipoprotein E have been linked to disorders of cholesterol metabolism and coronary heart disease (Saunders et al., 1993), this protein product has also been shown to raise the risk of AD. A number of studies have shown overrepresentation of the *APOE*-e4 allele in people with AD. Of individuals with AD 34%–65% carry the *APOE*-e4 allele, compared with only 24%–31% of people without AD of the same age (Jarvik et al., 1995; Myers et al., 1996; Roses et al., 1994). The number of *APOE*-e4 alleles is associated with earlier age of onset (Corder et al., 1993). The *APOE*-e2 allele, by contrast, may be protective against AD, but this finding has been challenged (Corder et al., 1994; Talbot et al., 1994; van Duijn et al., 1995).

Despite the association between *APOE* and AD, *APOE* testing is currently not recommended as a screening tool. A number of reasons have been advanced. First, the presence of an e4 allele is not necessary for the development of AD (35%–50% of persons with AD do not carry an e4 allele) (Roses et al., 1994). Second, the AD diagnosis is not difficult to make, and the extra predictive power provided by genetic testing would not add a great deal to clinical tools. Third, no treatment beyond tertiary symptomatic therapies is available in any case, so that awareness of AD risk before disease onset would not have practical benefit. And, finally, discrimination or other untoward effects are possible with such information, reducing the possible gain further.

A task force investigating the issue concluded:

> Because most patients presenting to physicians with dementia have AD, the additional information gained by genotyping would be useful only if it reduced the necessity for other more expensive or invasive tests. Individuals homozygous for epsilon-4 are the most likely candidates for disease, but they comprise only 2% to 3% of the general population; [and] even among AD patients, only 15% to 20% have this genotype. Most symptomatic epsilon-4 homozygotes will in fact have AD, but any uncertainty will oblige the physician to exclude other forms of dementia.

They go on to conclude: "Thus, although *APOE* genotype may be a risk factor for AD, it cannot yet be considered a useful predictive genetic test" (Farrer et al., 1995). The 2008 U.S. Task Force on Preventive Services concurred with this recommendation.

Socioeconomic Factors And Cognitive Reserve

Earlier we discussed lifelong cognitive resources as a predictor of Alzheimer's risk. The significance of cognitive resources early in the life span for this late-life outcome has become increasingly clear in studies that have linked risk of AD in late life to childhood IQ (Whalley & Deary, 2001; Whalley et al., 2000), educational accomplishments and leisure activities (Helzner, Scarmeas, Cosentino, Portet, & Stern, 2007; Scarmeas, Albert, Manly, & Stern, 2006; Wilson et al., 2004, 2009), occupational attainment and job demands (Stern et al., 1994), language skills in early adulthood (Snowdon et al., 1996), diversity of physical and cognitive engagement over the life span (Friedland et al., 2001), parental socioeconomic status, and literacy (Albert & Teresi, 1999; Manly, Jacobs, Touradji, Small, & Stern, 2002).

The case of childhood cognitive ability and AD risk is revealing. In a Scottish case-control study involving a match-back to childhood IQ tests, Whalley and Deary (2001) found that people who developed AD after age 65 had lower scores on this early measure of cognitive ability compared with people who did not develop AD. Differences in Alzheimer's risk, then, were already apparent at age 11. It is noteworthy that people who developed *early-onset* AD did not differ from other elders on the childhood IQ measure, suggesting an important difference in mechanism between early and late-onset AD.

What do these findings mean? One interpretation is that cognitive ability is similar to grip strength: differences (in muscle fiber density, in neuronal integrity or number) already apparent at birth or in the perinatal period (and which develop or set limits on development over the life span) provide variable reserves against depletions that occur with aging. These resources put one closer or further away from the threshold of disability associated with the loss of physical and cognitive function that occurs over the life span. In this view, development of AD is not so much a disease as one kind of aging, and some kind of early strengthening of cognition to build up reserve would be an appropriate intervention. The association between a cognitive resource and AD risk, then, is not evidence of an independent risk factor (as it is usually portrayed); instead, it is the identification of an early phase of the process that will ultimately result in AD.

Medical Morbidity: Hypertension and Vascular Disease, Diabetes, Bone Mineral Density Loss, Estrogen Deficiency, Depression

An increasing number of medical conditions have been shown to increase the risk of Alzheimer's disease. For the most part, these are considered secondary risks, in that they do not represent the primary mechanism for development of AD, but recent research suggests that the insulin pathway may have direct effects on the hippocampus. In any case, treatment of these secondary conditions may offer avenues for reducing Alzheimer's risk and may indicate points in the pathway of Alzheimer's neurodegeneration that may be amenable to intervention. The findings for these morbid conditions in some cases remain controversial.

Hypertension, Stroke, Diabetes, Cholesterol

Hypertension has been associated with cognitive performance, so it stands to reason that this condition might be associated with later risk of AD. However, one large prospective study failed to confirm this association (Posner et al., 2002). In this cohort, 731 of 1,259 subjects (58.1%), all free of AD at baseline, had a history of hypertension associated with diabetes, stroke, or heart disease. A history of hypertension was not associated with an increased risk for AD, but it did raise the risk for vascular dementia. The increased risk of vascular disease was evident only in respondents who had multiple morbidities. Respondents with hypertension and heart disease had a threefold increase in risk for vascular dementia, whereas respondents with hypertension and diabetes faced a sixfold increase.

These results stand in contrast to results from the double-blind, placebo-controlled Systolic Hypertension in Europe (Syst-Eur) Trial, in which randomly selected patients with hypertension were offered active study medication after the end of the trial for a further period of observation (Forette et al., 2002). In this add-on component, long-term antihypertensive therapy reduced the risk of dementia by 55%, from 7.4 to 3.3 cases per 1,000 patient-years, a finding that remained after adjustment for sex, age, education, and entry blood pressure. In a "number needed to treat analysis," the trial showed that treatment of 1,000 patients with hypertension for 5 years would prevent 20 cases of dementia.

Whether through an AD or vascular dementia process, diabetes is now increasingly recognized as a risk factor for cognitive decline. In the Study of Osteoporotic Fractures, women with diabetes ($n = 682$) had lower baseline scores than women without diabetes on a variety of cognitive measures (Digit Symbol, Trials B, MMSE). These women also faced greater likelihood of cognitive decline in models that adjusted for age, education, depression, stroke, visual impairment, heart disease, hypertension, physical activity, estrogen use, and smoking (Gregg et al., 2000). But, again, other research has shown only a modest association between diabetes and risk of AD (Luchsinger, Tang, Stern, Shea, & Mayeux, 2001).

Vascular risk factors may offer insight on mechanisms of AD. Wu and colleagues (2008) were able to show that diabetes and brain infarcts are each associated with hippocampal dysfunction, a key site for Alzheimer's pathology, but affect separate subregions and therefore may indicate distinct underlying mechanisms (Wu et al., 2008). "The hippocampal subregion linked to diabetes implicated blood glucose as a pathogenic mechanism, [while] the hippocampal subregion linked to infarcts suggested transient hypoperfusion as a pathogenic mechanism." This analysis suggests that elevations in blood glucose and hypoperfusion due to infarcts are separate sources of hippocampal degeneration. The implication is that Alzheimer's dementia may have different sources. We await studies that definitively establish the value of aggressive control of hypertension (a risk factor for strokes and brain infarcts) and glycemia for prevention of Alzheimer's.

Cholesterol may also be a risk factor for cognitive decline. Among people with Alzheimer's disease, higher prediagnosis low-density lipoprotein cholesterol and a history of diabetes was associated with faster cognitive decline (Helzner et al., 2009). This again points to the role of vascular factors in the course of AD and also as risk factors for the disease. This line of investigation is confirmed in other research showing associations between obesity earlier in life and risk of AD (Fitzpatrick et al., 2009) and the protective effects of the Mediterranean diet (Scarmeas et al., 2006).

Bone Mineral Density Loss and Estrogen Deficiency

Animal models and preclinical studies suggest that estrogen use may promote the growth and survival of cholinergic neurons and may also decrease cerebral amyloid deposition. Given the reduction in estrogen production that follows menopause, estrogen supplementation in women is a plausible strategy for delaying the onset of Alzheimer's disease. Hope for this approach was strengthened by prospective studies that showed a lower incidence of AD in postmenopausal women taking estrogen compared with women who did not. In a group of 1,124 older women who initially did not have Alzheimer's disease, Parkinson's disease, and stroke, the age at onset of Alzheimer's disease was significantly later in women who had taken estrogen. Alzheimer's disease was diagnosed in 5.8% of the estrogen users compared with 16.3% of nonusers, even after adjustment for such differences as education, ethnic origin, and *APOE* genotype (Tang et al., 1996).

Even a well-planned prospective study with statistical adjustment cannot rule out selection factors that are confounded with estrogen use (such as better education, income, and more proactive health behaviors). For this effort, randomized controlled trials are required. Confidence in estrogen replacement as a *treatment* strategy has been shaken by a series of negative clinical trials. A Cochrane Review (2002, and updated in 2009) assessed high-quality trials of estrogen use (selected from a review of all double-blind, randomized controlled trials on the effect of estrogen, alone or in combination with progestrin, for cognitive function in postmenopausal women with AD or other types of dementia). Meta-analyses showed no significant benefit and actually suggested that such treatment may be associated with worse outcomes in a number of cognitive domains.

The negative result for these treatment trials does not rule out a protective effect for estrogen as a *preventive* agent if given earlier to women who have not yet developed AD. A number of long-term prevention trials have been conducted or are underway to examine this potential benefit. However, expectations of success have been dampened by findings from the Heart and Estrogen/Progestin Replacement Study (HERS), a randomized, placebo-controlled trial involving 2,763 women with coronary disease. Participants at 10 of the 20 HERS centers (n = 517 estrogen, n = 546 placebo) completed a cognitive function substudy. At approximately 4 years of follow-up, the groups did not significantly differ on a variety of cognitive tests (modified MMSE, Verbal Fluency, Boston Naming, Word List Memory, Word List Recall, and Trials B) (Grady et al., 2002). This trial had only a single cognitive assessment at the end of the trial and did not examine incident Alzheimer's disease, so the question of the efficacy of estrogen replacement as a prevention strategy remains open. Still, these negative results are not reassuring. Combined with reports from the Women's Health Initiative of an increased risk of some cancers and stroke in women using estrogen replacement therapy (leading to early termination of the unopposed estrogen arm of the trial; Shumaker et al., 2003), estrogen replacement so far has not turned out to be useful as an anti-dementia agent. Meta-analyses suggest that "benefits of HRT include prevention of osteoporotic fractures and colorectal cancer, while prevention of dementia is uncertain. Harms include CHD, stroke, thromboembolic events, breast cancer with 5 or more years of use, and cholecystitis" (Nelson, Humphrey, Nygren, Teutsch, & Allan, 2002a). The Women's Health Initiative Memory Study and Women's Health Initiative Study of Cognitive Aging did not show clear benefit for hormone therapy (Asthana et al., 2009). The value of estrogen supplementation early in life remains an open question (Henderson, 2009).

Other evidence suggests that estrogen may turn out to be critical for cognitive health and risk of AD after all. For example, bone mineral density (BMD) is a marker of cumulative estrogen exposure and has been associated with cognitive function in older women without dementia (Yaffe, Browner, Cauley, Launer, & Harris, 1999b). In the Study of Osteoporotic Fractures (n = 8,333 older community-dwelling women not taking estrogen), women with low-baseline BMD had up to 8% worse baseline cognitive scores and up to 6% worse repeat cognitive scores.

For women who declined 1 *SD* in hip or calcaneal BMD, the risk of cognitive deterioration (defined as the most extreme 10% of those who declined) increased by about a third, compared with women with stable BMD. The same was true for women who had vertebral fractures. These women had lower cognitive test scores at baseline and greater odds of cognitive deterioration similar to those who declined 1 *SD* in BMD.

Thus, the relationship between estrogen and risk of AD remains unclear, but the preponderance of evidence suggests that it is not an appropriate therapy in old age. The effect of earlier use at or around menopause is still under investigation.

Depression

Depressed mood may be an early sign of AD or a risk factor in its own right. Prospective studies cannot settle the issue but do suggest that older people without dementia who have a depressed mood face an increased risk of AD. In one cohort study ($n = 478$ without dementia at baseline, mean of 2.5 years follow-up), depressed mood at baseline increased the risk of incident dementia nearly threefold. The effect persisted after adjustment for age, gender, education, language of assessment, and functional status (Devanand et al., 1996). The role of depression in subsequent cognitive decline has been confirmed (Yaffe et al., 1999a). However, a definitive treatment trial, in which depression would be treated to see if treatment response improves cognition or delays AD, remains to be completed.

Depression may also increase the risk of poor cognitive performance short of frank dementia. In one longitudinal cohort, depressive symptoms at baseline predicted declines in a number of memory domains (Panza et al., 2009).

OUTCOMES ASSOCIATED WITH ALZHEIMER'S DISEASE

Mortality

Table 6.4 presents U.S. mortality from AD by age and race strata in 1998. Approximately 50,000 deaths per year are attributed to AD, making AD the eighth most common cause of death in the United States. Mortality from AD is exceedingly rare in people under age 65: less than 1:100,000 per year. But AD very quickly becomes a prominent cause of

Table 6.4

MORTALITY AND ALZHEIMER'S DISEASE, UNITED STATES, 1998

AGE	TOTAL	WHITE MEN	WHITE WOMEN	AFRICAN AMERICAN MEN	AFRICAN AMERICAN WOMEN
45–54	0.1				
55–64	1.1	1.2	1.2		
65–74	10.4	10.6	11.1	7.4	8.1
75–84	70.0	69.3	74.8	50.2	59.2
85+	299.5	257.9	336.2	142.5	202.5

Table entries are deaths per 100,000.
From http://www.cdc.gov/nchs/datawh/statab/unpubd/mortabs/gmwk51.htm.

death at later ages. It is noted on death certificates in 10 (ages 65–74), 70 (aged 75–84), and 300 (aged 85 and older) of every 100,000 deaths. This is almost certainly an underestimate, because AD may be a contributory cause and not appear on the death certificate, especially if the certificate is prepared by a funeral home director, coroner, or doctor unfamiliar with the patient. The lower attribution of mortality to AD among African Americans may represent greater likelihood of death certificates completed in this way.

Alzheimer's disease increases the risk of mortality. Compared with older adults without dementia matched for age, drawn from the same community, and similar in socioeconomic features, these elders face a mortality risk 2–3 times higher. Figure 6.2 presents Kaplan-Meier plots of time to death in three groups first assessed in 1989–1992 and monitored for up to 10 years. These elders were recruited from a Medicare enrollee sample and AD registry, both in the Washington-Heights Inwood community, northern Manhattan, New York City.

In 1989–1992, people met criteria for AD when they were first seen (*prevalent AD*), or developed AD sometime in this period (no dementia at baseline visit, dementia at later visit over the follow-up period: *incident AD*), or never met criteria for AD over the entire follow-up period (*without dementia*). A convenient measure of mortality risk is

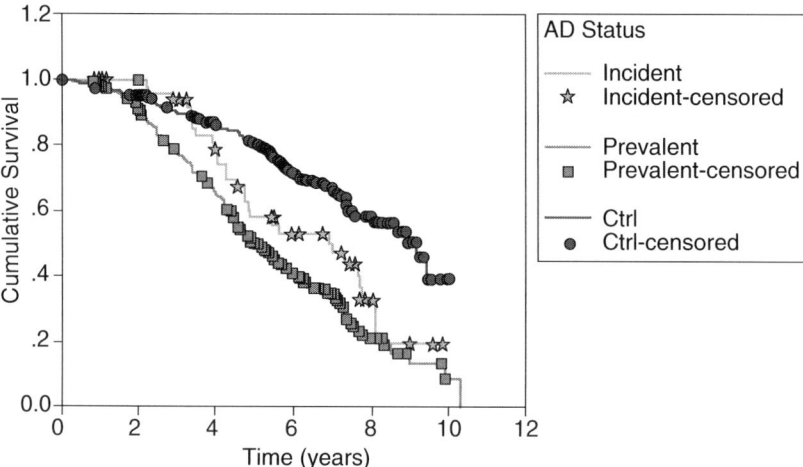

Figure 6.2 Survival in AD: prevalent, incident, and elders without dementia, New York City, 1989–1999.

to note the point in follow-up time when 50% of people in each of the three groups have died. As the figure shows, this point was reached in 5.2 years in the prevalent AD group, 7.0 years in the incident AD group, and 9.2 years in the without dementia group. Although an impressive difference, this approach does not adjust for differences in age or other factors, an important limitation, since age is related to AD risk, as we have already seen. To control for this confounding, proportional hazards models can be used to separate the effects of age and AD, as well as the influence of other factors. In such a model, we found that prevalent AD was associated with a twofold increase in mortality risk and incident AD was associated with a 1.7-fold increase, both highly significant effects.

It is not surprising that survival with AD depends heavily on the age at diagnosis. Results from the Baltimore Longitudinal Study of Aging show that median survival after diagnosis ranged from 8.3 years in people aged 65 to 3.4 years for people aged 90. Comparing this survival with elders without dementia showed that AD reduces life span by approximately two-thirds for people in whom AD is diagnosed at age 65 and by approximately 39% for people in whom AD is diagnosed at age 90 (Brookmeyer, Corrada, Curriero, & Kawas, 2002). These differences reflect the effect of competing risks of mortality, which increase at later ages.

Survival after a diagnosis of AD may in fact be shorter than these early estimates. A number of studies now suggest that AD is associated with a median survival of 4–5 years; (Helzner et al., 2008; Larson et al., 2004; Wolfson et al., 2001).

Nursing Home Care

Alzheimer's disease is a major risk factor for nursing home placement. In the Washington Heights-Inwood, New York City sample, described above, we tracked nursing home admission in up to 10 years of follow-up. This sample has the advantage of long follow-up and careful diagnostic assessment for AD, but it is probably atypical for estimating the absolute rate of nursing home use, because New York City offers an extensive alternative Medicaid-funded home care benefit. In addition, this study enrolled a largely minority sample, and research has shown that minorities are less likely to use skilled nursing home care than Whites.

In the Washington Heights cohort, 8.8% of prevalent cases entered nursing homes, compared with 3.5% of people who never met criteria for AD. Incident cases were intermediate, with 5% entering nursing homes. With this background of relatively low rates of nursing home placement, it is still impressive to see that incident AD was associated with a large increase in the risk of nursing home admission. Using a time-dependent approach, in which the date of AD diagnosis is used as a predictor of time to nursing home placement, we found that incident AD was associated with an eightfold increase in risk in models that controlled for age, race-ethnicity, and education.

In other settings, nursing home placement is more frequent. Among participants in a clinical trial of selegiline and tocopherol, all with moderate dementia and living in the community, two-thirds of the 341 patients followed up entered nursing homes over 2 years (Knopman et al., 1999). Dementia progression was the strongest predictor of placement, such that people progressing to severe dementia (CDR 3) were eight times as likely to enter nursing homes as people who had moderate dementia. Despite sociomedical determinants of nursing home placement (such as features of caregivers, e.g., caregiver burden, perceived skill or efficacy, presence of family support, and system-level features, such as availability of beds or alternative home-based services), nursing home placement remains an important outcome for assessing disease progression and treatment. To take these sociomedical factors into account, Stern and colleagues have developed a measure of "dependency" and "equivalent institutional care" that tracks need for services provided in institutional settings (Stern et al., 1994).

Nursing home placement is driven by exhaustion or depletion of caregiver resources, as well as by the progression of disease (Gaugler, Yu, Krichbaum, & Wyman, 2009). New research in this area has focused on assessment of risk domains that predict caregiver inability to manage Alzheimer's care at home. One promising approach involves screening of "caregiver risk" to identify domains amenable to support or intervention. The Resources for Enhancing Alzheimer's Caregiver Health (REACH II) Study has developed such a risk appraisal measure, which involves assessment of caregiver depression, burden, self-care and health behaviors, social support, safety, and patient problem behaviors (Czaja et al., 2009). We examine caregiver interventions in more detail below.

Hospitalization and Primary Care

Do people with Alzheimer's disease face an increased risk of hospitalization? This simple question is actually quite hard to answer. People with AD may enter the hospital for other reasons, and AD may not be recorded on the discharge diagnosis. Moreover, risk of hospitalization may be elevated in early stages of disease, when patients are likely to fall, fail to take medications, or have a psychiatric admission, and decline with more severe stages of dementia. Patients with the most severe dementia may reside in nursing homes, which provide medical care for many conditions, or may simply not be brought in for hospital care as part of a general strategy of less aggressive treatment. In addition, whereas the use of Medicare billing records, which include ICD-10 diagnoses of AD, can be used to establish hospital episodes and volume of costs, these sorts of analysis are prone to an observation bias, in which the most severe cases are overrepresented (Newcomer et al., 1999). Because AD is a terminal disease, it is hard to distinguish end-of-life care from AD care. Finally, the proper test would be a comparison between people with similar medical conditions and health status except for AD, but this comparison is difficult because AD may itself be associated with medical conditions, such as falls or injuries, wasting and dehydration, or pneumonia and infectious disease.

With these caveats, it is not surprising to see considerable variation in yearly rates of hospitalization in people with AD. The Consortium to Establish a Registry for Alzheimer's Disease (CERAD) reported a rate of 370 hospitalizations per 1,000 AD patients per year in a clinical cohort (Fillenbaum, Heyman, Peterson, Pieper, & Weiman, 2000). In a community cohort in New York City, the rate was 100 per 1,000 AD cases per year (Albert et al., 1999). In any case, what seems clear is the elevation of this risk relative to matched elders without AD. In the New York sample, 10% of AD cases had a hospitalization in a year, compared with 6.8% among elders without dementia. In logistic regression models that control for differences in age, gender, education, number of comorbid conditions, and death in the follow-up period, severe AD (CDR 3+) was associated with an elevated risk of 2.3. This study had the advantage of a large population-based cohort in which hospitalizations were tracked with an innovative electronic medical record. This risk was comparable with the added risk associated with the presence of two comorbid conditions.

The association between dementia and hospitalization has been confirmed in population-based studies. A large record-linked Australian study found that older people with dementia spent an average of 30 days in the hospital in the last year of life (Zilkens, Spilsbury, Bruce, & Semmens, in press). Among older people, in general, the length of stay in U.S. hospitals in the last year of life is 10–17 days (Fonkych, O'Leary, Melnick, & Keeler, 2008). However, variations across different health care systems make these comparisons difficult (Van den Block et al., 2007).

Primary care use and associated costs also seem to be elevated in AD. In the New York City cohort, people with recent diagnoses of AD were more likely to have more medical care encounters than people without AD, even 1–2 years before diagnosis (Albert, Glied, Andrews, Stern, & Mayeux, 2002b). Other studies have not found excess primary care costs in the prodromal period (Liebson et al., 1999).

Disability and Psychiatric Morbidity

The hallmark of progressive dementia is increasing dependency in ADLs and an increase in both "negative" (apathy, withdrawal) and "positive" (agitation, aggression, delusions, hallucinations, wandering) psychopathological symptoms. In the most severe stages of dementia, the prevalence of some symptoms declines (such as delusions), presumably because caregivers can no longer recognize these symptoms as patients become increasingly vegetative.

Cognitive performance in patients and ADL ratings from proxies (or from clinicians) are highly correlated in people with AD. For example, in one series of people with AD, correlations between the Blessed Memory-Concentration-Information Test, a mental status measure similar to the MMSE, and IADL and ADL (personal self-maintenance scale, PSMS) ratings were 0.83 and 0.78, respectively (Green, Mohs, Schmeidler, Aryan, & Davis, 1993). In this sample of 104 clinic patients with probable AD, PSMS scores were collected every 6 months and tracked for change. The PSMS items include toileting, feeding, dressing, grooming, indoor mobility, and bathing. These were scored on a scale of 1 (no difficulty) to 5 (maximum difficulty), so that total scores ranged from 6 to 30. In this sample, PSMS scores declined, on average, 2.44 points over 12 months, with a standard deviation of 3.87.

These numbers are important for gauging the clinical significance of changes in functional scales used in clinical trials in AD. A recent meta-analysis of the effect of cholinesterase inhibitors, the primary approved therapy for treatment of AD, showed a significant but small effect size of 0.1 SD favoring treatment. Using the standard deviation of 3.87, cited above, 0.1 SD is equivalent to 0.387, or about a 0.4-point change on the PSMS scale. Because the mean PSMS change over 12 months was 2.44, the 0.4 change is roughly equivalent to the decline patients can expect over a 2-month period (Trinh, Hoblyn, Mohanty, & Yaffe, 2003). Delaying decline by 2 months per year is a small but important benefit to patients and family caregivers.

A large trial of donepezil (Aricept) to assess preservation of ADL function in AD confirmed this benefit in an alternative way (Mohs et al., 2001). The trial sought to assess whether this cholinesterase inhibitor delayed "clinically evident decline in function," which was defined as progression to moderate or more severe levels of difficulty with particular ADL, or loss of 20% of instrumental ADL function, or onset of more advanced dementia, as assessed by the CDR. Fifty-six percent of patients receiving the placebo met the end point, compared with 41% of patients receiving donepezil. The median time at which patients met this end point was 208 days among patients receiving placebo and 357 days in patients receiving donepezil. The therapy, then, slowed progression by approximately 5 months in a 1-year period.

Cholinesterase inhibitors also showed benefit for the reduction in frequency of AD psychopathology. A meta-analysis showed that this class of therapies reduced Neuropsychiatric Inventory scores (NPI scores; Cummings, 1997), on average, by nearly 2 points, an improvement in the frequency or severity of one psychiatric symptom (Trinh et al., 2003). Because the presence of psychiatric symptoms is an important predictor of nursing home placement, not to mention caregiver distress and burnout, these therapies offer an important benefit, at least in the short run.

Thus, at this point, AD cannot be prevented and disease progression remains relentless. Available therapies offer benefit mostly as a holding action, delaying time to severe disability and nursing home placement. Schneider and colleagues have shown that when adverse events from antipsychotic medications are factored into assessments of benefit, differences between treatments and placebo are minimal and may actually favor placebo (Schneider et al., 2006).

Family Caregiving

Families provide the vast majority of Alzheimer's care. Although patients with Alzheimer's are common in nursing homes, accounting for perhaps half of the residents, these residents represent a minority of the population with Alzheimer's disease. As we discuss in Chapter 9, nursing home use has declined among older adults over the past decade in the United States as alternative residential care settings have expanded. Nursing home residence in people aged 65 and older declined from 54 per 1,000 in 1985 to 46.4 per 1,000 in 1995, and to 34.8 per 1,000 in 2004 (Federal Interagency Forum on Aging-Related Statistics, 2008). Most people with AD are cared for at home, use a variety of in-home (home attendant, allied health) and out-of-home services (adult day care, acute rehabilitation), and will enter nursing homes very late in the course of the disease, if at all.

In fact, people residing in nursing homes now are likely to be older and frailer than prior nursing home cohorts. They are also less likely to spend long periods of time in these institutions. The nursing home is becoming more of a short-stay rehabilitative or palliative care unit, funded by Medicare, than a long-term care residence (traditionally funded by Medicaid). The commonly cited estimate of a lifetime prevalence of 40% for nursing home residence (Kemper & Murtaugh, 1991), then, must be interpreted in this light.

How many people with Alzheimer's disease are cared for in the community? If we consider older people with three or more ADL limitations, we have an imperfect but reasonable indicator of dementia in the community. About half of these people relied exclusively on family and friends for assistance in 1994, a decline from two-thirds in the 1980s (Feder, Komisar, & Niefeld, 2001). This change reflects an expansion in financing for long-term care that occurred in the 1990s. Medicare spending for home health care grew from approximately $4 to $18 billion in the first half of the 1990s. Home care for Alzheimer's disease has benefited from this change. More recently, however, cost controls have been introduced into this health sector (Balanced Budget Act of 1997) that have reduced growth in Medicare-funded home care.

Estimates of the absolute number of family caregivers providing supportive care for older people, and also older people with Alzheimer's disease, are available in the 1996 panel of the Survey of Income and Program Participation (SIPP). In 1998, 6.7 million family members were providing help to some 4.5 million older adults with disabilities (Alecxih, Zeruld, & Olearczyk, 2000). This estimate is slightly lower than the estimate of 7.1 million derived from the National Long-Term Care Survey. The SIPP allows estimates of particular features of Alzheimer's caregiving. In 1998, approximately 473,000 family members or friends were serving as primary caregivers to people with diagnoses of Alzheimer's disease. These people were providing most of the nonpaid support received by people with dementia living in the community and were nominated as the person most involved in such care. They spent an average of 48 hours per week providing care and had been providing such care for a mean of 7 years. This compares with a mean of 24 hours per week and a mean duration of 5 years for all nonpaid caregivers in the community (Alecxih et al., 2000). Thus, Alzheimer's care is more demanding than standard care by this measure of caregiving intensity.

One investigation by Albert and colleagues (1998) tracked hours of care provided to people with Alzheimer's disease according to severity of dementia and also over a period of nearly 2 years. Family caregivers reported that more than half of the time they spent with these elders involved direct hands-on care, defined as help with ADL. Caregivers reported a mean of 7.2 hours per day of ADL care, or 50.4 hours per week. This report is quite close to the SIPP results. These informal, or nonpaid hours must be interpreted in light of the total hours of supportive care provided for these elders, which in this New York City sample were extensive. Total weekly hours were 56.7 for people with mild dementia, 81.2 for people with moderate dementia, and 112.0 for people with severe or greater dementia. Family contributions were 30.8 for people with mild dementia, 57.5 for people with moderate dementia, and 29.4 for people with severe dementia, suggesting substitution of formal for informal care in the most severe levels of dementia.

However, these cross-sectional findings can be deceiving. In longitudinal analyses, Albert and colleagues (1998) found that caregivers did not, in fact, reduce the number of hours they provided as elders progressed to more advanced dementia. Rather, formal hours increased, suggesting that these caregivers were already providing the maximum of hours they could provide.

What are the tasks of families who provide care for elders with dementia? Family caregivers certainly provide help with ADL, but providing ADL support at home to a family member is not well described by ADL measures. Although the ADL/IADL measures tell us that someone has a particular care need, satisfying that need takes place in a complex environment. Take bathing, for example. The ADL measure tells us that someone is dependent in bathing. It does not tell us the reason why the person cannot bathe independently, which may involve impairments in mobility and balance, or limb weakness, or cognitive incapacity, or psychiatric disorder, or some combination of these deficits. As a result, the ADL measure does not tell us if the person is cooperative during bathing, whether he or she helps wash parts of his/her body once in the tub, or whether he/she needs supervision throughout the entire course of bathing or only when getting in and out of the tub. Yet, these are the features that make caregiving for someone with bathing disability more or less difficult for families (Albert, 2004).

Thus, although a count of ADL/IADL needs will certainly be correlated with indicators of caregiving challenge (how many hours daily, reported burden and fatigue, risk of nursing home placement), these correlations will be low. Indeed, ADL status explains only a modest amount of the variance in caregiver reports of burden (Poulshock & Diemling, 1984).

The ADL/IADL measures also fail to capture the full context in which families provide care. What kinds of home modifications have family members made to facilitate caregiving? To return to our bathing example, providing bathing care will be easier if families have installed grab bars, or have a home with a walk-in shower or a flexible shower head. Similarly, what kinds of care arrangements have families put in place to ensure such care if they work, or wish to travel, or are themselves weak or ill? These too will determine how challenging ADL/IADL care may be. These sorts of care management tasks are a critical part of the work of caregiving, but are not considered in traditional ADL/IADL measures.

Thus, providing care is not simply the mirror image of the need for care, as expressed in ADL/IADL status (Albert, 2004). We have argued that ADL/IADL care should be subsumed within a wider, multidomain formulation that gives adequate scope to *how* people need ADL care and *how caregivers develop environments for providing it.* This is an especially salient issue in the care of people who have cognitive disorders, such as AD.

Even if we limit ourselves to traditional ADL tasks, we quickly see that caregivers who provide such care mention many additional factors that make ADL care easy or difficult, manageable or unbearable. One is *timing:* whether care is required rarely, frequently but in predictable ways, or frequently in unpredictable, unexpected ways (Hooyman, Gonyea, & Montgomery, 1985). AD care is characterized by great unpredictability in the timing of ADL care because of poor sleep hygiene, psychiatric complications, incontinence, inability to communicate care preferences, and noncooperation.

A glaring example of the central role of timing is nighttime care. People who routinely need to be taken to the toilet at night, disrupting a caregiver's sleep, are clearly more challenging than people who can be taken to the toilet during the day and sleep through the night, even though both equally need assistance in toileting (McCluskey, 2000). More generally, caregivers forced to adopt care receivers' schedules are likely to be the most burdened, because they are the most captive to caregiving.

A second dimension is *caregiver proximity* in the ADL task. Is it enough that a caregiver is in the house while someone eats a meal or bathes, or does the caregiver need to be in the same room standing by, or does the caregiver need to provide hands-on help? Stand-by help can be quite burdensome in that it limits caregivers to the home even if they do not have to provide hands-on help at all times. In fact, stand-by help, in some cases, may be more burdensome, because family members need to be available (and, hence, are prevented from doing other tasks) without a sense that they are providing care. This is a typical feature of caregiving to the elder with mild dementia.

A third dimension is the kind of *effort* caregivers need to exert to see that the ADL need is met. Someone with a need for help in bathing may only require supervision, or coaxing and support, or complete guidance and direction. It is possible that coaxing and support, in some cases, may be more challenging than complete guidance and control. For example, taking someone to the toilet every 2 hours may be more burdensome than complete continence care involving disposable diapers (Albert et al., 1999).

Finally, it obviously matters whether care receivers participate, actively resist, or are passive as receivers of ADL care (Feinstein, Josephy, &

Wells, 1986). Helping a person who is cooperative is far different from helping a person who is resisting assistance in bathing or eating (Reinhard, 2004). Unfortunately, care offered to people with severe dementia is often met with resistance.

The effects of providing care to a person with AD have been studied intensively. Marital discord and divorce, depression and anxiety, loss of employment, restriction of social life, invasion of privacy, impoverishment, and substance abuse have all been linked to caregiving stress. Buffering factors that mitigate these negative effects include support from family, religiosity, strong personal mastery and self-efficacy, satisfaction with caregiving, and adopting strategies to reduce the burden of care.

Caregiving strain has also been linked to mortality risk, as suggested in the Caregiver Health Effects Study, a study of the bereavement experience of people who cared for spouses who died during follow-up (Schulz & Beach, 1999). Spouses who provided care and reported burden from caregiving were more likely to die than noncaregivers, but caregiving spouses who did not experience burden did not face an elevated risk. Schulz concluded that mental or emotional strain is an independent risk factor for mortality among older spousal caregivers.

Caregiving is also associated with poorer work performance. In a study of a large employer database, employees reporting elder care responsibilities were more likely to report certain chronic conditions (such as diabetes), poorer attention to their own health (as evidenced in lower use of clinical preventive health services, less opportunity for physical activity), and greater overall medical care costs, in addition to greater absenteeism and poorer perceived productivity on the job (National Caregiver Alliance and MetLife Mature Market Institute, in press). We examine caregiving in more detail below, when we consider interventions to support families.

Quality of Life in AD

One central problem for people with AD is their inability, with later stages of the disease, to report on subjective states: their perceptions of pain, satisfaction, comfort, enjoyment, contentment, anxiety, or well-being. Because quality-of-life assessment is unthinkable without a patient's reports of such states (see Chapter 8), it would seem that assessment of quality of life in people with AD would be impossible. Severely affected patients (patients with MMSE scores below 12 or patients with more than moderate cognitive impairment) cannot reliably complete self-report questionnaires. Yet it is clear, even to the casual observer, that people with AD have good and bad days, that facial expressions and body posture reliably communicate information about internal states, and that these perhaps primitive indicators of mood or well-being are associated with changes in environment (Albert & Logsdon, 2001). If we can perceive mood changes and illness behaviors in animals, we can certainly recognize such changes in people with dementia. Thus, the challenge in advanced AD is to identify indicators of internal states that reliably convey information about mood and well-being.

What domains or aspects of daily life are important to patients in the presence of severely compromised cognition and function? The domains included in current measures vary considerably. Among other domains, Rabins includes "awareness of self" and "response to surroundings" (Rabins, Kasper, Kleinman, Black, & Patrick, 2001), and Brod includes "aesthetic sense" and "feelings of belonging" (Brod, Stewart, & Sands, 2001). Logsdon's QOL-AD measure includes items assessing "energy level" and "ability to do things for fun" (Logsdon, Gibbons, McCurry, & Teri, 2001). These are patient or proxy reports and face a variety of limitations. Proxy reports about patient quality of life are correlated with a caregiver's own mood or perceived caregiver burden. People impute moods or symptoms based on their own status. Patients' self-reports will be reliable only up to a point, although some patients are evidently able to complete questionnaires with MMSE scores as low as 10 (Logsdon et al., 2001).

Behavioral observation measures avoid these limitations. The Apparent Affect Rating Scale (APS) (Lawton, Van Haitsma, Perkinson, & Ruckdeschel, 2001), Multidimensional Observational Scale (MOSES) (Helmes, Csapo, & Short, 1987), Discomfort Scale (Hurley, Volicer, Hanrahan, Houde, & Volicer, 1992), and other observer ratings capture negative and positive behaviors in real time (Albert, 1997). "Behavior stream" technologies now allow clocking of the duration of mood or behavior states and the context in which patients express these states, such as "agitation during morning ADL care." Behavior stream measures are complicated by the need for extensive training of raters and limitation to institutional home settings.

One intermediate approach is to adapt behavior stream-like measures to proxy reporting. Albert and colleagues (1996, 1999a, 2001) asked proxies to report on affective states by use of APS items (i.e., facial expressions of the so-called "hot" affects: anger, anxiety, interest, pleasure) and patient activity over the prior 2 weeks (frequency of a series of in-home and out-of-home activities that could be completed with caregiving cueing and supervision). The measures were significantly correlated with dementia severity in both clinic and community samples (Albert et al., 1999a). This is important confirmation of the validity of the quality-of-life measures. Such measures should be correlated with stage of dementia (because dementia severity affects mood and opportunities for engagement) but should also show variance within stage (suggesting that there are other sources of pleasure or engagement relevant to dementia care).

This approach is also useful for specifying time to important quality-of-life milestones in the progression of AD. For example, in a group of people with moderate dementia at the start of follow-up, 50% no longer were leaving their homes at 20 months. In a group with mild dementia, this milestone was not reached until 30 months (Albert & Logsdon, 2001). This study was also able to show a hierarchy of quality-of-life (QOL) outcomes. Onset of home confinement preceded onset of null activity, which in turn preceded onset of null positive affect. Finally, this study showed that proxies identified states of pleasure even among patients with psychopathological behaviors. This finding reminds us that we must pay attention both to positive and negative behaviors if we are to understand dementia adequately.

One promising approach to assessing quality of life in people with AD involves more extensive "care mapping," in which detailed assessment of behavior streams is used for quality assurance purposes (Edelman, Fulton, Kuhn, & Chang, 2005). The premise of this approach is to supply supportive care personnel with real-time reports of environment-affect relationships. The hope is that personnel in skilled nursing facilities or adult day care settings can individualize the way care is provided and use this information to promote greater involvement of patients in activities or social interaction. A similar approach has been used by Schnelle and colleagues for training certified nursing assistants to deliver self-maintenance care and to improve other kinds of daily interactions, as well as to recognize resident pain or discomfort (Schnelle et al., 2009)

Dementia and the End of Life

Family caregivers face difficult decisions related to end-of-life care of relatives in the last stages of the disease (Meier, 1999). Should patients with pneumonia be treated aggressively with intravenous antibiotics, transferred to hospital, and intubated; or should they be treated symptomatically with analgesics, antipyretics, and oxygen? Should a patient with dementia who refuses food or who has trouble swallowing be tube fed? Little is known about the ways families make these decisions.

Persons with advanced dementia suffer serious medical problems, such as pneumonia, urinary tract infections, and fever (Fabiszewski, Volicer, & Volicer, 1990; van der Steen, Ooms, van der Wal, & Ribbe, 2002). Research suggests a high prevalence of intravenous antibiotic use and invasive procedures (Ahronheim, Morrison, Baskin, Morris, & Meier, 1996; Morrison & Siu, 2000). For example, despite the futility associated with aggressive care in end-stage dementia, Evers and colleagues (2002) found that more than 50% of the patients with dementia were treated with systemic antibiotics. Our own clinic series suggests similar trends. In a group of people with probable AD, 31% used intravenous antibiotics and 16% had feeding tubes placed in the 6 months before death. A series of studies have shown that feeding tube placement for people with AD in skilled nursing facilities is not associated with improved outcomes (Casarett et al., 2005; Morrison et al., 2005).

It is still unclear why some families opt for use of life-sustaining technologies in the case of older people with profound or terminal AD. It may be that family caregivers who score high on measures of distress (depression, caregiver burden, lack of social support) are less likely to develop medical care goals that limit aggressive end-of-life care. These families may also be at greater risk for emergency room use of life-sustaining technologies. To our knowledge, no research has investigated this issue. By contrast, AD patients may be less likely to be considered for life-sustaining technologies than other people with terminal conditions. The loss of cognitive ability and, hence, the loss of personhood associated with disease may allow families to "let go" of people who are in the last stages of life.

NON-ALZHEIMER'S DEMENTIAS

Vascular cognitive impairment (VCI), as opposed to Alzheimer's disease, is cognitive impairment related to cerebrovascular disease, such as stroke. VCI is mainly defined by neuroimaging, which allows further differentiation into subgroups that show cortical infarction, white matter changes, or some combination of the two. In cohort studies of incident dementia, such as the Cardiovascular Disease Study, approximately 70% of people meeting criteria for dementia can be classified as AD, another 10% as VCI, 15% as mixed AD and VCI, and the remaining 5% as some other etiology (such as hydrocephalus, metabolic disorders, or Korsakoff's syndrome) (Lopez et al., 2003).

VCI is a risk factor for mortality. In a Mayo Clinic record linkage study, patients with vascular dementia had a greater risk of mortality than matched controls without dementia. Among VCI patients, dementia related to stroke was associated with the highest mortality risk. Patients without stroke, but with imaging evidence of bilateral infarctions in gray matter structures, had a lower mortality risk (Knopman, Rocca, Cha, Edland, & Kokmen, 2003).

Another source of dementia in the older adults is Parkinson's disease (PD). The Parkinson's Foundation has reviewed a series of prevalence and incidence studies of dementia in PD and found that about a quarter of all patients with Parkinson's disease meet criteria for dementia. PD patients with dementia are older but do not differ in the duration of the disease (Lieberman, 2002). The annual incidence of dementia in patients with Parkinson's ranges from 2.7% (ages 55–64) to 13.7% (ages 70–79). Dementia risk in PD may vary according to whether patients have Lewy body inclusions in the brainstem or brain, or have Lewy bodies with Alzheimer's changes as well.

Mortality risk in PD is related to the presence of dementia. Incident dementia in PD increases mortality risk even when the motor effects of PD are controlled (Levy et al., 2002).

INTERVENTIONS TO PREVENT COGNITIVE DECLINE

If physical "prehabilitation" can retard disablement (Gill et al., 2002), could a program of preventive cognitive training have the same effect in the realm of cognitive decline? The Advanced Cognitive Training for Independent and Vital Elderly (ACTIVE) Trial investigated this question in the setting of a randomized clinical trial (Ball et al., 2002). A volunteer sample of nearly 3,000 older adults without cognitive or physical impairment was randomly assigned to one of three intervention groups or a no-contact control group. The three intervention arms involved 10 sessions devoted to training in memory skill (verbal episodic memory), reasoning (problem-solving strategies), or speed of processing (visual search and identification). The intervention program was delivered in small-group settings, with a focus on teaching strategies designed to improve memory, speed, or problem solving. Intervention groups were given exercises to practice and retain skills. In the memory-training arm, for example, participants "were instructed how to organize word lists into meaningful categories and to form visual images and mental associations to recall words and text." In this 2-year study, a subset of participants received booster training just before the 1-year evaluation.

Outcomes in the trial included ability on cognitive tests of these remediated skills, such as episodic memory, identification of patterns, and speed of processing. The trial also examined performance-based and self-reported everyday skills related to these cognitive domains. These included "everyday problem-solving" (for example, the ability to handle medication information), "everyday speed" (for example, the speed with which one looks up a telephone number), driving habits, and ADL and IADL limitations.

The trial showed that these cognitive interventions helped healthy older adults perform better on the specific cognitive skills for which they were trained. These benefits suggest that the slow cognitive declines reported for elders without dementia can be remediated. For example, ACTIVE participants receiving memory training improved by approximately 0.25 *SD* over 2 years, whereas the cognitive skills of older adults without dementia typically decline at about this rate over a 7-year period. However, these proximal cognitive benefits did not translate into improvements in everyday performance. The authors suggest that the absence of transfer to real-world outcomes is best explained by a ceiling effect in the everyday performance measures. Most subjects were not impaired in driving, in looking up telephone numbers, or in reasoning about medications. The pronounced ceiling effect may have obscured true benefit in this area. In fact, the control group did not decline on many of the everyday performance measures. The authors conclude, "it is not yet clear whether differential functional decline across treatment groups will be observed in the future as this select cohort enters more fully into an age of functional loss" (Ball et al., 2002).

More recent reports from the same trial indicate some generalization of benefit to self-reported quality of life (Wolinsky et al., 2006) and risk of depression (Wolinsky et al., 2009). However, the benefit in functional status has proven more elusive (Willis et al., 2006).

INTERVENTIONS TO SUPPORT FAMILY CAREGIVERS

Family caregiving, as we have mentioned earlier, is a major challenge in care of the elder with dementia. Families overwhelmed by the stresses of caregiving may resort to nursing home placement even when this is not a preferred choice. They may simply feel they have no other option once the stresses of caregiving and lack of respite have undermined coping resources and family function. A program of psychosocial support might strengthen caregiver resources and help them manage the stresses of care better. Would such a program, if effectively delivered, also reduce rates of nursing home placement? This difference in outcome would be a powerful demonstration of the effects of psychosocial support on vulnerable families, and in the case of spouse caregivers, highly vulnerable elders.

Mittelman and colleagues designed such a program for caregiving spouses of people with Alzheimer's disease and tested it in a randomized controlled trial of nursing home placement (Mittelman, Ferris, Shulman, Steinberg, & Levin, 1996). The intervention was designed to guide and support caregivers through the challenging period when spouses progressed to increasingly severe dementia. In the first 4 months of the study, spouses received two individual counseling sessions and four family sessions. "Counseling sessions were task oriented, promoting communication among family members, teaching techniques for problem solving and management of troublesome patient behavior, and improving both emotional and instrumental support for the primary caregiver." This phase was followed by participation in a support group and finally by continuing availability of contact with counselors. The control group received the usual follow-up and information and referral. Thus, "if control subjects asked about obtaining paid help at home, they were given the names of service providers, whereas treatment subjects were given as much help as they needed to find and appropriately use such services" (Mittelman et al., 1996).

After 3.5 years, 58.7% of patients in this sample of 206 families had entered nursing homes and 26.2% had died at home. In addition, not all caregivers in the intervention group agreed to support group participation; only 72% joined support groups. However, 42% of controls joined such support groups. Despite this combined drop-out and "drop-in" dilution of the experiment, patients in the treatment group remained at home significantly longer than patients in the control group. Treatment group patients entered nursing homes about a year later than controls. This difference was obtained in survival models that controlled for age and gender of caregivers, socioeconomic resources, caregiver mental health, and severity of dementia.

Mittelman and colleagues (1996) conclude that "continuously available support and information can enable spouse caregivers of AD patients to withstand the difficulties of caregiving and avoid or defer institutionalization of the patients." This conclusion is supported by the design of the experiment but also by the absence of differences in patient care between intervention and control groups. For example, patients in the two groups were equally likely to receive psychotropic medications and medical care. Thus, the intervention appears to have affected caregivers rather than patients. Patients were equally likely to develop urinary incontinence and equally likely to receive medical care for the condition, but intervention group caregivers, through support from training and counseling, were better able to manage the demands of care related to incontinence.

This finding is reassuring, given the absence or unclear benefit for a variety of other interventions involving patient and caregiver outcomes, including respite programs (Lawton, Brody, & Pruchno, 1991) and home attendant care (Weissert, Chernow, & Hirth, 2003). On the other hand, benefit has been reported for caregiver mental health, as in the Medicare Alzheimer's Disease Demonstration (Newcomer et al., 1999). As the United States moves toward increasing incentives for family caregivers (mostly in the form of tax breaks) and a greater diversity of services that can be provided in homes, it will become increasingly important to determine what kinds of resources families need to be effective caregiving units.

Results from REACH-II, Resources for Enhancing Alzheimer's Caregiver Health, show that training and low-intensity support can have a dramatic effect on caregiver health and well-being as well. This randomized controlled trial assessed the effects of a multicomponent psychosocial behavioral intervention designed to reduce burden and depression among family caregivers. The primary quality-of-life outcome comprised measures of caregiver depression, burden, self-care, and social support and care recipient problem behaviors at 6 months. The intervention group showed clinically significant benefit, which, however, was more pronounced among White and Hispanic caregivers than among African Americans (Belle et al., 2006). Institutional placement of care recipients did not differ over the 6 months. This linkage of targeted training and support to specific problem areas offers great potential for Alzheimer's caregiver support.

Finally, collaborative models to link family caregivers to dementia care consultants based in primary care practices show benefit for supporting caregivers and reducing the risk of nursing home placement (Fortinsky, Kulldorff, Kleppinger, & Kenyon-Pesce, 2009).

SUMMARY

Families confronting dementing disease face the very difficult problem of deciding when driving should cease, when supervision is required for safety, when elders can no longer live alone, and when parents or spouses are no longer competent to handle money, take medications, or manage their lives independently. They will likely have to contend with personality changes, psychiatric symptoms, and challenging behaviors as people reach more advanced stages of disease. Caregivers may have to perform ADL care, manage supportive care staff hired to assist the elder, or more likely both sets of tasks, possibly at a distance. They may face the difficult decision to admit the Alzheimer's patient to a nursing home. Or, as is increasingly common, older people themselves may choose residences (such as assisted living or continuing care retirement communities) that can accommodate Alzheimer's or nursing-home levels of care, should they need such services.

Definition of Dementia. A person meets criteria for dementia if he or she has memory impairment and one or more additional impairments in cognition, such as aphasia, apraxia, agnosia, or executive function deficits. These cognitive deficits must be severe enough to cause significant impairment in social or occupational function and represent a significant decline from a previous level of functioning. For Alzheimer's disease to be diagnosed, the course of this general cognitive disorder must, in addition, be characterized by gradual onset and continuing, progressive decline that is not attributable to other central nervous system conditions.

AD and Memory Decline in Aging. Research suggests that memory declines typical of Alzheimer's disease may be distinct from normal aging. In a cohort without dementia, declines in cognitive domains in people without the e4 allele, representing normal aging, were less pronounced than declines in people with the e4 allele, representing a likely early prodrome of AD.

Mild Cognitive Impairment. MCI is typically defined by subjective complaints of memory problems and memory performance below age- and education-referenced norms, with normal performance in other cognitive domains and absence of impairment in the instrumental and basic activities of daily living. Estimates of the proportion of older adults with cognitive impairment short of dementia range from 5% to as high as 22%. Dementia incidence in elders who report cognitive complaints and demonstrate mild deficits in cognitive assessment is much higher than that for elders as a whole, 5%–12% per year, compared with perhaps 1%–2% in the population of older adults as a whole. Consequently, mild cognitive impairment cannot be considered benign or a normal feature of healthy aging.

Prevalence and Incidence of Alzheimer's Disease. In a nationally representative sample of seniors aged 60 and older, the best estimate of AD prevalence is 3.3 million in 2002. Among elder aged 71 and older, 13.9% of Americans meet criteria for dementia. By 2015, we can expect 4.6 million cases of AD using a narrow definition and 5.3 million if we include mixed cases. About a third of these cases will have moderate or more severe forms of AD.

The incidence of AD is closely related to age. For people aged 65–74, annual incidence ranges from <0.5% to 1.3%. For people aged 75–84, the range is 1.5%–4.0%, and for people aged 85 and older the incidence is 4.7%–7.9% per year. Minority status is among the most important risk factors for AD. Given the increasing number of older adults in the minorities in the United States, this disparity has great public health significance.

Risk Factors for Alzheimer's Disease. Only approximately 7% of early-onset AD (< age 65) and less than 1% of late-onset AD have been linked to mutations on particular genes. For late-onset AD, attention centers on the *APOE* gene. A number of studies have shown overrepresentation of the *APOE*-e4 allele in people with AD. Despite this finding, the current recommendation is against use of *APOE* as a screening tool: "although *APOE* genotype may be a risk factor for AD, it cannot yet be considered a useful predictive genetic test."

The significance of cognitive resources early in the life span for dementia in late life has become increasingly clear in studies that have linked risk of AD to childhood IQ, educational accomplishment and leisure activities, occupational attainment and job demands, language skills in early adulthood, diversity of physical and cognitive engagement over the life span, parental socioeconomic status, and literacy. These findings suggest that cognitive ability is similar to grip strength: differences (in muscle fiber density, in neuronal integrity or number) already apparent at birth or in the perinatal period (and which develop or set limits on development over the life span) provide variable reserve against depletions that occur with aging. These resources put one closer or further away from the threshold of disability associated with the loss of physical and cognitive function that occurs over the life span.

A variety of medical conditions have been shown to increase the risk of AD, including hypertension and vascular disease, diabetes, loss in bone mineral density, estrogen deficiency, depression.

Outcomes Associated With Alzheimer's Disease. Compared to older adults without dementia matched for age and comorbid disease, drawn from the same community, and similar in socioeconomic features, elders with AD face a mortality risk 2–3 times higher than elders with normal cognition. AD is a key risk factor for nursing home admission. AD is also associated with greater risk of acute medical care in the hospital, as well as general medical care in the community.

Families provide the vast majority of Alzheimer's care. Although patients with Alzheimer's disease are common in nursing homes, accounting for perhaps half of the residents, these residents represent a minority of the Alzheimer's population. Most people with AD are cared for at home, use a variety of in-home (home attendant, allied health) and out-of-home services (adult day care, acute rehab), and will enter nursing homes very late in the disease, if at all.

The effects of providing care to a person with AD have been studied intensively. Marital discord and divorce, depression and anxiety, loss of employment, restriction of social life, invasion of privacy, impoverishment, substance abuse, and mortality have all been linked to caregiving stress. Buffering factors that mitigate these negative effects include support from family, religiosity, strong personal mastery and self-efficacy, satisfaction with caregiving, and strategies to reduce the burden of providing care.

Family caregivers and clinicians face difficult decisions related to end-of-life care of relatives in the last stages of AD. Should patients with pneumonia be treated aggressively with intravenous antibiotics, transferred to hospital, and intubated; or should they be treated symptomatically with analgesics, antipyretics, and oxygen? Should a patient with dementia who refuses food or has difficulty swallowing be tube fed? Little is known about the ways families make these decisions, but evidence suggests that use of life-sustaining technologies is common in this terminal population.

Investigation of quality of life in people with AD requires a judicious mix of patient, proxy, and observational measures. A useful QOL measure should be correlated with the stage of dementia (because dementia severity affects mood and opportunities for engagement), and it should show variance within stage (suggesting that there are other sources of pleasure or engagement relevant to dementia care). In this way, QOL investigation may be useful as a guide to clinical care and environmental modifications that will benefit patients and their families.

Interventions to Prevent Cognitive Decline. The ACTIVE trial showed that older adults can be successfully trained in specific cognitive skills. Whether such training reduces the risk of decline is at this point unclear, although some evidence suggests benefit.

Interventions to Support Family Caregivers. Randomized trials of targeted support show that both outcomes for elders (nursing home placement) and caregiver psychosocial status (burden, fatigue, depression) can be improved to mitigate the severe challenges of Alzheimer's care.

7 Affective and Social Function: Suffering, Neglect, Isolation

Symptoms of poor mental health may be different in older people than in younger people (Blazer, 2002). As we will see, older people are less likely to meet standard criteria for syndromal depression or anxiety disorders. Affective disorders are more likely to take the form of "subthreshold syndromes," symptom intensities and frequencies short of standard criteria for diagnoses of clinical disorders. Does this mean that older people are less depressed? Or should we draw the conclusion that depression needs to be redefined in this case because it is a different kind of clinical entity? The disability and excess morbidity associated with subthreshold disorders suggest the latter, as we will see below. These questions also suggest that we consider mental health in older adults within the broader context of emotional and social experience in old age.

Despite these difficulties in diagnosis and definition, late-life mood disorders, and in particular, depression, are highly prevalent and debilitating. Among the almost 35 million Americans age 65 and older in 2008, approximately 2 million experience depression (Reynolds, 2008). Seniors with depression, who often contend with other diseases and disability as well, are less likely to take medications reliably, seek appropriate medical care, or practice optimal disease self-management. Thus, psychiatric conditions which may result in increased risk of suicide, poorer function, and social isolation, carry with them more general threats to well-being. In addition, many seniors with subthreshold disorders also experience disability and are at high risk for developing syndromal clinical depression. Seniors with very mildly elevated depressive symptoms are more likely to have mild cognitive impairment as well (Bhalla et al., 2009). In addition, recognition and treatment of depression may be challenging in primary care settings because of lack of geriatric expertise, time pressure, and pressing concerns to handle more obvious physical illness.

Increasing recognition of these challenges has led to a new concern for bringing depression screening and treatment to community settings. These efforts include developing ways to link social service agencies and mental health care, training aging services staff to recognize and refer cases of depression, and training agency staff to deliver mental health interventions.

BURDEN OF MENTAL ILLNESS

The first Surgeon General's Report on Mental Health (1999) begins by recognizing the immense burden of disability associated with mental illness throughout the world. In more developed countries ("established market economies"), for example, mental health disorders account for approximately 15% of all disease burden, more, in fact, than the burden associated with cancer (Murray & Lopez, 1996). The rank of these diseases in terms of the burden they produce is shown in Table 7.1. Mental illness is exceeded only by cardiovascular disease in years lost to disability and early mortality. Cancer follows, showing that diseases of mental health, because they begin early in life and persist over the life span, produce a greater volume of morbidity and disability. Clearly, treatment and prevention of mental disorders would go a long way toward the reduction of disease burden.

The burden of particular diseases involving mental health relative to total disease burden is shown in Table 7.2. The table shows that the equivalent of 98.7 million person-years was lost to disability or early mortality in the more developed countries in 1990. Unipolar depression, the most prevalent mental illness, accounted for 6.8% of this total burden. Burden associated with depressive disorders exceeded burden associated with cardiovascular disease (more narrowly defined than above), alcohol use, and road traffic accidents.

Chapter 7 Affective and Social Function: Suffering, Neglect, Isolation **243**

Table 7.1

DISEASE BURDEN BY SELECTED ILLNESS CATEGORIES IN ESTABLISHED MARKET ECONOMIES, 1990

	TOTAL DALYs,[a] %
All cardiovascular conditions	18.6
All mental illness[b]	15.4
All malignant diseases (cancer)	15.0
All respiratory conditions	4.8
All alcohol use	4.7<
All infectious and parasitic diseases	2.8
All drug use	1.5

[a]Disability-adjusted life year (DALY) is a measure that expresses years of life lost to premature death and years lived with a disability of specified severity and duration (Murray & Lopez, 1996).
[b]Disease burden associated with "mental illness" includes suicide.
From "Evidence-Based Health Policy—Lessons From the Global Burden of Disease Study," by C. J. Murray & A. D. Lopez, 1996, *Science, 274(5288)*, 740–743.

Table 7.2

LEADING SOURCES OF DISEASE BURDEN IN ESTABLISHED MARKET ECONOMIES, 1990

		TOTAL DALYs (MILLIONS)	TOTAL, %
	All causes	98.7	
1	Ischemic heart disease	8.9	9.0
2	Unipolar major depression	6.7	6.8
3	Cardiovascular disease	5.0	5.0
4	Alcohol use	4.7	4.7
5	Road traffic accidents	4.3	4.4

From "Evidence-Based Health Policy—Lessons From the Global Burden of Disease Study," by C. J. Murray & A. D. Lopez, 1996, *Science, 274(5288)*, 740–743.

The measure of burden in these comparisons is the DALY, or disability-adjusted life year. This is a summation of years of healthy life lost to disability and early mortality. Whereas the DALY is similar in principle to other measures of health expectancy, discussed in Chapter 10, its calculation differs in an important way. It assigns weights to age, where these weights "reflect the relative importance of healthy life at different ages" (World Bank, 1995). These weights increase up to age 25 and then decline. They have also been designed to reflect the dependence of the young and older people on working age adults. One effect that this age-weighting factor in DALY calculations has is to decrease in the contribution of old age disability to the total years lost to disability. Be that as it may, the DALY approach to burden is useful for highlighting the greater morbidity and disability associated with mental illness.

An alternative indicator of the severe burden of mental illness, especially depression, is visible in self-reports of disability from people with different chronic health conditions. The Medical Outcomes Study examined adult outpatients with a series of sentinel conditions (hypertension, myocardial infarction, arthritis, gastrointestinal disorders, and depression), who did not have other comorbidities (Wells et al., 1989). The impact of each condition on six health-related quality-of-life domains (physical function, role function, social function, mental health, self-perceived global health, and bodily pain) was assessed relative to a nationally representative sample of adults ascertained outside the clinic setting. The differences in scores on each of the six domains, relative to the nonclinic sample, show important differences in disease impact. These findings are shown in Figure 7.1.

The dotted line represents scores from the nonclinic sample, assigned a zero value for purposes of standardization. The figure shows that hypertension has little effect on reported function and well-being. People with the condition reported only poorer perceived health and a greater number of mental health symptoms, both in keeping with the disease label and need to take medication (which may itself have a quality-of-life impact). Arthritis and gastrointestinal (GI) disorders were roughly comparable in their effects on physical function, but GI orders were more burdensome on role, social function, and mental health domains, whereas arthritis was more burdensome in the bodily pain domain. Myocardial infarction had primarily physical effects, with very low scores in the physical and role performance domains.

Wells et al. (1989) point out the perhaps surprising result that outpatients meeting criteria for depression performed worse, not just on

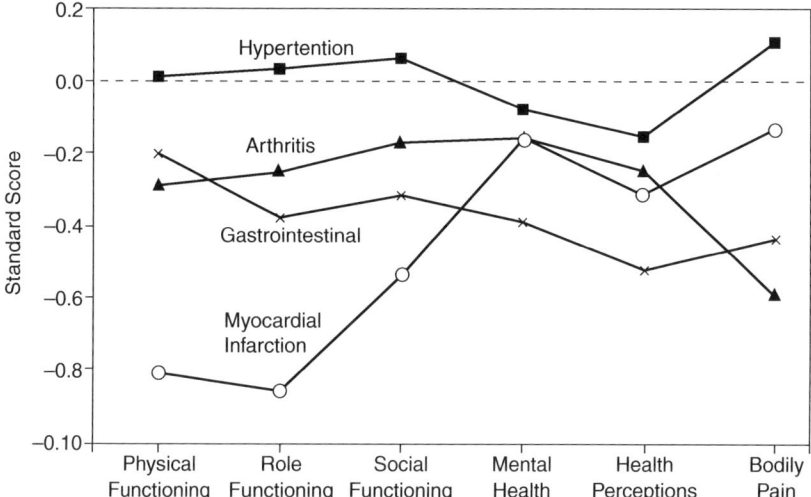

Figure 7.1 Health profiles for patients with four common conditions from Medical Outcomes Study.

Source: From "Functional Status and Well-Being of Patients With Chronic Conditions. Results From the Medical Outcomes Study," by A. L. Stewart, S. Greenfield, R. D. Hays, K. Wells, W. H. Rogers, S. D. Berry, et al., 1989. *Journal of the American Medical Association, 262*(7), 907–913. Reprinted with permission, *Journal of the American Medical Association.*

the mental health measures, as expected, but also on reports of physical function and role performance, in which they looked very much like the patients with myocardial infarctions. Wells concluded, "the functioning of depressed patients is comparable with or worse than that of patients with major chronic medical conditions."

Thus, the effect of mental disorders on daily life should not be underestimated. Below, we examine morbidity associated with depression and the role of depressive disorders in increasing the risk of future mortality and disability.

PRESENTATION OF MENTAL HEALTH SYMPTOMS IN LATE LIFE

Mental health symptoms seem to change with older age. For example, in later life depressive disorders fulfilling diagnostic criteria are relatively rare; "subthreshold disorders" are more common. Subthreshold depression, for example, includes symptoms of depression that are not severe, frequent, or disruptive enough to be labeled as clinical depression. In practice, people are said to have subthreshold depression when they report symptoms on a depression self-report measure that fall below standard thresholds for defining likely depression. In the case of the Center for Epidemiologic Studies-Depression Scale (CES-D), this would be a score above some minimum but below 16. In the case of the Geriatric Depression Scale (GDS) short form, this would be a score above 0 but below 10. In the case of the Patient Health Questionnaire (PHQ) (Spitzer, Kroenke, & Williams, 1999), it would be the endorsement of lack of interest and feeling down more than half the days of the week over the past 2 weeks, but endorsement of fewer than three other depression symptoms.

Rather than feeling depressed and reporting feelings of sadness or worthlessness, older people with depression may be more likely to report alternative clusters of symptoms, such as loss of interest in usual activities and somatic or cognitive symptoms, including fatigue, pain, sleep difficulties, and memory disorders. One study suggested that people at the oldest ages are more likely to report "delimited forms of distress," such as enervation, dysphoria, and sleep disturbances, rather than the anhedonia typical of younger cohorts (Newman, Engel, & Jensen, 1991). A similar process appears to be at work for anxiety, with greater likelihood of subthreshold anxiety disorders in later life.

Mossey and Moss (2002) reported a study of 600 community-dwelling elders aged 70 and older with a specific focus on subthreshold depression. They defined subthreshold depression by use of the CES-D (as well as additional questions assessing depressive symptoms) and found that 5.2% met criteria for depression and 22.2% for subthreshold depression. It was not surprising to find that people who met criteria for depression scored more poorly on measures of physical, functional, and social health, and were also likely to have more physician visits (22, compared with 13 in the group without depression) and spend a greater number of days in the hospital (12 versus 5.2 in the group without depression) during the previous year. An important result of this study was a set of similar findings for the subthreshold depression group. Older adults with subthreshold depression scored more poorly in measures of health and were also likely to have a greater number of physician visits and hospital days than the group without depression. Mossey and Moss (2002) conclude that "with a prevalence of 22%, the public health

Chapter 7 Affective and Social Function: Suffering, Neglect, Isolation 247

burden of an even modest impact of sub-threshold depression on life quality and functioning of older individuals is substantial."

It is also worth asking about the persistence and effect of mental health symptoms in older people after a diagnosis of depression. The natural history of depression in older adults was examined in the Longitudinal Aging Study, a cohort of older adults recruited in Amsterdam (Beekman et al., 2002). Within this large cohort, 277 were identified as depressed at baseline and were monitored for up to 6 years, with as many as 14 assessments in this period. Elders were assessed with the Diagnostic Interview Schedule (DIS), a clinical interview that allows diagnosis of depression and its subtypes. Use of the clinical diagnostic interview with such extensive follow-up is rare and allows insight on symptom duration, type of clinical course, and stability of diagnoses. In this group of older people who met criteria for depression at baseline, fewer than a fourth saw remission of their symptoms. On the whole, symptom levels remained high: 44% had an unfavorable but fluctuating course and 32% experienced a continuing severe chronic course. Older people with subthreshold disorders were at risk for progression to more severe forms of depression. In this community cohort, the natural history of late-life depression turned out to be poor, with persistence and increasing morbidity as the most common outcome.

This brief review of research on the presentation of mental health symptoms in older adults suggests that symptom profiles in depression may be different, with less affective symptoms (i.e., feelings of worthlessness or sense that life is not worth living, crying, thoughts of suicide) and more somatic and cognitive symptoms. The result is a profile of symptoms short of the standard clinical syndrome. But subthreshold mental illness can also be consequential, with significant suffering, great health impact, and lost opportunities for productive aging. Clinical and service delivery staff who work with older adults will need to recognize these differences if they are to provide effective care and referral.

Given the reduction in the most severe forms of depression and anxiety with age, one wants to know why symptoms of this sort decline and come to be replaced by milder forms. Jorm, Christensen, Korten, Jacomb, and Henderson (2000) suggest that "ageing is associated with an intrinsic reduction in susceptibility to anxiety and depression." They ask for caution in this conclusion, because we have few longitudinal studies covering the adult life span and therefore cannot yet reliably distinguish aging from cohort effects. If this difference in symptom expression turns out to be reliably associated with age, they suggest that the reason may be decreased emotional responsiveness with age, increased emotional control, and a kind of "psychological immunization" to stressful experiences. Supporting the first of these hypotheses, Lawton, Parmelee, Katz, and Nesselroade (1996) reported lower self-reported frequency of many affects in cross-sectional comparisons of young, middle-aged, and older adults. Carstensen (1992) has also demonstrated less interest in novel stimuli and greater social selectivity with age as a way of conserving psychological resources and promoting well being. These changes are aspects of "gerotranscendence" (Torstan, 2005). These findings provide some support for reduced emotional expression and greater emotional control in later life and the "selective optimization with compensation" noted in Chapter 1.

These last points deserve special emphasis because they show again the pervasive link between life span processes and health. Emotional life changes across the life span. As a consequence, the experience of depression may also change. Depression is not trivial in late life, but it may take on a less florid form because of changes in emotional makeup. If one talks to older people and asks about the emotions, one is likely to hear statements about the decline of emotion: "the highs are not so high anymore, but the lows are not so low either." In our research, we find that older people speak wistfully of their more intense emotional life at younger ages but also report a good deal of relief at getting off that treadmill.

PREVALENCE OF MENTAL ILLNESS AT OLDER AGES

As mentioned above, syndromal depression, that is, severity and duration of symptoms that meet criteria for clinical diagnosis, is less common among older people than younger people. This is apparent in population surveys that query respondents on symptoms of depression, such as the National Health Interview Survey, 2000 (NHIS). "Severe psychological distress" in the NHIS was measured according to the frequency of six distress symptoms over the past 30 days. The six items formed a scale with a range of 0–24 (so that each item was scored 0–4), and a score of 13 or greater was used to define severe distress.

As Figure 7.2 shows, less than 2% of people aged 65 and older reported "serious psychological distress." In people aged 45–64, approximately 4% reported this level of distress, nearly twice as many. In the youngest age group, aged 18–44, the proportion was also higher, ap-

Chapter 7 Affective and Social Function: Suffering, Neglect, Isolation

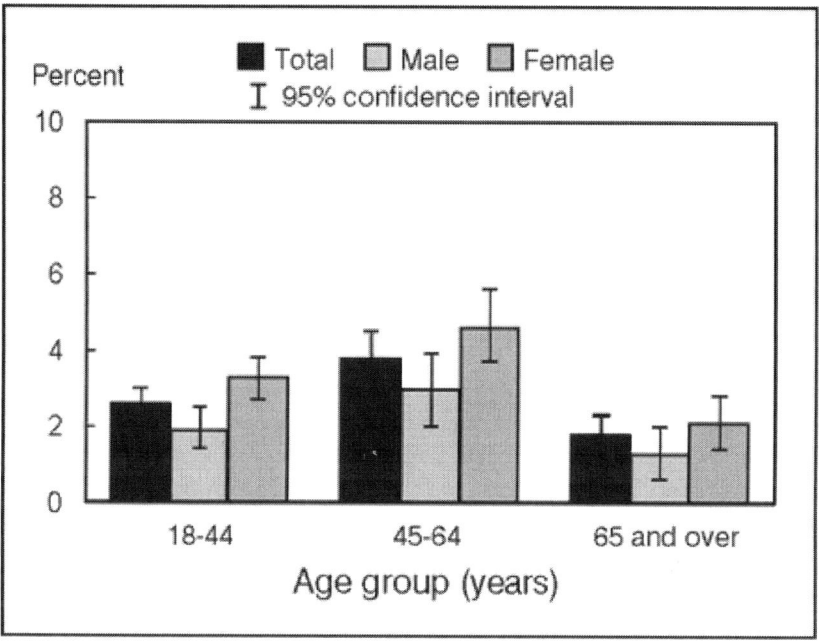

Figure 7.2 Percentage of adults aged 18 years and older who experienced serious psychological distress during the past 30 days, by age group and sex: United States, January–June 2002.

Notes: Six psychological distress questions are included in the Sample Adult Core component. These questions ask how often a respondent experienced symptoms of psychological distress during the past 30 days. The response codes (0–4) of the six items for each person are summed to yield a scale with a 0–24 range. A value of 13 or more for this scale is used here to define serious psychological distress.
Source: Based on data collected from January through June in the Sample Adult Core component of the 2002 National Health Interview Survey.

proximately 2.5%. Notably, in all age groups, women were more likely to report severe psychological distress than men.

A common measure of depression in late life, as mentioned earlier, is the Geriatric Depression Scale (Yesavage et al., 1983). The items cover dysphoria, sadness or lack of enjoyment (e.g., "Do you feel happy most of the time?" "Are you in good spirits most of the time?"); anhedonia, or lack of interest in activities that are usually sought out (e.g., "Have you dropped many of your activities and interests?" "Do you often get bored?"); somatic symptoms associated with depression (e.g., perceived memory problems, reduced level of energy); and demoralization or existential suffering (e.g., "Do you feel that your situation is hopeless?" "Do you feel that your life is empty?" "Do you often feel helpless?" "Do you feel pretty worthless the way you are now?") "Yes" responses to the 15 items are summed. In the short-form of the GDS, scores greater than 5 suggest possible depression and warrant follow-up. Scores greater than 10 are very sensitive for detecting syndromal depression.

Depression is usually assessed using self-report instruments of this sort, rather than clinical diagnostic interviews that allow for true diagnoses. This should be kept in mind when interpreting the diverse prevalence estimates of depression in older adults.

What then is the prevalence of depression in older people? A key consideration is what sort of older person: frail or hale, community resident or institutionalized, ascertained in a medical setting or not? Obviously, the prevalence of depression will be higher in people in medical settings or with extensive disability and chronic conditions than in a community sample of older people.

In one community study of people aged 65 and older, the Alameda County Study, 6.6% of men and 10.1% of women showed "symptoms of major depressive disorders." Once chronic conditions were controlled, the prevalence of depression of this severity did not increase with age. This is an important finding, consistent with what we have noted earlier. Depressive symptoms are much more closely associated with health status than with age. If the prevalence of depression appears to increase with age, it is entirely due to the increasing prevalence of chronic disease conditions with greater age (Roberts, Kaplan, Shema, & Strawbridge, 1997).

Compare this 5%–10% community prevalence with the much higher prevalence found in older outpatients. One study reported that 24% of an ambulatory care sample had "clinically significant depressive symptoms." However, even here, only 10% met criteria for major depressive disorder. Notably, only 1% of these people received treatment for a mental health problem (Borson et al., 1986).

The prevalence of depression in hospitalized and institutionalized older populations is even higher: 12%–45% in the hospital, and 15%–30% in skilled care facilities (Surgeon General, 1999). Likewise, the prevalence of depression in community-resident patients with the chronic diseases of late life is also quite high, 15%–20% in early Alzheimer's and perhaps 50% in Parkinson's disease.

MENTAL HEALTH IN A DISABLED OLDER POPULATION

The Women's Health and Aging Study, WHAS-I (Guralnik, Fried, Simonsick, Kasper, & Lafferty, 1995b) enrolled women with moderate to severe disability, representing the most disabled third of older women living in the community. Women were recruited from Medicare enrollee lists in the Baltimore, Maryland, area. Mental health in the sample was assessed with a variety of indicators, including the Geriatric Depression Scale (Yesavage et al., 1983), anxiety indicators from the Hopkins Symptom Checklist (Derogatis, Lipman, Riskels, Uhlenhuth, & Covi, 1974), the Perceived Quality of Life Scale (Patrick, Danis, Southerland, & Hong, 1988), and sense of control and efficacy from the Personal Mastery Scale (Pearlin & Schooler, 1978). The sample of over 1,000 women was divided into three age groups (65–74, 75–84, 85 and older) and three disability groups: women with "moderate disability" (limitations in upper extremity, lower extremity, or IADLs but no difficulty with ADLs), those with ADL difficulty without personal assistance, and those with ADL difficulty who received personal assistance.

Table 7.3 presents the mental health of women in WHAS-I. High levels of depressive symptoms, that is, symptomatology consistent with the clinical syndrome of major depression, were evident overall in 17.4% of the sample. Older people were less likely to report a high number of depressive symptoms: 14.3% of women aged 85 and older versus 18.6% of women aged 65–74. Disability, rather than age, was the stronger correlate. The proportion with symptomatology consistent with a diagnosis of depression was 13.1% in women with moderate limitations, 16.4% in women with ADL difficulty not receiving help, and 29.3% in women with ADL difficulty who received personal assistance.

Anxiety symptoms, unlike depression, increased with age: 2.8% in women aged 65–74, 4% in women aged 75–84, and 5.1% in women aged 85 and older. The relationship between disability and anxiety symptoms was less pronounced, increasing from 2.1% to 4.4% and 4.7% across disability severity categories.

Satisfaction with help received from family and friends was reported in approximately 80% of women, regardless of age or disability status (but note the gradient in satisfaction by severity of disability: 83.6%, 79.3%, and 74.8%). More pronounced are differences in the help these women feel they are able to provide to others. "Satisfaction with help

Table 7.3

MENTAL HEALTH INDICATORS: WOMEN'S HEALTH AND AGING STUDY, I

	AGE GROUP				DISABILITY STATUS		
	65–74	75–84	85+	MODERATE	ADL DIFFICULTY: NO HELP	ADL DIFFICULTY: HELP
High level of depressive symptomatology, %[a]	18.6	17.3	14.3	13.1	16.4	29.3
High level of anxiety, %[b]	2.8	4.0	5.1	2.1	4.4	4.7
Satisfied with help received from family & friends, %[c]	79.1	81.1	78.2	83.6	79.3	74.8
Satisfied with help you give to family & friends, %[c]	77.6	70.1	68.0	84.0	71.1	56.2
Satisfied with amount of variety in your life, %[c]	65.9	62.1	62.3	70.0	63.6	51.4
Satisfied with the meaning and purpose of your life, %[c]	76.4	75.8	75.7	79.7	74.8	72.1
I can do just about anything I really set my mind to do, % Strongly agree[d]	48.6	45.1	44.4	51.4	45.2	40.2
I feel helpless in dealing with the problems of life, % Strongly agree[d]	8.8	10.3	12.3	9.3	6.8	20.0

"Moderate disability": self-reported difficulty in two of three domains: upper extremity, lower extremity, or IADL. Summarized from tables 8-1 through 8-5, "Lower-Extremity Function in Persons Over the Age of 70 Years as a Predictor of Subsequent Disability," by J. M. Guralnik, L. Ferrucci, E. M. Simonsick, M. E. Salive, & R. B. Wallace, 1995a, *New England Journal of Medicine, 332*, 556–561.
[a] High level of depressive symptomatology: Score ≥ 14, Geriatric Depression Scale, long form (Yesavage et al., 1983).
[b] High level of anxiety: maximum score ("extremely") on "felt nervous or shaky inside" during past week, Hopkins Symptom Checklist (Derogatis et al., 1974).
[c] Items from Perceived Quality-of-Life scale (Patrick et al., 1988).
[d] Items from Personal Mastery scale (Pearlin & Schooler, 1978).

Chapter 7 Affective and Social Function: Suffering, Neglect, Isolation   **253**

provided to others" decreased from 84% in those with moderate limitations to 56.2% among women receiving assistance with ADL tasks.

"Satisfaction with variety in life" was also more strongly related to disability than age, approximately a 20% difference between women with moderate (70%) and severe disability (51.4%). But note also that half the women who received assistance with ADL tasks, and hence low scores on quality-of-life measures that emphasize function, still report satisfaction with variety in daily life. Note, too, that "satisfaction with the meaning and purpose of your life" was stable across age and disability categories; about three-quarters of these women, whatever their age or level of disability, reported satisfaction in this area.

Finally, this sample of women on the whole reported relatively low self-efficacy. Less than half reported confidence they could accomplish "anything I really set my mind to do." On the other hand, a minority of respondents reported "helplessness," less than 10% in the less severe disability groups and 20% in women receiving assistance with ADL tasks.

This inquiry suggests that disability has only a mild impact on mental health and general well being. This is an important result. Most of the women in this sample were able to maintain mental equipoise despite activity limitations. We should not underestimate the fundamental stability of mental health over the life span or the ability of older people to adapt to declines in the capacity to perform everyday activities.

OUTCOMES ASSOCIATED WITH MENTAL ILLNESS IN LATE LIFE

Depression in late life has been associated with an increased risk of mortality. The central question in this association is whether depression is a feature of disease and, for this reason, is artifactually associated with mortality, or whether depression is itself an independent risk factor for early death.

An accumulating set of evidence supports the latter hypothesis. For example, in the Cardiovascular Health Study (CHS), Schulz and colleagues showed that baseline depressive symptoms were associated with 6-year all-cause mortality in older persons (Schulz et al., 2000). The CHS consists of 5,201 people aged 65 and older from four communities across the United States. This study found a higher mortality rate (23.9%) in people with a greater number of depressive symptoms at baseline than in people with fewer depressive symptoms (17.7%). Depression in this study retained a significant association with mortality over 6 years of follow-up when controlling for sociodemographic factors, prevalent clinical disease, subclinical disease indicators at baseline, and biological or behavioral risk factors. In multivariate models that controlled for all of the factors, people with high depressive symptoms at baseline had a relative risk of 1.24 (95% CI, 1.06–1.46), about a 25% greater risk of mortality, compared with people with few or no depressive symptoms. Schulz (2000) suggests that "motivational depletion," lack of attention to self-care and treatment adherence and a more general loss of the will to live, may be responsible for this greater risk of death. Other research has confirmed this association, controlling as well for cognitive deficit (Rozzini, Sabatini, Frisoni, & Trabucchi, 2002).

Unutzer and colleagues (2002) reported a similar finding. They found that older adults with the most severe depressive symptoms had a significant increase in mortality risk, again after adjusting for demographics, health risk behaviors, and chronic medical disorders. The increased risk in mortality that was due to depression was comparable with mortality associated with such chronic medical disorders as emphysema and heart disease (Unutzer, Patrick, Marmon, Simon, & Katon, 2002b).

Mortality from suicide, in particular, is also a consequence of depression in late life. Suicide risk is highest in younger people and in people aged 85 and older. In fact, recent reports suggest that the highest suicide risk appears to be in White males aged 85 and older. The suicide rate for this group is 21 per 100,000, nearly twice the national rate of 10.6 per 100,000 (CDC, 2003).

One of the strongest tests of the clinical relevance of depression in older people is its role in predicting the onset of disability. In a review of 78 high-quality reports involving longitudinal studies (Stuck et al., 1999), depression was a consistently strong predictor of functional decline in older people. Depression predicted onset of activity limitations in studies that controlled for the presence of chronic conditions, behavioral risk factors, and cognitive status (Bruce, Seeman, Merrill, & Blazer, 1994). In one study, even the presence of depressive symptoms short of the severity or duration required for a diagnosis of depression ("subthreshold depression," described earlier) was a significant predictor of decline (Gallo, Rabins, Lyketos, Tien, & Anthony, 1997). Finally, there is also evidence that depressive symptoms are related to loss of underlying capacity in the pathway toward activity limitations (Penninx et al., 1998) (see Chapter 5).

These findings suggest that depression is a true cause of disability in older people, meeting many of the criteria for causality in epidemiology (Susser, 1997). Depressive symptoms can occur temporally prior to development of disability, appear to influence a link in the disablement pathway, and are consistently associated with disability across different age groups. Because treatment of depression is possible, this source of morbidity and disability should certainly be addressed in the care of the older person.

TREATMENT OF DEPRESSION IN LATE LIFE

We have already seen that depression is underappreciated and undertreated in older people, as it is younger people. The reasons for this neglect in late life are apparent from what we have already noted. The first reason has to do with the medical and psychosocial context of aging. Because most older people have a variety of medical conditions, it is tempting for physicians, families, and even elders themselves to assign symptoms of depression to these conditions. Similarly, it may be difficult, in some cases, to distinguish normal grief after the loss of a spouse, for example, from depression.

A second reason for underrecognition is the "softer" presentation of depressive symptoms, described above, and the greater prevalence of subthreshold disorders than of disease of accepted levels of clinical severity. The lack of affective symptoms in some cases, such as sadness, makes depression hard to diagnose for practitioners who do not have experience with geriatric mental health. The depressed elder may stress physical symptoms, reducing the likelihood of a mental health referral.

Finally, there is garden-variety ageism. Unfortunately, many providers and many older people themselves still think that misery is normal in late life. After all, the reasoning goes, late life is the time of decline in physical and mental health, so of course depression should be expected. This reasoning is absolutely fallacious, however, as we know from the studies of patients at the end of life. Depression is more common in terminal patients but far from universal. Even in these patients risk of depression appears to reflect life-long mental health more than illness and the dying process (Rabkin, Wagner, & Del Bene, 2000). Studies of people with severe neuromuscular disease approaching the end of life show only mild elevations in depressive diagnoses relative to primary care samples, and fewer than 20% express a wish to hasten dying (Albert et al., 2005; Rabkin et al., 2005). Most importantly, depression responds to treatment even in patients who are dying. Affective suffering should be considered a medical issue as significant as any other health indicator.

Treatment for depression in older people may rely on pharmacological agents, psychosocial interventions, or a combination of the two. Response rates in older people appear to be comparable with those in younger people, as both age groups respond in approximately 80% of cases (Surgeon General, 1999). However, older people may take longer to respond to therapy and may face a greater risk of relapse.

REDUCING THE RISK OF DEPRESSION AND ASSOCIATED MORBIDITY IN SENIORS

A pivotal randomized trial to improve outcomes among seniors with depression has provided important information on ways to reduce affective suffering in the primary care setting. PROSPECT (Prevention of Suicide in Primary Care Elderly-Collaborative Trial) examined whether a trained clinician can work in close collaboration with a primary care physician to implement comprehensive depression management and improve outcomes in older patients with depression (Mulsant et al., 2001). In PROSPECT, primary care practices in three regions were randomly assigned to either an intervention arm involving depression health specialists or an active control arm consisting of depression screening and assessment services without the health specialist. The choice of this control arm is important, because such screening and assessment is considered state-of-the-art but has been associated with high rates of suicide in older people related to untreated or undertreated depression.

One key outcome in the trial was "suicidal ideation," thoughts of suicide. Rates of suicidal ideation declined faster in intervention patients compared with usual-care patients. Resolution of suicidal ideation was faster among intervention patients. Intervention patients also had a more favorable course of depression relative to severity of symptoms and time to remission (Bruce et al., 2004). Further results revealed that the intervention offered more diffuse mental health benefits as well (Alexopoulos et al., 2005). Results from PROSPECT suggest that the integration of more active depression care in primary geriatric care is an important opportunity for addressing risk of depression and reducing morbidity from mental health disorders.

Chapter 7 Affective and Social Function: Suffering, Neglect, Isolation 257

Another productive area for intercepting depression among seniors is to harness community-based agencies that provide aging services. These agencies have regular contact with vulnerable elders and are sometimes the only source of such contact. For example, virtually all aging services providers (see Chapter 3) provide social visiting or other "check-in" services, in which agency staff or volunteers call seniors who receive services to stay in contact and unobtrusively determine new needs. These kinds of contact may uncover mental health needs and could be harnessed explicitly for assessment of depressive symptoms and, when needed, referral. But the challenges of developing such programs are not trivial. How should staff or volunteers, who often lack mental health training, be trained? What kind of supporting staff needs to be attached to agencies in case of need for mental health services? What kind of referral pipeline would best link aging services providers to mental health services?

A number of such programs have recently been developed and assessed in randomized trials. Three have achieved status as evidence-based approaches, according to the National Council on Aging Services. It is instructive to look at each program to distinguish alternative approaches to assessment and service delivery.

- PEARLS, the *Program to Encourage Active, Rewarding Lives for Seniors* (Ciechanowski et al., 2004) is designed for seniors with subthreshold depression. It involves problem-solving treatment, social and physical activation, and potential recommendations to patients' physicians regarding antidepressant medications. Patients receiving the PEARLS intervention were more likely to have reduction in depressive symptoms and to achieve complete remission from depression than patients in a control education condition. They were also more likely to report improvements in health-related quality of life. The program is delivered by trained counselors in a participant's home, and the cost to implement PEARLS is approximately $630 per patient.
- Healthy IDEAS (*Identifying Depression, Empowering Activities for Seniors*) (Quijano et al., 2007) delivers depression care through agency case managers who receive mental health training through the program. Depression care involves behavioral activation, promoting involvement in meaningful, positive activities. The start-up cost for an agency is approximately $2,500.
- IMPACT (*Improving Mood-Promoting Access to Collaborative Treatment for Late Life Depression*) (Lin et al., 2003) uses a team

approach designed to integrate treatment of depression within primary care. In the IMPACT model, a nurse, social worker, or psychologist works with the patient's regular primary care provider to develop a course of treatment. The cost of implementing IMPACT is approximately $500 per patient per year.

The three programs differ in their integration with medical providers, level of mental health training for agency staff, site of care, and combination of counseling and use of psychiatric medication. We are unaware of attempts to roll out these programs outside the confines of demonstrations or clinical trials. Thus, an important area for research would include investigation of the following issues:

- Whether treatment on site versus referral off site has greater benefit;
- How to tailor programs like IMPACT, designed for primary care, for social service agencies;
- How the organizational structures of agencies may lend themselves to different kinds of interventions;
- How sensitive and specific depression screening is in this setting;
- What sorts of follow-up are required to pre-empt depression among people who screen positive;
- How to ensure that mental health services offered by agencies are reimbursable; and
- How to build linkages between social service agencies and medical providers, such as federally qualified health clinics.

We anticipate increasing research and demonstration activity in this area, or perhaps a major community-based prevention trial that will harness aging services providers for this effort. This approach follows recommendations of the Institute of Medicine report, *Retooling for an Aging America* (2008), that emphasize the importance of new, flexible models to meet the public health burden of depression and other chronic illnesses in older Americans.

NEGLECT AND ABUSE

Victimization of older people takes many forms and extends across a continuum of behavior (Nerenberg, 2007). On one extreme of this con-

Chapter 7 Affective and Social Function: Suffering, Neglect, Isolation

tinuum we might place neglect of the older adults, whether self-neglect or inattention to an elder's needs by others. On the other extreme, we might place active physical abuse and exploitation. Somewhere in the middle lies purposeful neglect designed to injure or coerce. These are often lumped within a single category of "mistreatment," which is defined differently across surveys. Adult Protective Services, municipal agencies defined to assess and intervene in the case of victimization of older people, define three forms of mistreatment (Lachs, Williams, O'Brien, & Pillemer, 2002):

> *Abuse:* Willful infliction of pain or mental anguish, or purposeful withholding of resources necessary to meet basic needs;
> *Neglect:* Failure of an elder to satisfy basic needs (food, shelter, medication management, medical care) either because of incompetence in the elder or because another person charged with care for the elder fails to meet these needs (abandonment, poor supportive care);
> *Exploitation:* Taking advantage of an elder to steal or dispossess the elder of money, wealth, or valued goods.

Over an 11-year period, the cumulative incidence of abuse in the New Haven component of the Established Populations for Epidemiologic Studies of the Elderly (EPESE) was 7.2% (202 of 2,802). These 202 people came to the attention of the Connecticut Ombudsman and Elderly Protective Services. Of the 202, 44 were verified as cases of abuse and 120 as cases of self-neglect; 38 were nonverified allegations. Thus, the incidence of abuse was 1.6% (44 of 2,802) and self-neglect was 4.3% (120 of 2,802) over this 11-year period. If we take the total incidence of 7.2% and convert it to a yearly estimate, the annual incidence is about 6.5 cases per 1,000 per year (.072/11 per 1,000). We can compare this estimate with the 32 per 1,000 reported in a random sample prevalence survey (Pillemer & Finkelhor, 1998). This suggests that about one in five cases of abuse, neglect, or exploitation comes to the attention of protective services.

A variety of research is now available on the correlates of elder mistreatment. Using the merged EPESE-protective services dataset described earlier, Lachs and colleagues have shown that elders referred to protective services were at an increased risk of mortality, a threefold increase in the case of abuse and nearly a twofold increase in the case of self-neglect (Lachs, Williams, O'Brien, Pillemer, & Charlson, 1998).

This excess risk was calculated in models that adjusted for many predictors of mortality, including sociodemographic characteristics, chronic disease status, functional and cognitive status, social networks, and depressive symptoms.

Elders referred to adult protective services also face an increased risk of nursing home placement. In the same EPESE cohort monitored for 11 years, 31.8% of elders not referred to protective services were admitted to skilled care facilities. In elders referred to protective services for abuse, the rate was 52.3%; and for elders referred for self-neglect, the rate was 69.2% (Lachs et al., 2002).

What factors predispose elders to mistreatment? In the case of self-neglect, key risk factors are cognitive impairment and depression, although one study identified additional risk associated with living alone, poverty, male gender, and a particular profile of chronic conditions, such as stroke and hip fracture (Abrams, Lachs, McAvay, Keohane, & Bruce 2002). Elder self-neglect is associated with poorer physical function (Dong, Mendes de Leon, & Evans, 2009), whereas abuse may be more highly associated with cognitive impairment (Cooper et al., 2009).

Thus, abuse and self-neglect involve both elder and family features. Elders with cognitive impairment and greater needs in care because of disability are more likely to be abused or experience neglect (and less likely to report it). Family caregivers with substance abuse problems, mental and physical health symptoms, lower socioeconomic status, and poor coping and caregiving skills are more likely to abuse vulnerable elders.

SOCIAL ISOLATION

One result of poor mental health is social isolation, which, in turn, is associated with poor outcomes in a variety of areas, including greater risk of suicide, poor medication management, inferior nutrition, overuse of laxatives and other over-the-counter medicines, and poor living environments (i.e., greater risk of exposure to extremes of heat and cold). The connection between comorbid disease, poor mental health, social isolation, and these additional negative outcomes has been called a "spiral of deterioration" (Alexopoulos et al., 2002).

Yet, it also seems that social isolation in itself is a risk factor for poor outcomes. In one study, for example, poor health, physical disability, and social isolation were all independently associated with depression. Once

Chapter 7 Affective and Social Function: Suffering, Neglect, Isolation   261

controlling for these factors, the association between depressive symptoms and lower socioeconomic status was no longer significant, leading the authors to suggest that "money cannot buy happiness" in older adults (West, Reed, & Gildengorin, 1998).

Social isolation and loneliness also increase the risk of nursing home admission, even when the effects of other predisposing factors (such as age, education, income, mental status, physical health, morale, and social contact) are controlled (Russell, Cutrona, de la Mora, & Wallace, 1997). Why should loneliness or social isolation predict nursing home admission? Russell and colleagues suggest that this association may indicate that some lonely and isolated older adults in this rural Iowa sample may have sought out nursing home admission as a strategy to gain social contact.

BROADER CONSIDERATIONS OF ENVIRONMENTAL INFLUENCES ON HEALTH

Exposure to extreme heat and cold causes more deaths among older people than the natural disasters that usually make the headlines, such as earthquakes and floods. An important study by Klinenberg (2004) shows the critical role of social isolation for risk of hyperthermia, that is, heat death. Isolation, which we usually think of as problems for individuals, turns out to depend heavily on features of communities. Findings from the Chicago heat wave described by Klinenberg have unfortunately been replicated in France, Italy, and other countries over the past two decades.

How many people died of hyperthermia as a result of the July 1995 Chicago heat wave? The answer is not an obvious one. The official heat-related death toll was 465 for July 14–20, the week where the heat reached its maximum, and 521 for the month as a whole. But this count depends on the integrity of case ascertainment and a particular definition of heat death. A more careful look at mortality for the week of July 14–20 relative to deaths in prior years showed an excess of 739 deaths among older people. This is the more likely toll of this terrible heat wave. Beyond mortality, we are unaware of studies that have quantified excess hospitalizations, emergency room visits, or other morbidities in the weeks of the heat wave.

Mortality among older adults was not uniform across socioeconomic status or community residence. Victims were primarily older, poorer, African American, and isolated. In age-adjusted analyses, three

African American elders died for every two Whites, just as men were more likely to die than women. Figure 7.3 shows mortality by race, stratifying by age. Among people aged 85 and older, nearly twice as many African Americans were likely to die compared with Whites.

Klinenberg (2004) reviews the many arguments city and health officials made to explain this disparity. Differences in individual health status, such as the presence of cardiovascular disease, is one possibility. And, indeed, CDC case-control studies did note that cardiovascular disease was more prevalent among decedents relative to age-matched elders living in the same buildings. But this does not account for the racial difference. Socioeconomic factors are also likely to be relevant, but Klinenberg shows that similarly impoverished communities did not bear the same brunt of heat mortality. For example, North and South Lawndale, contiguous communities with equal proportions of both older people and older people living below the poverty level, differed by a factor of 10 in heat deaths. The difference, Klinenberg argues, is in community social capital, of health resources related to social ties. South Lawndale's predominantly Latino community was economically vibrant, less crime-ridden, more densely populated, and had active civic organizations. North Lawndale, predominantly African American, stood out among Chicago communities for loss of population over the prior 30 years, crime, decaying housing stock and, most critically,

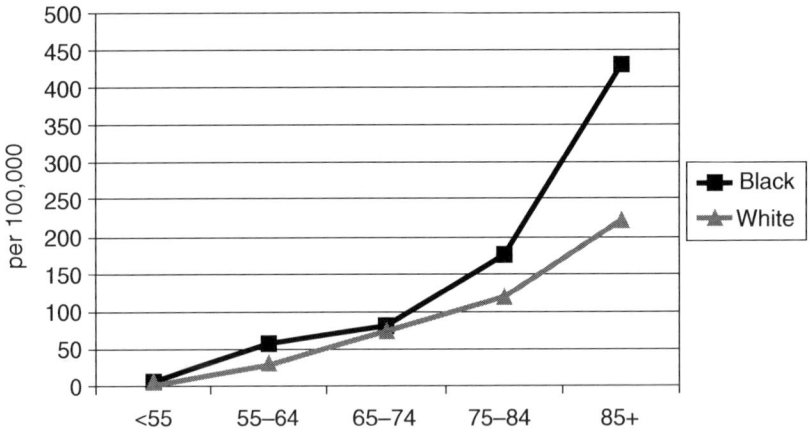

Figure 7.3 Heat mortality: Chicago, 1995.

Source: From *Heat Wave: A Social Autopsy of Disaster in Chicago,* by E. Klinenberg, 2004, Chicago: University of Chicago Press.

Chapter 7 Affective and Social Function: Suffering, Neglect, Isolation

absence of economic activity and civic organization. Isolated elders in North Lawndale were most at risk of heat death. They lived in fear of crime and nailed windows shut. They feared opening doors to city social workers sent to check up on them. Even if they ventured outside, they had no place to go because there were few stores, parks, or community gathering places to seek cooler air or information about services. Most critically, they had no one to check up on them as part of the normal course of daily life.

As with this contrast in communities, so went the city. Figures 7.4 and 7.5 show the relationship between risk of heat death among older people and broad macrosociological factors, such as proportion of population lost over the prior 30 years and crime rank. We plot the position of the 12 communities with the highest heat mortality and the 12 with the lowest. The patterns are striking. Weak neighborhoods lead to greater risk of isolation, which in turn increases the risk of a wide variety of negative health outcomes, including risk of heat death. The Chicago heat

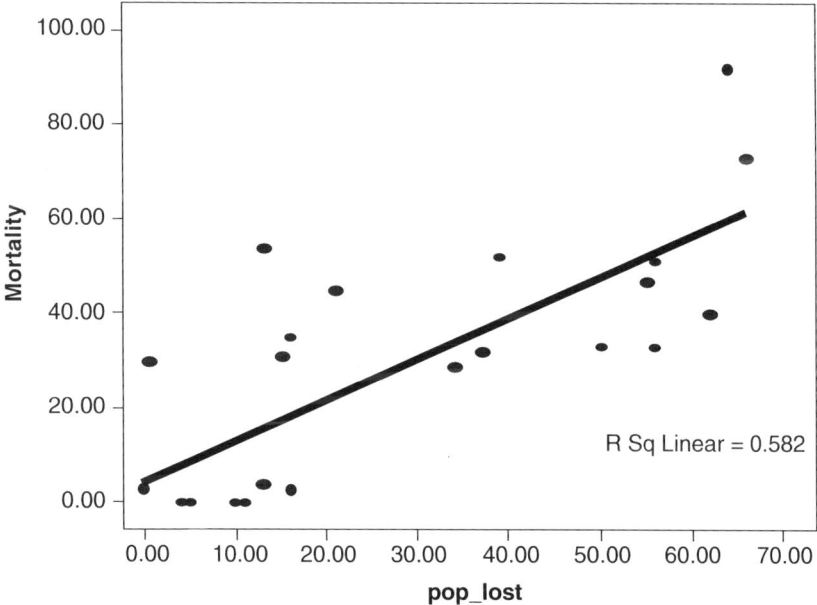

Figure 7.4 Heat mortality in communities by proportion of population lost over prior 30 years.

Note: Twenty-four communities with lowest and highest heat mortality deaths.
Source: From *Heat Wave: A Social Autopsy of Disaster in Chicago*, by E. Klinenberg, 2004, Chicago: University of Chicago Press.

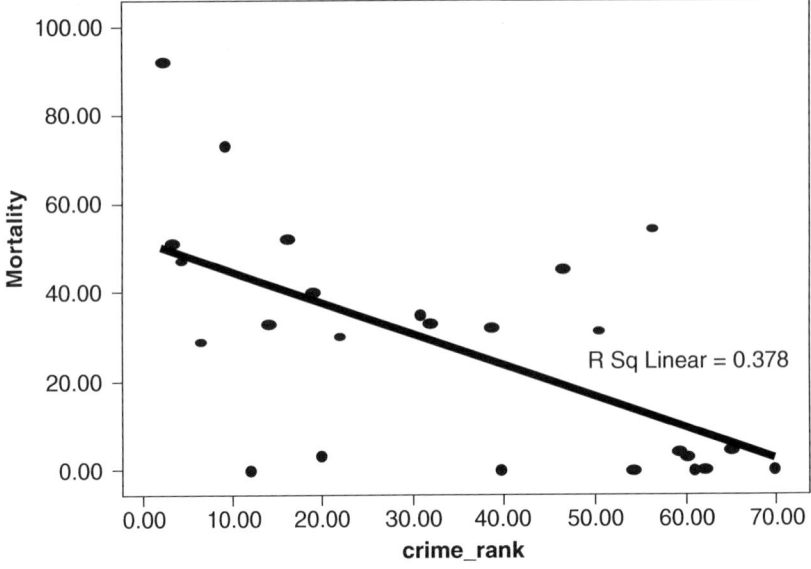

Figure 7.5 Heat mortality in Chicago communities by Community Crime Rank

Note: Twenty-four communities with lowest and highest heat mortality deaths.
Source: From *Heat Wave: A Social Autopsy of Disaster in Chicago*, by E. Klinenberg, 2004, Chicago: University of Chicago Press.

deaths make clear the health protective properties of social networks and more diffuse community solidarity.

These aspects of social capital are an active area of research in aging and public health. Social capital may be involved in quite distal health processes, such as likelihood of recovery from coronary disease (Scheffler et al., 2008). Similarly, measures of community integration that appear quite remote from health processes, such as the proportion of people in a community performing volunteer service, may turn out to be critical resources for healthy aging. Even more striking, what we see in risk of heat death or other extreme health events may apply to a far more general range of health behavior and outcome. Wight and colleagues (2006) used data from the Health and Retirement Survey, merged with community ecological indicators (i.e., census tract indicators of median levels of education or income) to show that community status and individual cognitive health are related. Levels of community educational attainment, apart from individual education, may explain variance in MMSE scores. This relationship is shown in Figure 7.6.

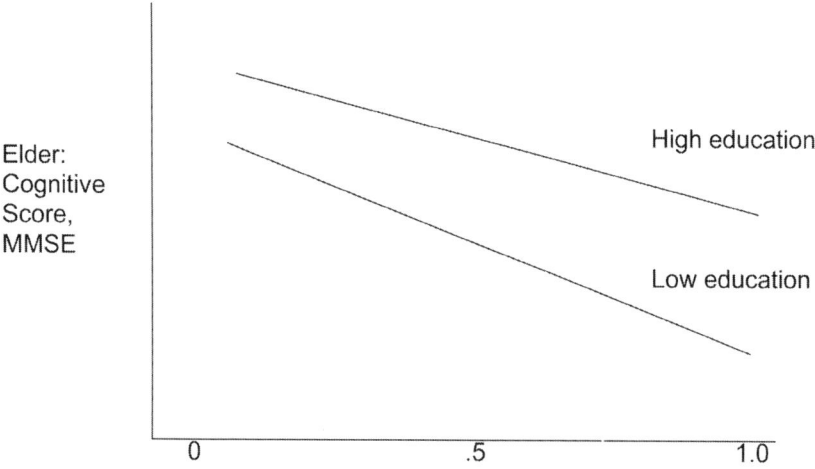

Figure 7.6 Neighborhood effects on relationship between individual education and cognitive performance.

Source: Adapted from "Urban Neighborhood Context, Educational Attainment, and Cognitive Function Among Older Adults," by R. G. Wight, C. S. Aneshensel, D. Miller-Martinez, A. L. Botticello, J. R. Cummings, A. S. Karlamangla, et al., 2006, *American Journal of Epidemiology, 163*, 1071–1978.

The proportion of people in a community with a high school education helped predict individual MMSE performance independently of individual education. Thus, although people with greater education performed better on the test, people with the same educational achievement did better if they lived in communities where most people had completed high school. Wight et al. (2006) advance a number of potential explanations. Low-education communities have (a) greater exposure to chronic stressors and low social resources that hinder engagement in physical and cognitive activities (walking places, social support); (b) fewer cognitively stimulating or supportive resources (physicians, libraries), and (c) higher tolerance for illness and untreated chronic disease that may affect cognition. These are productive areas for further research and suggest that community-level interventions to improve social resources may offer strong benefit to elder cognitive and physical health.

SUMMARY

Burden of Mental Illness. The effect of mental disorders on daily life should not be underestimated, in the young as in the old. By any measure, whether a national estimate of lost productivity or reports of daily symptoms, mental illness is as debilitating as physical illness.

Presentation and Prevalence of Mental Health Symptoms in Late Life. Mental health symptoms appear to change with older age. In later life, depressive disorders fulfilling diagnostic criteria are relatively rare; "subthreshold disorders" are more common. Subthreshold depression, for example, includes symptoms of depression that are not severe, frequent, or disruptive enough to be labeled as clinical depression. In the National Health Interview Survey, 2000, less than 2% of people aged 65 and older reported "serious psychological distress," less than half that reported by people aged 45–64. However, evidence is now available to suggest that subthreshold depression is a risk factor for poor outcomes, including declining function, increased disability, cognitive impairment, and death.

Mental Health in an Older Population With Disability. In the most limited subsample of women in WHAS-I, mental health is related to severity of disability, but mental health is, on the whole, well preserved. This speaks to adaptation in late life and psychological resiliency, and reminds us again that mental and physical health are separate but related spheres.

Outcomes Associated with Mental Illness in Late Life. The Cardiovascular Health Study showed that people with pronounced depressive symptoms were at risk for higher mortality (23.9% versus 17.7% in people with few depressive symptoms). This finding persisted when analyses controlled for other factors that increase mortality risk. Similar findings have been reported for depression, and risk of disability, cognitive decline, nursing home placement, suicide, and a host of other negative public health outcomes.

Treatment of Depression in Late Life. Evidence suggests that older people respond to treatment at rates comparable with younger people, although differences in metabolism, polypharmacy, and the presence of other chronic conditions complicate treatment. A major obstacle is an ageist expectation that affective suffering is a part of late age and frailty.

Neglect and Abuse. Despite difficulty in defining these domains, it is now clear that self-neglect is more common than outright abuse, that the most vulnerable older adults are most often victims, and that both forms of mistreatment have major public health consequences.

Chapter 7 Affective and Social Function: Suffering, Neglect, Isolation **267**

Social Isolation. Older people desire less novelty in social life than younger people do and may be more comfortable with a smaller set of friends. Yet isolation is a public health issue to the extent it is associated with medication misuse, poor nutrition, and greater risk of depression and suicide.

Broader Considerations of Environmental Influences on Health. Social capital, the health benefit associated with social networks and strong communities, may have powerful effects on health risk at old ages, ranging from risk of heat death to cognitive performance.

9 Aging, Public Health, and Long-Term Care

Is long-term care an appropriate topic for public health and aging? We think so, although some investigators limit public health and aging efforts to healthier elders who do not make use of supportive care services. This limitation is artificial for a number of reasons. First, older people increasingly move between states of ability and disability, in which they may require long-term care services for some period of time and later recover function. Early work from the National Long Term Care Survey showed substantial movement over 5 years toward both decline and improvement in elders with limitations in household competencies (the IADLs: cleaning, cooking, shopping, laundry, medication management, handling money, using the telephone) and isolated ADL limitations (such as limitations only in bathing) (Manton, 1992). More recent work has shown great dynamism in states of disability in old age (Gill et al., 2002; Hardy & Gill, 2004). Second, it is artificial to truncate public health efforts according to elder function or disability. A theme running throughout our account of the field is the need to acknowledge the full spectrum of health and function in old age, as well as the unity of risk factors and the potential for intervention across the life span. Finally, an increasing body of research shows that prevention of excess morbidity is critical among even the most frail and that the potential for gain through population-based prevention efforts is as strong here as in other populations.

Given the focus on allowing people with disabilities to live in maximally integrated settings (a step beyond the former goal of "the least restrictive setting"), we use "long-term" or "supportive" or "residential" care rather than "custodial care," a term that has appropriately and increasingly dropped out of the professional lexicon. This chapter reviews what long-term care is, provides an overview of recent trends in use and spending, and delves into the major types of long-term care: home- and community-based services, personal assistance services, family caregiving, and residential care settings. We then take up the question of how public health efforts might enhance long-term care and review several research topics that have recently gained interest: recognizing older people's care preferences, upgrading home attendant and nursing assistant care, and expanding options for supportive care and housing for older adults.

WHAT IS LONG-TERM CARE?

"Long-term care" includes the complete spectrum of services and supports required to meet health and personal care needs over an extended period of time. It is distinguished from medical care in that it is supportive rather than curative and is designed to maximize independence in daily living among people with health limitations. It is distinguished from acute or subacute care in that it is not rehabilitative. Rather, long-term care provides services that allow older people to meet personal self-maintenance needs (such as bathing, dressing, using the toilet, and the other ADLs; (see Chapter 6). Older people receiving long-term care are not expected to improve in function (although this may occur), and, in fact, elders receiving long-term care are likely to require increasing levels of supportive care, moving from help initially with transportation and household tasks (such as cleaning or cooking), to help with medication management and ADLs, and finally to help with the most basic ADL tasks, such as toileting, transfer, and feeding. The latter are supportive care needs consistent with skilled nursing facility care.

Thus, long-term care covers a wide spectrum of services and settings. It may involve activity programming for elders with dementia in an adult day program, ADL support from a home care agency, medical supplies or assistive technology from a vendor that contracts with a local Area on Aging, residence in a nursing home, home-delivered meals from a church, congregate meals in an assistive living facility, or case management to secure such services.

Chapter 9 Aging, Public Health, and Long-Term Care

Consistent with the preference to maintain vulnerable seniors in their homes and a health-financing system that favors medical rather than supportive care (see Chapter 6), family members necessarily provide the vast bulk of long-term care services. However, with the increasing availability of home- and community-based services, family caregivers are now more likely to share long-term care with formal paid providers. Families thus have increasing contact with a wide variety of providers and payers. These include Medicare in the case of ADL support linked to rehabilitation following a hospitalization, Medicaid for nursing home care, paraprofessional or informal nonfamily caregivers who are paid out-of-pocket, Medicaid waiver programs that allow payment to family caregivers for ADL support, and Medicare-Medicaid programs that link medical and long-term care, such as the Program for All-Inclusive Care for the Elderly (PACE). Medicaid waiver programs allow states increasing latitude in bundling long-term care services for lower-income elders and younger people with disabilities.

Finally, in some cases, it is genuinely difficult to tell where long-term care services begin and end. For example, visiting nurses and other home health care rehabilitative services are normally linked to posthospital care and are limited by Medicare to 90-day cycles. But in many cases these services serve as long-term care placeholders until families are able to put other services in place, as families recognize that the discharged elder can no longer function independently in the home. Likewise, programs that combine medical and supportive care blur these boundaries. In some municipalities, as in New York City, Medicaid-eligible seniors can receive home health care nursing services along with separate paraprofessional ADL-based home care on a long-term basis. Even families may be unclear whether they are providing long-term care. Although family members can identify when they began to provide ADL support (Albert & Brody, 1996), they are not always able to distinguish when they stopped providing occasional help and became "caregivers."

OVERVIEW: TRENDS IN LONG-TERM CARE USE AND SPENDING

Spending on long-term care in the United States for all ages reached nearly $200 billion in 2004; approximately half of this amount was paid by Medicaid. Approximately 20% was paid by Medicare, another 20% through out-of-pocket payments, and the remainder through health insurance (including long-term care insurance) and other public sources (Komisar & Thompson, 2007). From 1990 to 2004 national long-term care expenditures grew at an annual rate of 7.4%, somewhat higher than the 7.0% average annual growth rate for all personal health care spending. Two important trends in long-term care payments include a growing share of public funding and a shift away from spending on institutional care toward home- and community-based services. These trends show increasing public sector commitment to long-term care and recognize the public's preference for care in the home or community, whenever possible. Spending on noninstitutional care was 19% of Medicaid's long-term care spending in 1995, but it reached 37% in 2005 and continues to increase (Komisar & Thompson, 2007).

Approximately 9 million people over age 65 need assistance with one or more personal self-maintenance activities, such as bathing or dressing (ADLs) (U.S. DHHS National Long Term Care Clearinghouse, www.longtermcare.gov/LTC/Main_Site/index.aspx). As we analyze in more detail (Chapter 6), these 9 million represent approximately 25% of older adults. In 2005, approximately 1.5 million of these people received care in nursing homes (approximately 4.6% of people aged 65 and older), again pointing to the many other components of the long-term spectrum and the many different ways older adults manage to meet these most basic needs.

Skilled nursing home use is clearly only the tip of the iceberg of long-term care. Even among older adults with ADL limitations, for every one receiving nursing home care, seven others receive long-term care in the community. Of course, nursing home care is reserved mostly for the oldest and most severely dependent elder, but it is notable that residence in skilled nursing homes among older adults continues to decline. The rate per 1,000 was 54.0 in 1985, 46.4 in 1995, and 34.8 in 2004 (Federal Interagency Forum on Aging-Related Statistics, 2008). Still, the need for long-term care is a feature of aging. Approximately 70% of individuals over age 65 will require some type of long-term care services during their lifetimes, and over 40% will spend at least some time in a skilled nursing facility (Kemper, Komisar, & Alecxih, 2005). Someone aged 65 in 2005 is likely to need long-term care services for 3 years of his or her remaining life span.

As mentioned earlier, families provide the bulk of long-term care services. Approximately three of four caregivers of older adults with long-term care needs are family members. Half of these family members provide help daily, and two-thirds live with care recipients. Although the hourly investment in caregiving is linked to elder needs, most of these informal, unpaid caregivers provide 1–5 hours of care daily (Johnson, Toohey, & Wiener, 2007). Important emerging trends in family caregiving include increases in the proportion of husbands and sons providing care, and reductions in the proportion of households in which a middle-generation caregiver is "sandwiched" between the demands of elder and child care.

HOME- AND COMMUNITY-BASED SERVICES

For an appraisal of access to paid or "formal" home- and community-based services, it is helpful first to examine the residential arrangements of older people, because people living in supportive housing may receive some services by virtue of residence. Table 9.1 shows the proportion of older adults living in different kinds of residential settings in 2005. Data on older people living in "naturally occurring retirement communities" (NORC), which may also be a site for long-term care services, are harder to come by because their definition is less clear and they vary greatly in access to long-term care services (Ormond, Black, Tilly, & Thomas, 2004). In Table 9.1, "community housing with services" includes assisted living, board and care homes, and senior citizen housing that provides support for household maintenance activities. Long-term care facilities are Medicare- or Medicaid-certified entities that provide full-time personal assistance care.

Table 9.1

RESIDENTIAL ARRANGEMENTS OF OLDER ADULTS, 2005

	65+	65–74	75–84	85+
ALL SETTINGS (1,000'S)	33,394	16,116	12,703	4,575
Residential type, %				
Traditional community	93.0	98.0	92.6	76.3
Community housing with services	2.4	0.7	3.1	6.8
Long-term care facilities	4.6	1.3	4.3	16.9

From *Older Americans 2008: Key Indicators of Well-Being,* by Federal Interagency Forum on Aging-Related Statistics, 2008, Table 37a. Retrieved September 15, 2009, from http://www.agingstats.gov/chartbook2008/default.htm.

As expected, we see a clear association between age and residence in supportive housing. Whereas nearly all elders aged 65–74 reside in traditional community housing, only three fourths of people aged 85 and older live in the community. Use of nursing home care increases from 1.3% in people aged 65–74 to 16.9% in people aged 85 and older. The proportion without disability is 63.6% among community-dwelling elders, 39.6% in people living in community housing with services, and 5.8% in people living in long-term care facilities (the latter include spouses of more impaired elders and people who reside in these facilities for lack of alternative housing). In the group residing in community housing with services, over 80% receive prepared meals and housekeeping services and nearly half receive help with medications.

For elders living outside supportive housing settings, in-home services are provided by both Medicare and Medicaid, as noted earlier. The rate of Medicare home health care visits in 2005 was 2,770 per 1,000, or about 2.8 home health care episodes for each older adult. This is in keeping with the high rate of hospitalization among older people (350 per 1,000) (Federal Interagency Forum on Aging-Related Statistics, 2008, Table 29a). Use of Medicare home health care is again strongly related to age. The rate per 1,000 in 2005 was 1,333 for people aged 65–74, 3,407 for people aged 75–84, and 6,549 for people aged 85 and older (Federal Interagency Forum on Aging-Related Statistics, 2008, Table 29b).

Medicaid home- and community-based services are far more extensive and vary considerably by state and, in some cases, by county. Medicaid provides personal care services through an optional state plan benefit (Title XIX) and the more common 1915(c) waiver. For further information on the relevant Medicaid services, see the Web site of the Centers for Medicare and Medicaid Services (http://www.cms.hhs.gov/MedicaidStWaivProgDemoPGI/). State commitment to personal care services for the elderly and adults with disabilities varies dramatically. In 2001, Medicaid personal care participants per 1,000 people ranged from 7.33 to 0.04 per state, and per capita expenditures ranged from $91.21 to $0.02 (LeBlanc, Tonner, & Harrington, 2001).

The diversity of Medicaid home- and community-based services is impressive. In New York City, 10 different programs are available. These include Traditional Personal Care, Consumer-Directed Personal Assistance, Long-Term Home Health Care, Medicaid Managed Long-Term Care, the Program for All-Inclusive Care for the Elderly (PACE), Certified Home Health Agency Services, Medical Adult Day Health

Care, the Traumatic Brain Injury Waiver, the Nursing Home Transition and Diversion Waiver, and Medicaid Advantage Plus. Two-thirds of these programs require nursing home levels of need for eligibility. In New York City in 2007, approximately 166,000 people received in-home services through Medicaid programs (compared with 81,000 receiving nursing home or assisted living services). Of the $12.3 billion spent on Medicaid long-term care services in New York City 47% went to these home- and community-based services (Hokenstad & Shineman, 2009).

A survey of older adults receiving Medicaid waiver personal care services in Virginia suggests that the program meets the needs of recipients, and that recipients are on the whole very satisfied with aides and care delivery (Glass, Roberto, Brossoie, Teaster, & Butler, 2008–2009).

PERSONAL ASSISTANCE SERVICES AND PUBLIC HEALTH

Across the different programs that deliver formal, paid home- and community-based services, 1.2–1.5 million Americans receive personal assistance services (PAS) (LeBlanc et al., 2001). Recipients receiving PAS require long-term help with bathing, dressing, and other activities of daily living, receive this support from nonmedically trained providers, and would otherwise require nursing home residence to meet their needs (Kitchener, Carrillo, & Harrington, 2003; LeBlanc et al., 2001). PAS is not designed to manage a client's clinical needs, but rather to manage disability and support independence at home. Thus, PAS is *not* a skilled care intervention, as in the case of the Medicare home health benefit, which stresses rehabilitation, but it may have beneficial health consequences by effectively managing disabilities that would otherwise put people at risk for poor outcomes. We have shown that PAS is associated with a potential health benefit, even though its primary purpose is to provide support for independent living at home (Albert, Simone, Brassard, Stern, & Mayeux, 2005b). Thus, PAS may have important public health significance. However, little research is available on the measurement of effective PAS delivery and its health and quality-of-life consequences.

Increases in the prevalence of PAS are expected, given the substantial growth in Medicaid programs that provide PAS, an aging population, declines in the nursing home population, and legislative efforts (e.g., the *Olmstead* decision, in which the Supreme Court in 1999 upheld elements of the Americans With Disability Act that mandate the most integrated setting for people with long-term care needs; see *Olmstead v. L. C.* (98-536) 527 U.S. 581, 1999). In addition, consumer-directed PAS is now a popular option, with elders and their families taking control of the hiring and training of PAS providers or, in some cases, serving as paid PAS providers themselves. Thus, examination of outcomes associated with PAS is critical for an accurate appraisal of the conditions under which elders and their families can best benefit from the program.

Studies of PAS outcomes are complicated by two key factors. First, the number of PAS hours per week that elders receive (service intensity) is based on the severity of disability (need). More severe disability will be associated with unfavorable outcomes, even when PAS is delivered effectively. Second, informal care arrangements complicate assessment of PAS outcomes. Family caregivers may supplement paid PAS to different degrees (or develop variable kinds of division of labor), making it difficult to assess the effect of PAS on outcomes. Careful designs will be required to disentangle these confounding factors.

Some initial evidence in this area is available from "cash and counseling" demonstrations. Medicaid has allowed waiver programs for PAS that encourage consumer-directed care, in which families may hire (and fire) home care providers. In these programs, certified home care agencies may vet home attendants or handle payroll and other administrative duties, but families supervise PAS and work out hourly arrangements with home care attendants. The Arkansas Cash & Counseling Demonstration (Independent Choices) suggests that suboptimal delivery of PAS is a concern (Foster, Brown, Phillips, Schore, & Carlson, 2003).

In this demonstration, Medicaid-eligible elders were randomly assigned either to a consumer direction arm, in which they were able to use a monthly allowance to purchase PAS services (as well as assistive equipment), or to standard agency care. Elders able to direct PAS care were more likely to report that providers completed tasks and that household and transportation needs were met. But these simple indicators reveal considerable variation in how effectively PAS was delivered, even when families were able to hire relatives or friends as PAS providers. For example, 65.8% of elders in the consumer direction arm reported that PAS providers "always" completed mandated care plan tasks, compared with 47.2% in the standard agency care arm. Thus, PAS delivery by this simple measure was effective in only about half to two-thirds of cases across the two groups.

Despite only partially effective delivery of PAS, elders in the consumer direction arm were more likely to report they were "very satisfied with the way they spend their life these days" (55.5% vs. 37.0%).

Also, "treatment group members were somewhat less likely than control group members to report some kinds of health problems that might indicate they received inferior or insufficiently frequent personal assistance" (Foster et al., 2003). These findings suggest that effective delivery of PAS may be associated with health benefit.

Thus, an important area for public health inquiry in home- and community-based services is direct investigation of features of PAS delivery that promote desired outcomes. Does PAS allow elders to meet basic provisioning, hygiene, mobility, and nutrition needs? And does effectively meeting these needs in turn promote desired short-term health and functioning outcomes, such as fewer falls, better skin integrity, weight maintenance, and lower extremity strength, which may in turn influence well being?

It is clear as well that personal assistance care does not occur in a vacuum. Whereas family care without paid assistance is still the most common caregiving arrangement, the proportion of families that combine formal and informal care has grown to encompass about a third of caregiving arrangements (Federal Interagency Forum on Aging-Related Statistics, 2008). Thus, a second line of inquiry should be to examine the relationship between family caregivers and paid providers because this might affect PAS delivery and outcomes.

Table 9.2 illustrates a public health approach to assessment of PAS and suggests linkages between delivery of PAS and relevant indicators of health and functioning.

Table 9.2

DOMAIN-SPECIFIC INDICATORS OF EFFECTIVE PAS DELIVERY AND OUTCOMES

PERSONAL ASSISTANCE TASK	INDICATOR OF EFFECTIVE DELIVERY	CLINICAL STATUS INDICATOR
PAS provider report: ADL		
Bathing: frequency, comfort performing task, difficulty	Personal cleanliness	Skin integrity
Dressing: frequency of clothing changes, elicitation of elder preferences	Clothing comfort, variety	

(Continued)

Table 9.2

DOMAIN-SPECIFIC INDICATORS OF EFFECTIVE PAS DELIVERY AND OUTCOMES (*Continued*)

PERSONAL ASSISTANCE TASK	INDICATOR OF EFFECTIVE DELIVERY	CLINICAL STATUS INDICATOR
Toileting: presence of toileting schedule; comfort with task	Availability of commode; report of availability of prompt toileting & cleanliness	
Grooming: frequency	Satisfaction with appearance	
Eating: recognition of dietary restrictions & limitations posed by dentition	Foods appropriate to dentition & swallowing status; verbal/physical prompting; report of variety & satisfaction	Weight maintenance, dehydration; appetite
PAS Provider Report: Mobility		
Transfer & mobility support: frequency, difficulty	Presence of assistive devices, provider ability to lift elder; report of fear of falling during transfer, opportunity to move, access to rooms	Lower extremity strength & balance performance; opportunity to change environment
PAS Provider Report: IADL		
Meal preparation: concern for elder meal preference and schedule	Regularity of meals and snacks, sufficient food in home; enjoyment of social and physical setting of eating	
Laundry: frequency	Cleanliness of clothing & linens	Relocation of elder over follow-up
Housework: frequency	Cleanliness of household, clutter; appliances in good repair; trash removal; comfort, satisfaction with living quarters	
Shopping, errands: frequency	Adequate food & household supplies, timely replacement	

FAMILY CAREGIVING

In its most expansive definition as unpaid help with household tasks and care management for a chronically ill, disabled, or aged family member or friend, more than 50 million Americans can be considered caregivers in any given year (National Family Caregivers Association, www.thefamilycaregiver.org). Limiting the definition to people who provide unpaid ADL or IADL care lowers the yearly prevalence (in 2004) to 44.4 million (National Caregiver Alliance and AARP, 2004). With these definitions, family caregivers are active in approximately 20% of U.S. households. Note that these estimates do not separate caregiving to older and younger adults with disabilities.

These surveys suggest the following profile of the typical family caregiver: she is 46, married, and employed; and she is caring for a widowed mother who does not live with her (National Caregiver Alliance and AARP, 2004). This profile is in keeping with the greater likelihood of women as caregivers (60%) and the lower likelihood of spousal caregiving (30% of family caregivers are themselves aged 65 or older). The economic value of family caregiving is substantial and has been estimated at over $300 billion yearly, nearly twice as much as the total costs incurred by the formal long-term care sector of paid home care and long-term care facilities (AARP, 2006). Given the growing rate of people over age 65 (projected to increase at 2.3% annually) and much slower rate of growth in younger people likely to provide care (0.8% annually), shortfalls in family caregiving can be expected, along with a greater cost burden for the formal long-term care sector (Mack & Thompson, 2001).

The high prevalence of such caregiving has led the CDC to develop a caregiver module for its ongoing Behavioral Risk Factors Surveillance System (BRFSS). In the BRFSS, caregiving is established with the following question. "People may provide regular care or assistance to a friend or family member who has a health problem, long-term illness, or disability. During the past month, did you provide any such care or assistance to a friend or family member?" The module will be fielded nationally in 2009 and will provide the first state-level estimates of caregiver prevalence.

In an initial statewide survey in North Carolina using the BRFSS module, the prevalence of caregiving was 15.4% (DeFries, McGuire, Andresen, Brumback, & Anderson, 2009). Approximately 75% of caregivers were providing help to people aged 60 and older. By respondent self-report, 41.5% of care recipients were cognitively impaired. Caregivers in this survey provided a mean of 20.2 hr/wk in the case of cognitively impaired care recipients and 16.6 hr/wk for other care receivers. Mean duration of caregiving was just under 4 years for people with cognitive impairment, and just under 3 years otherwise. Not surprisingly, care recipients with cognitive impairment were older, as were their caregivers.

The associations between family caregiving and various outcomes, both negative and positive, have been extensively documented. On the negative side, family caregiving is associated with lost wages and work absenteeism, lower work productivity, and greater risk of poverty (Schulz & Martire, in press). Strained caregivers face an increased mortality risk (Schulz & Beach, 1999) and an increased risk of depression, anxiety, substance abuse, and other chronic conditions (Cannuscio et al., 2002). On the positive side, caregiving is associated with gains in personal mastery, family continuity, and, in some cases, new careers in aging and health services.

While only 17% of family caregivers provide 40 hr/wk of care or more (National Caregiver Alliance, 2004), less intensive caregiving can be associated with a variety of negative outcomes, in particular, with the caregiver's health. These associations were explored in a sample of 17,000 U.S. employees from a large corporation who completed health risk appraisal questionnaires on the job (National Caregiver Alliance and MetLife Mature Market Institute, in press). In this sample, 11.6% of employees reported they provided care to an older person. Employees reporting elder care responsibilities reported poorer health than noncaregivers in a variety of domains:

- Caregivers were more likely to report fair or poor health. For example, among female employees aged 50 and older, 17% of caregivers reported fair or poor health compared with 9% among noncaregivers.
- Employees providing elder care were significantly more likely to report depression symptoms and diagnoses of diabetes, hypertension, and pulmonary disease. For example, in models adjusting for age, gender, and work type, caregivers were 26% more likely to report diagnoses of diabetes.
- Female employees with elder care responsibilities reported more stress at home than noncaregivers in every age group. Stress at home appears to affect younger female employees most. Caregivers were more likely to report negative influences of personal life on work.

- Elder care demands were associated with greater health risk behaviors. For example, smoking is higher among male caregivers, especially among young men. Smoking is also higher among caregivers relative to noncaregivers among white collar employees. Among blue collar workers, alcohol use is higher among caregivers.
- Employee caregivers find it more difficult than noncaregivers to take care of their health. For example, among women, caregivers were less likely to report annual mammograms.
- Employees with elder care responsibilities were more likely to report missed days of work. Overall, 8.5% of noncaregivers missed at least 1 day of work over the past 2 weeks because of health issues compared with 10.2% of caregivers. Differences were mostly driven by the much higher absenteeism among younger caregiver employees.

In addition, this study found that the greater prevalence of chronic disease among caregivers and related challenges to health maintenance is costly. Imputing the average cost of a series of sentinel health conditions, employees with elder care responsibilities cost employer health plans 8% more per year more than noncaregiver employees. Excess employee medical care costs associated with elder care were highest among younger, male, and blue collar employees.

A recent study (Amirkhanyan & Wolf, 2006) raises questions about whether these associations are the result of the stress of caregiving per se, or from having a parent who needs care, irrespective of one's role in providing care to that parent. Using panel data from the Health and Retirement Study, the authors estimated models of mental symptoms of 3,350 men and 3,659 women. They found that female, but not male, caregivers whose parents needed care exhibited adverse mental health symptoms. However, both male and female noncaregivers whose parents needed care were also more likely to report such symptoms than noncaregivers. In other words, adverse psychological outcomes related to having a parent with care needs may be dispersed throughout the family and not just to those providing hands-on care. The authors conclude that the focus on caregivers, and not other family members, may be underestimating the social burdens of disability at older ages.

This brief treatment of family caregiving shows the central public health significance of this component of long-term care. First, families provide perhaps two-thirds of the supportive care elders with disabilities require. Even when formal paid care is involved, as in nursing home care or home health care, family caregiving does not end. Families are nearly always partners in these efforts. The contribution of family caregiving to elder health, hard to quantify, is clearly substantial, as are the effects of caregiving on other family members of having an older relative with care needs, including both caregivers and noncaregivers. Second, family caregivers face the substantial health consequences of caregiving, visible in virtually every domain of health and well-being. Finally, family caregiving affects the ramifying networks of these caregivers: employers, children, spouses.

A productive area for public health and aging is better coordination of formal services and family caregiving. In a study of the end of paid home health care for people discharged from hospitals with stroke, we found substantial family caregiving involvement during this period, which lasted, on average, approximately 7 weeks. Between a third and a half of these family caregivers were not adequately prepared for the case closing. Although clinicians reported that they informed patients and family caregivers that the service would be limited and short-term, agencies did not have a systematic or consistent way of preparing caregivers for case closing and referrals to community resources (Levine et al., 2006).

LONG-TERM RESIDENTIAL CARE ARRANGEMENTS

In 2005, the United States had approximately 16,000 certified nursing homes and 35,000 assisted living residences (Alecxih, 2006; U.S. DHHS National Long-Term Care Clearinghouse). These serve approximately 1.5 million and 900,000 people, respectively. The difference between the two is slowly disappearing. Despite the requirement that new admissions to assisted living sites be mobile or not meet criteria for dementia, these people age in assisted living sites and develop such disabilities, and they are now often maintained on site without transfer to skilled nursing facilities. Assisted living facilities are now likely to offer dementia-specific services, such as Alzheimer's special care units. Research suggests that the prevalence of disability and cognitive impairment in the two settings is not as different as might be expected (Zimmerman et al., 2005). Nursing homes are far more regulated than assisted living facilities are, and this convergence in services and populations suggests that assisted living will ultimately need to be similarly monitored and regulated.

Chapter 9 Aging, Public Health, and Long-Term Care

Variation within the two residential settings is important. Skilled nursing facilities may be freestanding or linked to hospital systems; also, the national and state Veterans Administration and now even prison systems administer nursing homes. Physicians may or may not be based on site. Nursing facilities may or may not offer hospice beds and differ in the proportion offering "Medicaid beds." Almost all now contain wings for subacute rehabilitative care, short-stay posthospital care for people unable to return to their homes even with home health care.

Assisted living facilities may contain skilled nursing units on site, as in the case of continuing care retirement communities. They also differ in their opportunities for community integration, privacy, likelihood of aging on site given increasing disability, and spectrum of services offered.

Concern for the quality of residential long-term care services is longstanding. After exposure of the industry's inadequacies in the 1980s, the Institute of Medicine proposed quality standards that were later incorporated into the 1987 Nursing Home Reform Act. This legislation aimed to ensure that residents of nursing homes receive high-quality care designed to promote the "highest practicable" physical, mental, and psychosocial well-being. To achieve this aim, nursing homes were required to provide a consistent and wide spectrum of services, including nursing, social services, rehabilitation, pharmacy, and nutrition. Larger nursing homes were required to have a full-time social worker, and many now include additional staff, such as activity therapists. The 1987 Nursing Home Reform Act also required periodic assessment and a linked comprehensive care plan for each resident. These were formalized in the Resident Assessment Instrument (RAI), which includes a Minimum Data Set (MDS) that is now collected by all nursing homes, and which is transmitted electronically to the Centers for Medicare and Medicaid Services. MDS information is used to generate Resident Assessment Protocols (RAPs) that are used to personalize care. Initial versions of the MDS involved only nurse and therapist ratings, which were ideally integrated and qualified in quarterly (and sometimes monthly) meetings with families and, when possible, residents. The newest version of the MDS (3.0) now includes an opportunity to collect information from residents themselves on key quality-of-life domains.

A 2001 Institute of Medicine report reexamined quality of care in long-term care settings and noted some improvements in nursing homes (such as declines in chemical and physical restraints for agitated residents), but continued concerns for undertreatment of pain, high rates of pressure ulcers, under- and malnutrition, and other shortfalls in quality supportive care (Wunderlich & Kohler, 2001). Assisted living facilities came under fire for inadequate concern for resident privacy and inadequate staffing. The IOM report also stressed the need for greater consumer access to information about particular long-term care sites to make informed choices.

This review led to the launch of Nursing Home Compare in 2002, a Web site in which consumers can examine quality and staffing indicators for any certified nursing home according to region or other search criteria. The Web site integrates data from the Online Survey, Certification and Reporting system (OSCAR), which captures complaints, facility-level staffing, and MDS resident-level information. Quality indicators currently tabulated in Nursing Home Compare include the proportion of residents who fail to meet particular benchmarks, such as receiving a flu vaccination, having moderate to severe pain, being physically restrained, feeling depressed or anxious, using an in-dwelling catheter, losing mobility, having a urinary tract infection, or losing a significant amount of weight.

This model was later expanded to cover Medicare home health care agencies in the Home Health Compare Web site. Again, consumers choosing home health care providers can examine performance of particular agencies on a variety of quality indicators, such as the proportion of clients who gain in mobility, who see progress in restoration of ADL function, and who are readmitted to hospitals. Home Health Compare is based on data collected in OASIS, the Outcome and Assessment Information Set, used in all Medicare-certified home health care agencies.

Access to real-time information about the performance of nursing homes and home health care agencies represents an important step in promoting empowerment of consumers and accountability of providers. One may quibble with the appropriateness of particular indicators or the reliability of data, insist on the need to visit sites or make personal inquiries in any case, or question whether consumers appreciate the limitations of such information. This level of engagement in long-term care choice and planning is a central development likely to lead to important change in how families obtain long-term care services. We can expect to see expansion of this approach to Medicaid services and perhaps aging services, in general, as the aging services system adopts a common dataset (SAMS, see Chapter 3) and a new focus on outcomes and quality indicators.

Finally, it is important to note that disparities extend to long-term care services. Evidence suggests that nursing home care is currently a two-tiered system (Mor, Zinn, Angelelli, Teno, & Miller, 2004). The bottom tier consists of facilities that provide care to Medicaid residents almost exclusively. This 15% of nursing homes has fewer nurses, lower occupancy rates, and more health-related deficiencies. As a result, these nursing homes face a greater risk of decertification from the Medicaid-Medicare program. They are mostly found in poor counties and are more likely to serve African American residents. This disparity is of a piece with disparities in access to high-quality medical care and requires appropriate changes in financing and policy.

ENHANCING LONG-TERM CARE

Kane and Kane (2000) have specified goals for supportive care populations, such as people with Alzheimer's disease or severe psychiatric illness, or people dependent on extensive medical technologies. For these populations, rehabilitation or cure is not a reasonable goal, nor, in some cases, is extended survival. That is, for an individual with severe dementia receiving formal home care services, or the older patient receiving ventilator care in a nursing home, excellent supportive care should be the goal but will most likely not extend survival or lead to regained function. What, then, are the goals for enhanced supportive care? What outcomes would be reasonable targets for interventions in these populations? Table 9.3 shows supportive care goals for these populations.

These goals, for example, dignity, privacy, a sense of security, or the opportunity to participate in meaningful activity or reciprocal social relationships, are the essence of sensitive treatment of any person. The goals are no different than ones we set for ourselves and expect in daily activity. Thus, an important conclusion from research with supportive care populations is that the same goals apply. Privacy is as important in the nursing home as anywhere else. Allowing someone to maintain individuality, perhaps through the use of personal objects or "memory cases," is appropriate in institutions just as it is in homes. "Meaningful activity" is a goal even for someone with severe memory impairment and even if attempts at such activity strike the observer as terribly primitive or unsatisfying.

In fact, one additional conclusion from Kane's approach is that we cannot presume to know, without detailed investigation, the valence of behaviors for people with severe dementia. Agitation is almost always a negative behavior (patients appear distressed, risk injuring themselves, and elicit negative responses both from caregivers and other patients). Likewise, a patient's demonstration of a preference, or assertion of continuity with the past, or clear pleasure in activity is easily recognized as positive behavior (as indicated by facial expressions of happiness, contentment, or interest) (Lawton et al., 2001). But the valence of other behaviors is less clear (see Chapter 7). Wandering, perseveration, delusions, and vocalizations are disturbing to observers but may represent sources of pleasure or engagement to the person with severe dementia (Albert, 1997).

For supportive care populations, the following areas have recently become topics of research: recognition of older people's care preferences and designing care regimens that respect such preferences; upgrading home attendant and nursing assistant care; developing special care units for people with Alzheimer's disease; expanding options for supportive housing; and supporting family caregivers. We examine each below.

Table 9.3

GOALS FOR ENHANCED SUPPORTIVE CARE

- Sense of security and order
- Enjoyment
- Meaningful activity (opportunity to accomplish goals)
- Social relationships (opportunity for reciprocity)
- Dignity
- Privacy
- Individuality (identity with past)
- Autonomy (opportunity to express preferences)
- Spiritual well-being
- Functional competence
- Physical comfort

From "Expanding the Home Care Concept: Blurring Distinctions Among Home Care, Institutional Care, and Other Long-Term Care Services," by R. A. Kane, 1995, *The Milbank Quarterly, 73*(2), 161–186.

Recognizing and Taking Older People's Care Preferences Seriously

Are family caregivers, even when they are in daily contact with patients with dementia, good judges of patient preferences? Reason for doubt on the accuracy of caregiver perceptions is evident in Logsdon's finding of high correlations between caregiver mental health, particularly depression, and caregiver ratings of a patient's quality of life (Logsdon, Gibbons, McCurry, & Teri, 2001). Depressive symptoms in caregivers were associated with lower ratings of patient quality of life, suggesting that caregivers are not accurate reporters, but rather transfer their own negative perceptions on to patients.

A related result is shown in Figure 9.1, which displays patient reports of enjoyment in activity, caregiver perceptions of patient enjoyment in activity, and the relationship between each of these reports and *patient* reports of depressive symptoms. The figure is based on reports from 161 patient-caregiver pairs in a clinical cohort of Alzheimer's patients with mildly dementia. Patient reports of enjoyment in activity were correlated with patient depressive symptoms. Caregiver reports of patient enjoyment were less clearly related to patient depressive symptoms. Thus, at least in the case of enjoyment of activity, patient reports may be more accurate than caregiver reports.

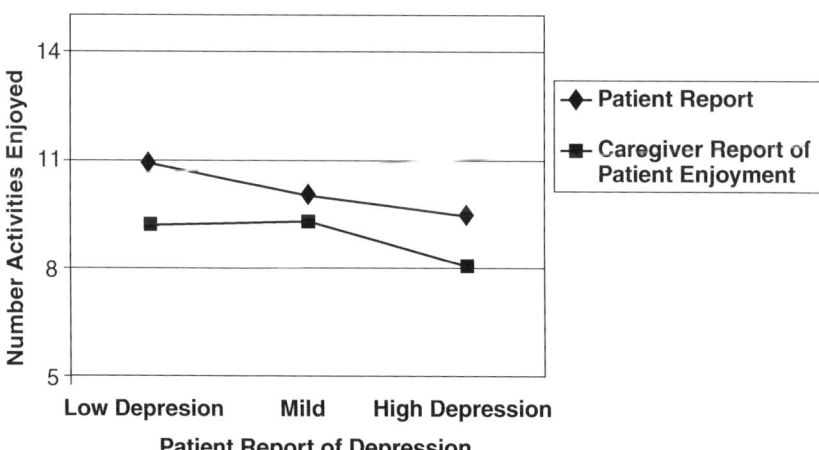

Figure 9.1 Mild dementia: Patient reports of enjoyment in activity correlated with patient-reported depressive symptoms. $n = 161$, ratings from patients with mild dementia and caregivers.

This situation contrasts with other domains of patient experience, in which caregiver reports may, in fact, be more accurate than patient reports. In the same Columbia clinical cohort, for example, caregiver reports of the *frequency* of patient activity were significantly correlated with the patient's Mini-Mental State Examination score. Patient reports of activity frequency were not related to patient cognitive status. Thus, for these elders with mild dementia, reports of affective experience (enjoyment in activity) are likely to be more accurate than reports of the frequency of behaviors or symptoms.

Examining the care and more general psychosocial preferences of community-dwelling elders has become an important focus of research. As Carpenter and colleagues point out, "just as people have unique wishes about the medical care they receive, they may have unique wishes about the personal care they receive as they become more dependent" (Carpenter, van Haitsma, Ruckdeschel, & Lawton, 2000). Documenting these preferences is useful for the concurrent delivery of care, but may also be useful for establishing an "advanced psychosocial directive," a statement about preferred care delivery and living situation that can be consulted when a person is no longer able to state these preferences. This approach would likely encourage individualized care planning rather than current standard service plans.

In a pilot concept-mapping approach to psychosocial preferences, Carpenter and colleagues (2000) found that preferences for care and caregiving formed a well-defined cluster, distinct from other domains (such as "growth activities," "leisure," or "self-dominion"). On a scale of 1–5 to indicate importance, preferences in this domain ranged from 4.35 ("caregivers should know about my medical conditions and treatment") to 1.90 ("caregivers should address me by my first name"). Midrange preferences included "having friends involved in my care," "using alternative medicine providers," "having caregivers call me by a particular name," and "accepting restrictions for my safety." The investigators have developed an extensive inventory to assess daily preferences, the Preferences for Everyday Living Inventory, and fielded it in a large sample of elders in different care settings.

One of us (SA) used a modified version of this preference inventory to examine concordance between family and formal caregivers on the perceived preferences of people with dementia for particular activities. For this study, patients with mild to moderate dementia who were attending an adult day care program at a senior center were enrolled. The primary family caregiver (the person making sure the needs of the patient were met, either directly or by arranging services) was identified. The formal caregiver in every case was a home attendant who provided care in the patient's home and also accompanied the elder to the adult day care program. The families and home attendants in this study spoke Spanish. Concordance between the two different types of caregivers was assumed to be an indicator that patients with mild to moderate dementia were able to communicate preferences (even if they could not state them in an interview or research questionnaire). Each type of caregiver was asked to rate how important particular behaviors or activities were to the patient on a 4-point Likert scale (very, some, little, or no importance).

Concordance between family and formal care providers was quite good. The proportion of patients for whom family caregiver and home attendant maximally disagreed (i.e., where one said the activity was "very important" and the other said "no importance") was low. For activities with low frequency, pairs were discordant in less than 15% of instances. These preferences included the wish to be left alone, to have a challenging task, to talk about worries, and to keep to a particular routine. For more commonly preferred activities, such as choosing what clothes to wear, hearing the news, spending time outside, and having visitors, discordance was also relatively uncommon and was again about 15%. This level of agreement between different types of caregiver suggests that patients with mild to moderate dementia can express preferences, as evident in the joint recognition of such preferences by people who spend time with these elders.

Upgrading Home Attendant and Nursing Assistant Care

As we have seen, home care paraprofessionals are an important element in the long-term care spectrum. They provide in-home support for elders with ADL needs severe enough to require nursing home levels of care. These paraprofessionals do not have medical training and are barred from providing help with prescriptions or medical equipment. In New York City's Home Care Services Program, a Medicaid waiver program, 65,000 low-income elders received ADL support from home attendants in 2005, and the number is increasing each year. New York City continues to have the highest percentage of Medicaid recipients using home care services and the highest expenditures for such services, as well as the highest state spending for Medicaid services (Centers for Medicare and Medicaid Services/Office of Research, Development, and Information [ORDI], 2008).

Nearly a third of the elders receiving home care through the New York City program have moderate to severe dementia and have some degree of cognitive impairment (Hokenstad, Ramirez, Haslanger, & Finneran, 1997). In fact, in a study of elders with Alzheimer's disease living in the community, more than half of the sample received ADL support from home care paraprofessionals. Moreover, a quarter of the sample received *all* ADL care from such paraprofessionals (Albert et al., 1998).

Home care paraprofessionals are typically referred to as "home attendants" (HAs). Older adults with disabilities who meet income requirements are eligible, and an algorithm used by the New York City Health Resources Administration assigns blocks of hours according to severity of ADL limitation, medical conditions, and availability of informal care. Home attendant time is allocated in 4-, 8-, 12-, or 24-hour blocks, with weekly visits from a visiting nurse service and quarterly reevaluation of the elder by the subcontracted home care agency. Home care agency care coordinators supervise groups of attendants, and HAs are required to meet in-service requirements on a regular basis.

The difficulty of the HA-client relationship is apparent in a number of ways: HAs are family and not family; they perform roles typically assumed by family but are also performing a job. They may care for more than one client at a time, sometimes in "cluster care" arrangements. They are often asked to perform tasks outside the scope of their duties. They have to get along with other family members. They are isolated for a large part of the day with a person who has some authority over them but is also dependent on them.

Albert's interviews with 70 home attendants from two home health care agencies provide insights into their situation. These were seasoned paraprofessionals; inclusion criteria required that they had at least 1 year of experience. The interviews revealed that HAs in New York City were almost exclusively female, members of minority groups, and largely immigrants. Their median age was 49 years, and the median length of time they had been in the United States was 17 years, suggesting that these women were well-established breadwinners for their families. They had worked as HAs for a median of 9.5 years, and most were working full-time (with overtime) in this capacity. The median number of clients they had been assigned over time was 12, and one of every four clients was reported to have dementia.

In their current situation, the median number of hours spent with the index client was 55.0 per week over a median of 4 days per week.

The high number reflects the large number of HAs spending 24 hr/day with clients for 3–4 days per week. (More recently, the NYC Human Resources Agency that administers the program has begun to reduce 24-hour shifts.) The large number of hours per HA also reflects the low-wage nature of the work and the need for these women to work extremely long hours. In fact, 44% of the HAs had another client, and the median number of hours for such second clients was 12.0 per week.

The median age of their clients was 82, of whom 86% were women. HAs reported that more than half the elders showed signs of depression and that approximately 40% had Alzheimer's disease or stroke. Symptoms of poor health were highly prevalent among clients. About a third were reported to have dyspnea, difficulty swallowing, or severe pain. Cognitive symptoms were also highly prevalent: 62% were reported to have a memory problem, 32% were said to be disoriented, and 5% were said to be vegetative. HAs provided help with bathing, dressing, and outdoor mobility in almost every case, and the majority of clients were also receiving aid in toileting, indoor mobility, and bed/chair transfer. Half of the client sample was incontinent, a third were limited to bed or chair, and 16% could not be taken outside. Thus, these elders were receiving support equivalent to nursing home care.

Home attendants were also asked to rate how difficult it was to provide care for their clients so that correlates of these ratings could be examined. The strongest correlate of perceived "easiness" was client emotional status. "Easy" clients were reported to demonstrate positive affects more frequently than other clients ($r = 0.40$, $p < .01$). They were also seen as more satisfied with the care provided by the HA ($r = 0.30$, $p < .05$). The presence of daily medical symptoms was associated with greater difficulty in providing care ($r = -0.27$), but none of the other indicators of poor function or general medical status achieved statistical significance. Severity of functional deficit was not strongly associated with HA judgments of client difficulty, suggesting that HAs view this aspect of their work as a "job," without the emotional valence family caregivers attribute to such care.

Almost all training sessions ("in-services") for home attendants stress the physical demands of care, and not help with practical issues that might mitigate the more emotionally charged challenges of home care. Albert and colleagues have developed a manual, based heavily on their interviews with home attendants, to remedy this gap (Albert, 2002). To give the flavor of this approach, Table 9.4 provides an excerpt from the manual.

Developing training in this practical approach to the dilemmas of home care would go a long way to improve the experience of home care

Table 9.4

EXCERPT: HOME ATTENDANTS SPEAK ABOUT HOME CARE

WHAT YOU DO . . . WHEN YOU FEEL YOU CAN'T HANDLE THE JOB BUT FEEL YOU CAN'T GIVE THE JOB UP

Sometimes conditions in a home or with a particular client are just not acceptable. You can notify the agency and complain, or give up the job. But because of the wait to get a new long-term client assignment, you may be reluctant to complain or leave.

One home attendant reported that she did put up with a terrible home situation, where they would not even let her use the toilet, because she did not feel she could afford to give up the job. Another mentioned that she did not report neglect of the client to the agency for the same reason. She was afraid the agency would call the family, and that the family would dismiss her. As she put it, "You cannot tell them. You have to walk into that house everyday. You don't know what they will do to you."

But other home attendants disagreed. "If you feel the family might threaten you or something, you don't want to be there. You don't go back there." Or, as another said, "I am not going to put myself in that kind of predicament. I will tell the agency that they better take me out of there." Even home attendants who had put up with terrible conditions in the past because they felt they needed a job now agreed that it was not a good strategy. Better to quit the job than face abuse.

One complication, though, is concern for neglected or abused clients. "If I see something like that, I don't stay on the job but you feel sorry for the client." Still, no one benefits, neither you or the client, if you keep quiet about a situation of neglect or abuse. The welfare of clients requires that you report the problem to the agency. This allows the agency to arrange for the proper intervention.

How do you let the agency know about a problem with a client or home? Using the telephone in the home may be a problem because of privacy. Clients and families may listen in. One solution is to call while you are out doing errands: "When I call the agency to speak to the coordinator, I always try to call when the client sends me to the store. So I call when I am out in the street."

From Speaking from Experience: Home Attendants Speak about Home Care (Albert, 2002)

---

for both caregivers and care receivers. A second approach would be to "credentialize" paraprofessional care, that is, make it more of a profession, with standardized training, licensure, and opportunity for continued training leading to nursing degrees. This would likely result in wage increases and improvement of work conditions.

Similar challenges appear to be at work among certified nursing assistants (CNAs), who provide the bulk of care, as we have seen, in nursing homes. They provide almost all "bed and body work" for residents and, as a result, have the most daily contact with residents. New efforts are underway to take advantage of the CNA's greater contact with residents to improve resident care, especially in the setting of special care units for people with Alzheimer's disease (see below).

Do CNAs view residents in the same way as nurses or nurse managers? Or does their greater contact with residents lead them to rate residents differently? Albert and colleagues examined this issue in a pilot study. Forty CNAs were asked to nominate a "difficult" and an "easy" resident under their care. They then completed eight questions regarding these residents' behaviors, which were drawn from the nursing home Minimum Data Set form (see above). CNA ratings were compared with the nurse-rated MDS record within the same month.

On the whole, agreement between CNA ratings and MDS scores was low. For example, in the case of verbal abuse, 24 of 40 CNAs reported verbal abuse from the resident, which was recorded in only one MDS chart for this set of residents. On almost every indicator, CNAs reported more symptoms (depressive mood, memory problems, dependence in daily tasks, and physical abuse) than the MDS record. These findings need to be investigated further. It may be that CNAs use different criteria when completing MDS questions, or, more likely, daily contact with residents allows them to identify greater deficits. If CNA ratings were incorporated into MDS records, different resident assessment protocols would be triggered and perhaps more intensive care plans initiated.

Schnelle and colleagues (2009) have developed standardized training and observation protocols to demonstrate that opportunities for more effective care delivery are often missed in the nursing home, and also that specific training for nursing home staff in ADL care, mobility, and psychosocial support result in improved outcomes. Standardized observation protocols also show that many MDS measures recorded by staff do not fully capture resident experience. For example, in one study of standardized observation of ADL care, staff failed to offer residents choices for at least one of three care activities in all 20 nursing homes in the study. In morning ADL care, staff did not offer choices to residents in when to get out of bed (11%), what to wear (25%), and location of breakfast dining (39%). Only two of the 20 nursing homes were cited for this deficiency in formal surveys (Schnelle et al., 2009). In randomized trials of carefully designed training protocols for care delivery by

CNAs, a feeding assistance intervention led to increases in caloric intake and weight gain (Simmons et al., 2008). Similar benefit was evident for continence, mobility, and pain recognition interventions, in some cases with family members noting benefit (Cadogan et al., 2004; Levy-Storms, Schnelle, & Simmons 2007). Related efforts have shown that training CNAs in behavioral management techniques may reduce agitation episodes during ADL care (Burgio al., 2002). These interventions require careful attention to behavior streams to establish relationships between resident and aide behavior (Roth, Stevens, Burgio, & Burgio, 2002). Relationship building is especially relevant for "culture change" efforts in nursing homes, that is, a movement in which nursing homes are attempting to increase the quality of care provided and quality of life for their residents by shifting the focus from being solely responsive to regulatory requirements to placing the resident and staff's needs at the center of care concerns.

Special Care Units for People With Alzheimer's Disease

Freiman and Brown (1996) point out that "today's nursing home population is more functionally and cognitively disabled and requires more skilled and/or specialized care than ever before." Special care units (SCUs) for Alzheimer's disease have been developed to meet this need. The 1996 Medical Expenditures Panel Study (MEPS) found that over 10% of nursing homes in the United States had an Alzheimer's unit, at that time a total of 73,400 SCU beds in just over 2000 homes. SCUs tend to be relatively small, in keeping with the greater staff time and more specialized staff assignments typical of the units. The MEPS survey found that Alzheimer's units contained a mean of 34 beds (Freiman & Brown, 2001).

Despite the growth in specialized care for Alzheimer's disease, at this point there is still no standard definition of an SCU. Units called "SCUs" differ considerably in environmental design, physical separation from other units in nursing homes, specialized dementia care training for staff, staffing ratios, and activity programming (Morris & Emerson-Lombardo, 1994; Teresi, Holmes, Ramirez, & Kong, 1998). This variation has posed difficulties for the assessment of the SCU as a superior approach in Alzheimer's care.

Outcome studies have not found an SCU benefit in slowing the trajectory of functional or cognitive decline (McCann, Bienas, & Evans, 2000; Phillips et al., 1997). The SCU setting, however, may offer benefit in promoting participation in activity (as measured by behavior stream real-time observation) and resident well-being (as observed in ratings of resident affective expression) (Holmes, Teresi, & Ory, 2000). SCU care differs in important but unexpected ways from non-SCU care in residents with similar physical and cognitive status. SCU residents in one study were less likely to be tube fed and more likely to have more extensive care plans, but did not differ in physical restraints and actually were more likely to be prescribed psychotropic medications (Gruneir, Lapane, Miller, & Mor, 2008).

Although results to date have been mixed for SCU evaluations, the evaluation effort has been useful in drawing attention to features of environment and staffing that affect resident well-being. One finding of interest is that environmental simplification for residents with Alzheimer's disease, in the absence of increased staffing, may have negative effects (van Haitsma, Lawton, & Kleban, 2000). On the other hand, changes in lighting may affect sleep patterns, which in turn may affect agitation behaviors (Kutner & Bliwise, 2000). Low levels of light, excess glare, and noise may be environmental sources of excess morbidity for patients with Alzheimer's disease that can be altered easily (Sloan, Mitchell, Calkins, & Zimmerman, 2000). Changing staff assignments so that particular CNAs are assigned to particular residents may also promote resident participation in organized activity (Lindeman, Arnsberger, & Owens, 2000).

The role of nursing home staff, in particular, the CNA, as an agent of resident well-being is only now being fully appreciated. Innovations in the delivery of nursing home care are now underway, and undergoing evaluation, to see whether giving staff greater latitude to change the way they deliver care offers benefit to residents. For example, in one labor-management partnership in New York City, staff on certain demonstration units is free to assign more time to certain activities (such as bathing or feeding), based on their understanding of resident needs and unit dynamics. In another nursing home, CNAs are being encouraged to upgrade clinical skills, communicate information they have obtained about resident health, and participate in comprehensive care-planning meetings for residents. The role of labor-management partnerships in this effort is critical.

Expansion of Options for Supportive Care and Housing

Kane (1995) has identified a series of policy challenges for home care that would give adequate scope to the preference of frail older people to live in homes, rather than institutions, and that would also give greater flexibility to service providers to cross current, fixed service categories. She urges policymakers to think beyond the rigid service categories that have been linked to particular living environments, such as home care, board and care or assisted living care, and nursing home care.

This change has already begun. "Home care" paraprofessionals now assist clients outside the home, as they travel, shop, go to physician appointments, attend adult day care, or simply go outside for exercise or entertainment. "Home care" paraprofessionals also provide ADL care and housekeeping support to frail older people who do not live in "homes" in the traditional sense, but who instead reside in group settings, such as board and care homes, low-income housing, or single-room occupancy hotels (that have become de facto sites for long-term care). This is a welcome development, for it suggests that people can hold on to "home" despite severe ADL needs, and that providing ADL support can be made flexible enough to accommodate different kinds of home settings and preferred personal lifestyles.

Implicit in this expansion of the home care concept is recognition that the nursing home is mostly a residence rather than a site for medical or nursing care. The 24-hour care designation of nursing home care is a fiction. As Kane (1995) points out, "These prescribed settings provide remarkably little nursing care." One study of nursing home care, reported by Kane, showed that 39% of residents received no care from a registered nurse in a 24-hour period. The mean duration of nursing care over this 24-hour period was quite small: for RN care, 7.9 minutes; for LPN care, 15.5 minutes; and for CNA care, 76.9 minutes. Thus, the nursing home is mainly a residence, and care of this sort or degree could be brought into homes, although not necessarily in as cost-effective a manner. "This modest amount of care cannot be replicated at home for the same price because the nursing home efficiently provides stand-by assistance and can meet unscheduled, quickly arising needs" (Kane, 1995). PACE has developed models, however, that allow cost-effective home care service in lieu of nursing home care, provided that housing services are altered to create more easily serviced groups of elders.

While extending what we mean by "home care," it is also worth thinking about ways to extend the flexibility of "service provision." A number of such efforts are underway. One is to allow greater delegation of nursing skills in home care settings. Traditionally, only nurses could administer medications, care for wounds, monitor vital signs, perform catheter or ostomy care, or suction patients who are on ventilators. Kane (1995) reminds us that families have always performed these tasks, and that family members learn these skills from nurses. There really is no reason why less skilled formal caregivers, such as home care paraprofessionals, cannot take on these tasks. It would mean an upgrading of their skills, a boon to family members, and a significant cost savings.

A second development in the expansion of services is a shift in the balance of authority between home care providers and families. The "consumer-directed care" movement, as mentioned earlier, allows elders and their families to use funds assigned for a home care benefit (such as the Medicaid personal assistance home care benefit) to hire, train, and employ home care aides as they think best. In practice, families are helped by home care agencies in this process. The agencies suggest lists of potential workers, provide training and counseling on how to be an employer, and usually manage disbursement of funds.

Finally, families are now being trained to take a more active role in planning for hospital discharge or the end of home health care services. New Web sites, "caregiver navigation programs," and greater emphasis on family involvement in discharge planning will probably place greater emphasis on improving care transitions, which have proven to be one of the greater challenges in long-term care.

SUMMARY

What Is Long-Term Care? "Long-term care" includes the complete spectrum of services and supports required to meet health and personal care needs over an extended period of time. Long-term care primarily provides services that allow older people to meet personal self-maintenance needs, such as bathing, dressing, using the toilet, and the other activities of daily living.

Trends in Long-Term Care Use and Spending. Need for long-term care is best indexed by the proportion of older people with ADL limitations who require personal assistance services. These services are provided in a variety of settings, ranging from the certified nursing assistant in a skilled nursing facility to unpaid family in their homes. In the United States, Medicaid is the primary payer, accounting for about half of these costs for the 9 million older people with ADL limitations and the 1.5 million receiving paid personal assistance services.

Home- and Community-Based Services. In between skilled nursing homes and family care is the wide spectrum of services and providers elders need for supportive care. These include home health care, personal assistance care, adult day care, provision of assistive and medical equipment, and even home modification. States continue to innovate in bundling long-term care services by use of Medicaid waiver options.

Personal Assistance Services and Public Health. Personal assistance services may have beneficial health consequences by effectively managing disabilities that would otherwise put people at risk for poor outcomes. An important area for public health inquiry in home- and community-based services is direct investigation of features of PAS delivery that promote desired health and functioning outcomes. Does PAS allow elders to meet basic provisioning, hygiene, mobility, and nutrition needs? And does effectively meeting these needs, in turn, promote fewer falls, better skin integrity, weight maintenance, and increases in lower extremity strength? Do these outcomes in turn influence well being?

Family Caregiving. Fifteen to 20% of U.S. households provide family caregiving support. Family caregivers face severe challenges in maintaining their own health and well-being under this strain, with consequences on employment and other spheres of life. Yet the contribution of families to elder supportive care is central to elder health and forms the backbone of long-term care delivery in the United States.

Long-Term Residential Care Arrangements. In 2004–2005, the United States had approximately 16,000 certified nursing homes and 35,000 assisted living residences, which served approximately 1.5 million and 900,000 people, respectively. Nursing homes have a national standard for data recording and quality assurance, and this information is available to consumers who need to choose nursing home care. Similar standardization and public access is available now for home health care and may extend to other aging services as well.

Enhancing Long-Term Care. For the individual with severe dementia receiving formal home care services, or the older patient receiving care in a nursing home, dignity, privacy, a sense of security, and the opportunity to participate in meaningful activity or reciprocal social relationships are the essence of sensitive treatment. To reach this goal, we need to take the care preferences of older people seriously, upgrade home attendant and certified nursing assistant care, continue to redesign care environments (such as special care units for people with Alzheimer's disease), and introduce greater flexibility in home care and service delivery, making families partners whenever possible.

Physical Change & Aging

A Guide for the Helping Professions

FIFTH EDITION

SUE V. SAXON, PhD

MARY JEAN ETTEN, EdD

ELIZABETH A. PERKINS, PhD (c), RNMH

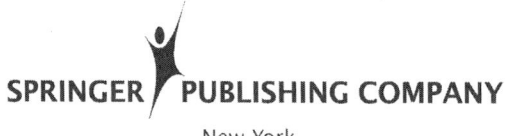

SPRINGER PUBLISHING COMPANY

New York

Copyright © 2010 Springer Publishing Company

All rights reserved.

No part of this publication may be reproduced, stored in a retrieval system, or transmitted in any form or by any means, electronic, mechanical, photocopying, recording, or otherwise, without the prior permission of Springer Publishing Company, LLC, or authorization through payment of the appropriate fees to the Copyright Clearance Center, Inc., 222 Rosewood Drive, Danvers, MA 01923, 978-750-8400, fax 978-646-8600, info@copyright.com or on the web at www.copyright.com.

Springer Publishing Company, LLC
11 West 42nd Street
New York, NY 10036
www.springerpub.com

Acquisitions Editor: Sheri W. Sussman
Project Manager: Megan Washburn
Cover Design: Mimi Flow
Composition: Publication Services, Inc.

E-book ISBN: 978-0-8261-0447-2

10 11 12 13/5 4 3 2 1

The authors and the publisher of this Work have made every effort to use sources believed to be reliable to provide information that is accurate and compatible with the standards generally accepted at the time of publication. Because medical science is continually advancing, our knowledge base continues to expand. Therefore, as new information becomes available, changes in procedures become necessary. We recommend that the reader always consult current research and specific institutional policies before performing any clinical procedure. The author and publisher shall not be liable for any special, consequential, or exemplary damages resulting, in whole or in part, from the readers' use of, or reliance on, the information contained in this book. The publisher has no responsibility for the persistence or accuracy of URLs for external or third-party Internet Web sites referred to in this publication and does not guarantee that any content on such Web sites is, or will remain, accurate or appropriate.

Library of Congress Cataloging-in-Publication Data
Saxon, Sue V.
  Physical change & aging: a guide for the helping professions / Sue V. Saxon, Mary Jean Etten, Elizabeth A. Perkins. — 5th ed.
    p. cm.
  Includes bibliographical references and index.
  ISBN 978-0-8261-0441-0 (pbk. : alk. paper)   ISBN 978-0-8261-0447-2 (ebook)
 1. Aging—Physiological aspects.   2. Geriatrics.   I. Etten, Mary Jean.
 II. Perkins, E.A. (Elizabeth A.)   III. Title.   IV. Title: Physical change and aging.

QP86.S29   2009
618.97—dc22   2009039611

Printed in the United States of America by the Hamilton Printing Company

Sue V. Saxon, PhD, is Professor Emeritus, the School of Aging Studies, University of South Florida. She received her PhD in Developmental Psychology and Counseling from Florida State University and pursued additional graduate work in Physiological Psychology at the University of Wisconsin. She was a Research Psychologist for the National Institutes of Health and for the Laboratory of Perinatal Physiology at the University of Puerto Rico Medical School, before joining the faculty in Behavioral Sciences at the University of South Florida. As a charter faculty member in the Aging Studies program, she has developed and taught numerous courses in aging as well as presented workshops, given in-service training, and authored a number of books and book chapters on aging. She has been designated a Gerontological Pioneer for outstanding achievement and exemplary contributions to the field of Gerontology by the Southern Gerontological Society.

Mary Jean Etten, EdD, was a tenured full professor in the College of Nursing at St. Petersburg College, where she taught nursing, gerontology, and thanatology, and developed innovative curricula teaching hospice care and gerontological nursing. She is currently an adjunct lecturer in thanatology in the School of Aging Studies at the University of South Florida. Dr. Etten received her doctoral degree in Education from Nova Southeastern University. She received an M.A. in Gerontology, an M.A. in Counseling, and an M.S. in Nursing from the University of South Florida and is a gerontological nurse practitioner. She is a fellow in thanatology and is board certified as a music practitioner. She has authored several books and manuals, as well as journal articles, and lectures throughout the United States. She was named Florida Nurse Educator of the Year in 2002 and received the National Association of Gerontology in Higher Education Part-Time Faculty Recognition award.

Elizabeth A. Perkins, PhD (c), RNMH, is a doctoral candidate in the School of Aging Studies at the University of South Florida, where she also completed a BA (summa cum laude) in Psychology. In addition, Ms. Perkins is an RNMH—a registered nurse who is trained specifically to care for people with intellectual and developmental disabilities (IDD). She received her nurse training from the Hereford and Worcester College of Nursing and Midwifery, England. Her clinical nursing and managerial experience has centered on both the general aging population and persons with IDD in nursing homes and residential long-term care settings. She taught the Physical Change and Aging undergraduate course for several years at the University of South Florida, where she has twice received awards for her outstanding teaching. Ms. Perkins' national leadership activities include being the current president of the Gerontology Division of the American Association on Intellectual and Developmental Disabilities. She is also the present co-convener of the Formal Interest Group on Developmental Disabilities for the Gerontological Society of America.

Contents

Preface 285

1 Perspectives on Aging 289
  Basic Concepts in Physical Aging 290
  Patterns of Disease 292

2 Theories of Aging 297
  Stochastic Theories 297
  Nonstochastic Theories 299
  Psychosocial Theories of Aging 301

4 The Musculoskeletal System 309
  The Skeletal System 309
  Age-Related Changes in the Skeletal System 312
  Age-Related Skeletal System Disorders 313
  The Muscles 324
  Specific Age-Related Disorders in Muscles 328

7 The Sensory Systems 333
  Vision 335
  Age-Related Changes in Vision 337
  Age-Related Disorders of the
      Visual System 342
  Audition (Hearing) 345
  Age-Related Changes in Hearing 348
  Age-Related Disorders of Hearing 352
  Vestibular System 353
  Age-Related Changes in the Vestibular
      System 354
  Age-Related Disorders of the Vestibular System 354
  Taste (Gustation) 356
  Age-Related Changes in Taste 356
  Smell (Olfaction) 357

viii Contents

    Age-Related Changes in Smell 357
    Age-Related Disorders in Taste and Smell 358
    Skin (Cutaneous) Senses 358
    Age-Related Changes in the Skin Senses 358
    The Importance of Sensory Changes in Aging 359

8 The Cardiovascular System 361
    Anatomy and Physiology of the Cardiovascular System 362
    Age-Related Cardiovascular Changes 368
    Age-Related Disorders of the Cardiovascular System 371
    Vascular Disorders 385

17 Health Promotion and Exercise 389
    Health Promotion 390
    Disease Prevention 390
    Strategies for Change 394
    Barriers to Health Promotion 395
    Exercise 395
    Age-Related Changes Modified by Exercise 396
    Exercise Programs 398
    General Recommendations for Exercise Programs for Older Adults 400

19 Nutrition 405
    Psychosocial and Cultural Aspects of Nutrition 407
    Physiological Aspects of Nutrition 409
    Water and Body Fluids 410
    Protein 411
    Carbohydrates and Fiber 412
    Fats 413
    Vitamins and Minerals (Micronutrients) 414
    Water Soluble Vitamins 415
    Fat Soluble Vitamins 417
    Minerals 419
    Malnutrition 423
    Undernutrition 423
    Overnutrition 425
    Failure to Thrive 425
    Food Labels 426
    Older Adults and Institutional Diets 427
    Basic Food Groups 428
    The Food Guide Pyramid 429

Nutritional Recommendations for Older Adults   431
Education   432
Supplemental Nutrition   433
Community-Based Nutrition Programs for
   Older Adults   434

20 Medications and the Elderly   439
Cultural Responses to Drugs   441
Older Adults' Responses to Drugs   441
Over-the-Counter (OTC) Drugs   444
Generic Drugs   445
Adverse Drug Reactions   446
Drug Therapy   452
Commonly Prescribed Drugs   453
Attitudes Toward "Pill Popping"   469
Prevention of Drug Accidents   469

Preface

As we are educators in gerontology, it continues to be our experience that many available texts on physical changes associated with aging either present their material in highly technical terms beyond the comprehension of those without extensive basic science backgrounds or else skim over this area superficially. In the years since the fourth edition was published, substantial research on the physical changes that occur with aging has become available. However, it continues to be difficult to separate "normal" aging from pathology, even though it is widely recognized that such a distinction is both useful and necessary in fully understanding the impact of the aging process on the human body and its functions. Data from healthy older adults clearly show that the aging process is not necessarily as devastating as earlier research had indicated, and more effort is currently being directed to the prevention or moderation of age-related changes previously thought to be inevitable. This presents a much more positive and realistic view of aging and allows for greater personal control over our individual aging process by directing attention to significant lifestyle modifications and preventive health care strategies.

Although this book focuses primarily on physical changes and the common pathologies associated with aging, it also considers the psychological and social implications of such changes for human behavior. Since aging is a complex process, it is impossible to consider biological or physical aspects without a comparable concern for the psychological, emotional, and social factors involved.

In this edition we have rewritten, updated, and expanded material throughout the text. We have also included additional material on diagnosis and treatment when relevant, because those who work with older adults will almost always become involved to some extent in their medical care. Major references for additional reading about aging in the various organ systems are located at the end of each chapter, and in Appendix B.

Appendix A includes practical hints for improving safety for older adults. A glossary of medical terms used in the text is also included.

This book was written primarily for those in the helping professions—gerontologists, nurses, social workers, psychologists, rehabilitation specialists, clergy, counselors, and others who seek a better understanding of the physical aspects of aging and their implications for human behavior. It can be used as a textbook for academic courses, for workshops and in-service education, or as a resource for those who would simply like to know more about the aging process. We hope readers will find this book helpful in understanding both the human aging process and ways to improve quality of life in the later years.

S.V.S. M.J.E. E.A.P.

We are especially grateful to Sheri W. Sussman, our editor, whose continued guidance and support made this book a reality.

We appreciate and thank Robert Singer, Jr., who provided technical computer assistance and great patience throughout this project.

Kathy Coughlin, Mary Kate Haver, and Laura Steinmetz of St. Petersburg College have been invaluable in assisting with library research and support for which we are grateful.

We thank them and all others who in any way contributed to the completion of this book.

1 Perspectives on Aging

Demographic changes in the United States have long indicated we are becoming an aging society. In 1900, 4% of the American population was age 65 or older; now approximately 13% of Americans are 65 or older. By 2030, nearly 20% of Americans will be over 65. The fastest growing segment of the older population is those over age 85, the oldest-old. In 1900, life expectancy was 47.3 years; in 2000 it was 76.9 years. Americans who reach 65 today have an average life expectancy of 82.9 years. Many gerontologists, thus, argue that it is necessary to differentiate between those who are "young-old" (65–74), those who are "old-old" (75–84), and the "oldest-old," those over age 85.

Most service providers agree that since needs are generally different in the young-old and older-old groups, services and programs should be planned, oriented, and delivered in different ways for each group. In general, the young-old need more programs and services to reintegrate them into meaningful roles and activities after retirement, whereas the older-old tend to need supportive and protective programs and services. The aging process is, however, so highly individualized that some young-old need supportive and protective services while other older adults prefer reintegrative programs and services. Although chronological age is not an accurate predictor of physical condition or behavior, it is used for convenience and for certain legal purposes (such as voting, Social

Security eligibility, etc.). Using the distinctions "young-old," "old-old," and "oldest-old" serves to focus attention on the enormous diversity in the group we call elderly and suggests differentiations must be made in this large segment of the population if we are to provide effectively for all its needs.

People become more unique as they grow older, not more alike. Because of this, and because aging is a distinct part of the life cycle not yet personally experienced by most of those who work with older adults, understanding older persons is difficult for many in the helping professions. In our attempts to understand others, we often lean heavily on our own personal experiences and can, therefore, empathize reasonably well with a child, adolescent, or young adult. To understand the behavior and perspective of older adults, however, it is necessary to project ourselves into an age context with which we have no personal experience. This is not easy to do and is one of the challenges in working effectively with older adults.

The academic study of the aging process includes gerontology, the broad study of the aging process, and geriatrics, a specialty concentrating on medical problems associated with growing older. Gerontology utilizes multidisciplinary concepts and approaches in an attempt to understand all aspects of the complex aging process. Three academic areas have contributed substantially to gerontology: biological aging, concerned with longevity and how (and why) the body changes as aging occurs; psychological aging, concerned with adaptive capabilities including memory, intelligence, and how individuals cope with their own aging; and social aging, concerned with social roles and expectations for older adults in a particular culture or society.

BASIC CONCEPTS IN PHYSICAL AGING

Research continues to indicate a much more optimistic picture of the aging process than previously presented. There are now increased efforts to differentiate "normal" aging from disease or pathology. It is clear that aging is not synonymous with illness or disease. Certain aspects of the aging process make individuals more vulnerable to illness and disease, but no pathology is inevitable with age. Numerous physical changes historically attributed to aging are now recognized as more likely to be caused by lifestyle variables. For example, aches and pains traditionally attributed to aging are more likely due to a sedentary life style or disuse of abilities rather than to aging per se. "Use it or lose it" is a common adage in gerontology and applies to physical, psychological, and social aging. We will maintain those skills and abilities we continue to use well into older age (barring accident or disease), whereas those we do not use, we will lose.

Obviously, some factors associated with aging are non-modifiable (i.e., genetics, gender, and age), but others can be modified by lifestyle (i.e., exercise, nutrition, smoking, and stress management). Since a substantial part of the aging process depends on lifestyle, we as individuals can make significant choices to increase the probability of healthy, positive aging. Three lifestyle factors having a major impact on the manner in which we age are regular exercise, proper nutrition, and stress management. These, and others, will be discussed in this book.

Lessened Reserve Capacity

The major age-related change in the body is a lessened reserve capacity. All organ systems of the body have a substantial reserve capacity available to deal with high-demand or high-stress situations. With aging, there is a lessened reserve capacity in all the organ systems. Behavioral implications of lessened reserve capacity include:

1. Slowness. Although the aging process varies between one person and another, we all become slower with age. Most older adults are somewhat slower than they once were at taking in, processing, and acting on information. A fast-paced younger person will probably be a fast-paced older person, but will be slower than when he or she was younger. Being slower in a fast paced society is difficult, but it is important to realize that slowness is not synonymous with incompetence. Older adults who are allowed to pace themselves according to their own preferred schedule generally perform exceedingly well, whereas those who are forced into a schedule that is faster than they prefer are likely to perform much less well.
2. Stress. The body calls on its reserves to deal with high stress or prolonged stress situations. The impact of stress tends to be greater on older adults because of their lessened reserve capacity. Being able to pace stressful situations appropriately helps older adults offset the impact of lessened reserve capacity.

3. Homeostatic Equilibrium. Homeostatic equilibrium becomes more precarious as reserve capacity decreases with age. Homeostasis refers to a dynamic equilibrium that must be maintained in the body's internal environment. All the body cells depend on a constant internal environment in order to function properly. Although there is a range of variation possible in the internal environment, if homeostatic processes such as blood pressure, blood gases, acid-base balance (acidity or alkalinity of blood), and blood sugar become too high or too low, the individual will not survive. Highly complex regulatory mechanisms in the body help maintain homeostatic equilibrium. With age and a lessened reserve capacity, it is easier for homeostatic balance to be disrupted, and once disrupted it is difficult to restore. For this reason, older adults are more vulnerable to illness, disease, and accidents. Biological aging is sometimes considered to be a decline in the ability to maintain homeostatic equilibrium, leading to impaired function and ultimately to death. It is, therefore, necessary for older adults to be particularly attentive to health maintenance behaviors and healthy lifestyles.
4. Pacing. Being able to pace oneself, or doing things in one's preferred way and time frame, becomes increasingly important in older age as one way to decrease the impact of lessened reserve capacity. Those who work with older adults need to allow for pacing if they wish to help those older adults perform effectively and competently.

PATTERNS OF DISEASE

Illness and disease are common in older adults, although no specific disease is inevitable in older age. As research becomes more concerned with the dynamics of normal aging, and as health promotion and education for older adults becomes more available, many diseases currently associated with aging may be prevented. If not prevented, they may at least be delayed until extreme old age by healthy lifestyle choices and greater attention to health maintenance.

Diagnosing and treating illness/disease in older adults becomes complex because:

1. Many older persons have several health problems that need to be treated concurrently (comorbidity). An already existing problem

may mask a new one, and medications desirable for one health problem may exacerbate an existing health condition.
2. The symptoms older persons describe may not be the classic symptoms characteristic of younger individuals. For example, older adults may have a "silent" heart attack and not experience the classic or usual symptoms. A ruptured appendix may be reported as an upset stomach or abdominal cramps.
3. Older adults tend to expect pain and discomfort as they age, and may not report symptoms until a medical problem is far advanced. Those who work with older adults need to encourage them to report unusual symptoms that arise and not assume they are just signs of "old age."

Because greater numbers of people are living into older age than ever before, an accurate understanding of how body functions change with age and the implications of those changes is becoming increasingly important for all who work with older adults and for those who wish to know more about the best kind of preparation for their own old age. The aims of this book can be summarized by four major perspectives:

1. **Aging is a highly diverse process.** Chronological age is not a reliable predictor of specific organ system efficiency. There is enormous variation in the rate of aging both among individuals of the same chronological age and in the body systems of a given individual. This is because some organ systems age more rapidly than others depending upon heredity, diet, exercise, and stresses caused by past illnesses and the environment.
2. **Importance of reserve capacity.** In spite of individual variations, the body organ systems, unless stressed, generally continue to function quite adequately in older age although there is some loss of reserve capacity. Stress results in reduced efficiency and/or inability to cope. Proper nutrition, exercise, pacing one's self, and regulating the environment to be maximally supportive are all positive ways to help offset the impact of physical aging in the body.
3. **Accident Prevention.** Age-related physical changes increase the possibility of accidents and injury. Older persons and those working with them need to become extremely sensitive to and aware of situations that may contribute to accidents. Recovery time from accidental injury is usually longer for older adults, and

often accidents are the first step in the transition from independence to dependence. Consequently, accidents have profound physical, psychological, and social significance for older adults' lives. Every effort should be directed toward preventing accidents.
4. **Increase health promotion and health maintenance activities.** Older adults are more susceptible to disease than younger adults. Some physical changes associated with age lead to the loss of body reserves. These changes increase the older person's vulnerability to illness. Greater emphasis on health promotion and health maintenance education for older adults allows them to become more actively involved in their own health and to feel they have more control over aging.

We do not intend by the recitation of the physical changes and diseases associated with aging to overemphasize decline and deterioration as an inevitable part of growing old. Indeed, many individuals are not drastically handicapped by age-related changes in their body systems. We believe others would be less impaired if they knew more about health promotion and health maintenance along with ways to adapt more efficiently to their individual aging process. The detrimental effects of age are a threat to self-image, to feelings of self-worth, and to independence, all of which are crucial to a satisfying and enjoyable life. Although physical changes are a reality of growing old, there are numerous ways to mitigate their impact and cope with them so as to at least partially offset the disabilities or limitations they impose. We suggest that gerontology and other helping professions place more research and educational efforts in helping older adults cope and adapt most effectively.

Although there are many different formulas for "successful aging," most include the following:

1. Admit and accept the reality that aging imposes some limitations. Conserve energy, keep involved with life, make appropriate choices about use of time, and pace life realistically in accordance with needs, desires, and abilities.
2. Be willing to change or modify lifestyle as necessary, especially physical activities and social roles. Remain flexible both mentally and emotionally. Reduce stress whenever possible. Plan a lifestyle to minimize disabilities and maximize remaining abilities.

3. Develop new standards for self-evaluation and new goals. Measure self-worth by inner values, such as the quality of human relationships, spirituality, and the appreciation of life, and not just by how much one can produce and achieve. Be a graceful receiver as well as a graceful giver. Older age can be a time of creativity and self-actualization if we choose to make it so.

Theories of Aging

There is no consensus as to how or why biological aging occurs, and although numerous theories have been proposed, no single theory is accepted as an adequate explanation of the complex aging process. Much of the available research in this area has involved subhuman species and thus generalizations to humans is problematic; in addition, all of the current theories are in need of further research verification. Explanations of biological aging range from genetic influences, to changes at the cellular level, to a consideration of entire organ system changes. Some of the better known theories of biological aging, as well as selected relevant theories of psychosocial aging, are included in this brief overview of the topic. Biological theories can be grouped into two types: stochastic and nonstochastic (Meiner, 2006; Mauk, 2006; Jett, 2008).

STOCHASTIC THEORIES

These theories view aging as caused by a series of adverse changes in the cells that lead to replicative errors. These changes occur randomly and accumulate over time. Four theories of this type are the wear and tear theory, error theory, cross-linking theory, and free radical theory.

Wear and Tear Theory

The wear and tear theory is one of the earliest attempts to explain biological aging changes. It is based on the assumption that continued use leads to worn out or defective parts of the body. This process is presumably further affected by the accumulation, over time, of by-products in cells and tissues that are detrimental to the tissues' normal functioning. This theoretical perspective ignores the various repair mechanisms available in the body, and the fact that, in some cases (such as the muscles), use contributes to increased strength and improved functioning.

Error Theory

This theory is primarily concerned with cumulative mistakes in DNA (deoxyribonucleic acid) and RNA (ribonucleic acid) with age. If random errors occur in the "copying" functions of RNA, inaccurate genetic information is copied and transmitted, impairing cell functions. Thus, aging and death are presumed to be the result of errors that occur and are transmitted at the cellular level. Research has not provided adequate support for this theory; however, it has stimulated a great deal of research.

Cross-Linking Theory

Elastin and collagen (connective tissue proteins that support and connect body organs and structures) figure prominently in this theory. Collagen is the most variable and widespread of all body tissues. With age, both elastin and collagen tissues change from molecules that are loosely associated with each other (making the tissues flexible) to molecules that become more closely associated, or cross-linked (making the tissues less flexible and more rigid). Cross-linking not only lessens the flexibility of these tissues, but also affects the accessibility of white blood cells to fight infection, decreases access to nutrition, inhibits cell growth, and reduces the ability to eliminate toxins that are by-products of metabolism. Age-related changes in skin tissue are a good example of cross-linking. Although cross-linking occurs in some other proteins besides collagen and elastin (in DNA, for example), most of the available research has focused on these two particular tissues. Research on cross-linking continues to some extent, but how to prevent cross-linking and its actual impact on aging has yet to be explained.

Free Radical Theory

Free radicals are chemical by-products of normal cell metabolism involving oxygen. Ozone, pesticides, and radiation may also produce free radicals. It is also possible that gasoline and by-products of plastic production produce free radicals. Free radicals are extremely unstable and last only a brief time (a second or less), but they are highly reactive chemically with other substances, especially unsaturated fats. Protective enzyme systems or natural antioxidants in the body usually quickly destroy free radicals. Nevertheless, some may escape and accumulate, damaging cell membranes, altering normal cell activity, and ultimately causing the death of cells. With age, the body's ability to neutralize free radicals decreases. Vitamins E and C are naturally occurring antioxidants in the body, and research on prevention of free radicals has focused on these as well as other vitamins and dietary supplements. Melatonin, coenzyme Q10, niacin, and food additives BHT and BHA are all being investigated for their possible antioxidant roles. The free radical theory is still an active research area.

NONSTOCHASTIC THEORIES

These theories view aging as caused by replicated errors in cells that are intrinsic and predetermined or programmed. Theories in this category are programmed aging theory and immunological or immunity theory.

Programmed Aging Theory

Hayflick and Moorehead (1961) raised the possibility that a biologic or genetic clock may determine the aging process. Noting that human fetal fibroblastic cells (connective tissue cells) maintained in tissue cultures outside the body (in vitro) were able to divide approximately 50 times before deteriorating, they deduced that this is a form of programmed aging at the cellular level. Life expectancy was thought to be preprogrammed in a species-specific range.

Immunological Theory, Also Referred to as the Immunity Theory

This theory deals with the immune system of the human body, which is composed of a series of responses that protect it against invasion of foreign materials, viruses, and bacteria. The bone marrow, spleen, thymus gland, and lymph nodes are the major organs of the immune system. Since the thymus gland, which is significant in the development of the immune system, decreases in size with age, and since immune system functioning declines with age, considerable research activity has been directed toward understanding the significance and implications of thymic developmental changes. The thymus gland is of maximum size in late childhood or early adolescence. It begins to atrophy (shrink) in the teens, and by middle age only remnants of the thymus remain. In old age the thymus is probably still functional, but the amount of thymic tissue remaining is quite small.

Materials that initiate an immune response are called antigens. The body responds to antigens by producing antibodies (complex proteins) that combine with antigens to inactivate and destroy the invading material. The immune system is designed to recognize and ignore its own tissues, and to attack and destroy invading foreign substances. With age, the immune system becomes less effective in warding off these invading substances, a process called immunosenescence. In addition, it loses the ability to distinguish between its own tissues and the invading materials and begins to attack and destroy its own tissues (an autoimmune response). Therefore, if cells of the body are somehow changed with aging, these changed cells may not be recognized as body tissue and an autoimmune response will be triggered to destroy them. Autoimmune antibodies tend to increase with age. Older adults often have a decreased immune response, as evidenced by decreased resistance to disease, decreased ability to initiate the immune response, and, very likely, more autoimmune disorders. There is currently considerable research interest in the relationship of the immune system to aging.

Emerging Areas

Of particular interest are the role of DNA in the aging process and the specific role of genetics in an individual's aging process. The mapping, or identification, of the human genome will certainly add to our understanding of biological aging. Another research development of particular interest is the role of telomeres in determining the process of aging. Telomeres are areas at the ends of chromosomes that may act as "biological clocks." Each cell division in normal human cells results in a loss of part of the telomere; they shorten with age. In "abnormal" cell production, such as cancer, an enzyme, telomerase, is produced which adds telomere sequences to the ends of chromosomes at each cell division. Research is currently focused on attempts to prevent the production of telomerase to stop cancer cells from multiplying. Other new theories of biological aging include the neuroendocrine control (pacemaker) theory and the caloric restriction theory. The neuroendocrine theory is in the early stages of development and assumes that changes in the brain and endocrine system cause aging. Specific hormones under investigation include estrogen, growth hormone, and melatonin. The hypothalamus-pituitary-endocrine gland feedback mechanisms are also currently under scrutiny for their roles in the aging process. The caloric restriction (metabolic) theory is based on earlier research indicating that caloric restriction in diet increases life span, slows metabolism, and at least delays the onset of a number of age-related diseases. A final theoretical view of aging is the apoptasis theory, which studies cell death as a noninflammatory, gene-driven process occurring normally in the body. When regulated properly it is beneficial to the body, but dysregulation may cause aging (Miller, 2009).

PSYCHOSOCIAL THEORIES OF AGING

Theories of psychosocial development consider the ways in which the experiences of earlier years contribute to behavior in later years. Even though there is a dearth of empirical data for these views, a few attempts have been made to devise a series of developmental tasks encompassing the entire life span. These attempts are based on the assumption that specific tasks are expected to be encountered and learned at certain points or stages in the life cycle. Failure to master developmental tasks at the appropriate time presumably interferes with personal-social adaptation and with adjustment to the next stage and its specific tasks. Although these age-stage approaches are not acceptable to all, and supporting research is generally lacking, a developmental perspective does provide guidelines to society's expectations for individual behavior at different ages. This perspective may be useful in working effectively with older adults.

Maslow's Hierarchy of Basic Human Needs

Abraham Maslow (1968) proposed a hierarchy of basic human needs that motivate human behavior. As the needs of one level are met, the individual strives to meet the needs of the next level. According to the hierarchy, those needs necessary for survival are the most basic. Maslow's hierarchy of needs includes:

1. Physiological or survival needs—food, water, and oxygen—that must be met in order to live. These take priority over all other needs.
2. Safety and security needs are met after physiological needs are satisfied.
3. If physiological and safety and security needs are met, needs for belonging or affiliation become important. According to Maslow, humans have basic needs to belong, to be loved, and to be accepted.
4. Esteem needs are next in this hierarchy. Once the previous needs are met, individuals need to develop a sense of self-esteem, or self-worth.
5. The final and highest level of Maslow's hierarchy is the need for self-actualization. This is the need to develop one's potential to the fullest. Some characteristics of self-actualization are acceptance of self and others, effective problem solving, self-direction, appreciation of new experiences, identification with and concern for others, creativity, and strong personal values.

Maslow's hierarchy could conceivably be useful in planning programs and services for older adults. For example, if an older person is having difficulty meeting his or her safety and security needs, that person will have little energy or motivation to invest in a program promoting self-esteem or self-actualization. In this theoretical perspective, it is necessary to address each individual according to the personal needs that are the most pressing at the moment. This strategy will facilitate that person's growth and development toward the satisfaction of higher needs.

Erikson's Stage Theory of Development

Erik Erikson (1963) was one of the first theorists to suggest a psychosocial stage approach to the entire life cycle. He proposed a series of developmental "crises" that the individual resolves in either a predominantly positive direction or a predominantly negative direction. For instance, the developmental crisis in a child's first year is to develop a sense of basic trust rather than mistrust. Obviously, few if any children are going to develop a sense of total trust, but children who have a preponderance of positive experiences with others rather than a preponderance of negative experiences will undoubtedly develop a stronger sense of trust. The adjustments or attributes a person chooses at any stage may be reversed or altered later, depending on the nature of his or her interpersonal relationships and the environment. It is important not to view Erikson's stages as either-or phenomena or as adjustment choices that irrevocably determine the future direction of development. We will only consider middle age and older age stages here.

Middle Age: Generativity vs. Ego Stagnation

Middle age involves a changing time perspective in which individuals become more aware of the finiteness of life. The desire to leave a legacy or to leave some tangible evidence that one's life was lived becomes an important developmental concern at this time. Interests and concerns broaden to include social issues and/or succeeding generations rather than a focus on self and contemporaries. Failure to resolve earlier psychosocial demands, however, may result in increasing preoccupation with self and rigid adherence to the familiar.

Late Adulthood: Ego Integrity vs. Despair

In older age the major developmental task is to review one's life, reconcile successes and failures, and put it all into perspective. If this process is accompanied by feelings of self-worth and satisfaction in knowing one did the best one could in various life circumstances, ego integrity will be achieved. If life is viewed as a series of failure experiences, and the individual feels he or she was inadequate to meet most of life's demands, despair may well follow. How one met earlier life challenges or psychosocial crises will have a bearing on the resolution of this final stage.

Peck's Tasks of Middle and Old Age

Although Erikson covered the entire life cycle in his system of eight stages, the last two stages included the final 40–50 years of adult life. In an effort to address significant issues of later adulthood, Robert Peck (1968) subdivided Erikson's last two stages into seven specific tasks. One difference between Erikson's and Peck's positions is that Peck proposed four specific tasks for middle age and three for older age. According to

Peck, the tasks for each age may be dealt with simultaneously rather than in a specific order. Sequence is not necessary.

Peck's four tasks for middle age are:

1. Valuing Wisdom vs. Physical Powers. As physical strength and endurance decrease in middle age and the later years, it becomes necessary to shift one's value system to gain satisfaction and a sense of ego competence from mental activities rather than relying strictly on physical competence. Mental or intellectual abilities hold up well with age (barring accident or disease), whereas physical abilities peak in young adulthood and begin to decline gradually thereafter.
2. Socializing vs. Sexualizing. In middle age, Peck suggests people redefine their relationships with both sexes to stress friendship and companionship rather than "playing the sexual game" and relating to others primarily on the basis of physical attractiveness or sexual desirability. Obviously, Peck does not suggest that sexual relationships should be replaced by companionship roles, but urges the broadening of criteria for meaningful relationships to include other personal qualities as well as those specifically related to sexuality.
3. Cathectic Flexibility vs. Cathectic Impoverishment (Emotional Flexibility vs. Emotional Rigidity). Emotional flexibility involves the ability to reinvest emotional energies in new relationships and new roles as older, well-established emotional attachments undergo changes with age. Those who are unable or unwilling to continue investing emotionally in new friendships, new social roles, or change in general may find themselves isolated since change is a prime ingredient in life.
4. Mental Flexibility vs. Mental Rigidity. As in emotional flexibility, it is also necessary to remain mentally or intellectually flexible in order to cope and adapt effectively.

Peck's three tasks for older age are:

1. Ego Differentiation vs. Work Role Preoccupation. Older adults who cling to previous lifestyles or work roles as measures of their self-esteem find these criteria inadequate if they are removed from such lifestyle roles or are unable to perform them satisfactorily. Older adults who value themselves as worthwhile, however,

can enhance their self-esteem through a variety of continuing positive interactions with others.
2. Body Transcendence vs. Body Preoccupation. Those older adults who are able to rise above preoccupations with their health or the physical changes associated with their own aging process are better able to maintain an interest in, and derive personal satisfaction from, life in the later years than those who become preoccupied or obsessed by evidence of poor health or physical changes.
3. Ego Transcendence vs. Ego Preoccupation. Older adults who are able to see beyond themselves and maintain an active interest in society and people are more likely to see themselves and their lives in a positive perspective.

Other Developmental Views

Adolescence is still extremely significant in our culture since the transition from child to adult generally occurs (or is expected to occur) during this stage. Unfortunately, our culture has no clearly defined and universally accepted guidelines for determining when the transition is complete. Therefore, adults, especially parents, may not behave consistently toward the adolescent, who is considered to be an adult in one situation but may be treated as a child in another. Neither parents, friends, society, nor the adolescent know when the transition to adult status has been completed. This uncertainty increases the possibility of conflict. In addition, many important life decisions are made at this time, such as career choice, education, marriage, parenthood, and establishment of an independent lifestyle and personal identity. Establishing a firm sense of personal identity and independence becomes paramount.

Early adult years are an experimental stage in which young people test their ideas against reality. The young adult begins to establish him or herself as an independent person testing self against the realities of work, home, civic, religious, recreational involvements, and interpersonal relationships.

Middle age is a consolidation stage, which for many is a time for intensive reevaluation of self and life. Middle age involves a changing time perspective with the realization that half of one's life is over and that one needs to set priorities for the last half of life. Emphasis here is specifically on coping with the physical and psychological implications of impending old age. Menopause in women, climacteric changes in men, gray hair, wrinkles, and less energy and stamina are all physical signs of age. Some middle-agers experience depression as a number of psychologically significant events often cumulate at this point in the life cycle: children leave home, career and financial abilities peak, parents and friends begin to die, and one's time perspective changes to time left to live. For those who fear old age and death, depression and psychological problems are more likely to occur. Some make drastic changes in their lifestyle (divorce after 20 or 30 years of marriage is not uncommon); others have a "last fling" of infidelity to substantiate their sexual prowess and attractiveness; and some experience actual emotional breakdown.

On a more positive note, however, middle age can be a highly satisfying period of life. Many find new interests, intensify current interests, and set new priorities for the meaningful use of time. Middle age is for many a time of competence and mastery, the prime of life, and a very comfortable stage.

Older age tends to be a time for evaluating one's life. A major task is to work through a life review—a purposeful, constructive effort to review one's life and put it into perspective—and to cope with cumulating losses that usually occur with advancing age. A sense of personal integrity and the comfort of believing that one's life was well-lived and was generally satisfying are important achievements during this period.

SUMMARY

Human behavior involves complex interrelationships among physical, psychological, and social factors. Both the nature and significance of bio-psycho-social interrelationships change as aging occurs. Each individual remains a unique and complex being throughout life and can only be properly understood from a holistic perspective.

REFERENCES

Erikson, E. (1963). *Childhood and society* (2nd ed.). New York: Norton.
Hayflick, L., & Moorehead, M. (1961). The serial cultivation of human diploid cell strains. *Experimental Cell Research, 25,* 585–621.
Jett, K. (2008). Theories of aging. In P. Ebersole, P. Hess, T. A. Touhy, K. Jett, & A. S. Luggen (Eds.), *Toward healthy aging* (7th ed., pp. 26-42). St. Louis: Mosby Elsevier.
Maslow, A. (1968). *Toward a psychology of aging* (2nd ed.). Princeton: Van Nostrand Reinhold.

Mauk, K. L. (2006). *Gerontological nursing*. Boston: Jones & Bartlett.
Meiner, S. E. (2006). Theories of aging. In S.E. Meiner, & A.G. Lueckenotte (Eds.), *Gerontologic nursing* (3rd ed., pp. 19–32). St. Louis: Mosby Elsevier.
Miller, C.A. (2009). *Nursing for wellness in older adults* (5th ed.). Philadelphia: Wolters Kluwer/Lippincott Williams & Wilkins.
Peck, R.C. (1968). Psychological developments in the second half of life. In B. Neugarten (Ed.), *Middle age and aging* (pp. 88–92). Chicago: University of Chicago Press.

4 The Musculoskeletal System

The musculoskeletal system allows us to actively respond to the ever-changing demands of the environment. A complex system consisting of bones, cartilage, joints, muscles, tendons, ligaments, and bursae, its significance is often not appreciated until musculoskeletal limitation or impairment occurs. Mobility and independence depend, in large part, on the integrity of this system. Although age-related changes are not usually life-threatening, musculoskeletal disorders and limitations cause substantial physical and psychological suffering and thus greatly impact the quality of life in the later years. The skeletal and the muscular systems will be discussed separately.

THE SKELETAL SYSTEM

Components and Functions

The skeletal system is composed primarily of bone, although joints, cartilage, and ligaments are also part of it. *Joints,* the junctures between two or more bones (articulations), make possible the wide range of movements and flexibility characteristic of the skeletal system. *Cartilage,* a nonvascular, tough, flexible connective tissue, assists in supporting the skeleton. *Ligaments,* bands of flexible connective tissue, bind bones together and reinforce joints. *Tendons* are fibrous connective tissue connecting muscle to bone, or muscle to muscle.

Bones contain both organic and inorganic components, and are classified according to structure or shape. Bone shape includes four types: long bones, short bones, flat bones, and irregular bones. All these bones contain varying proportions of compact or cortical (hard, dense) bone, and cancellous (spongy) bone. Cancellous bone contains small cavities filled with marrow that are usually enclosed by compact bone. Human bones range in size from the size of a pea (a small bone in the wrist) to the femur (thigh bone), which is almost two feet long. Bone, an active and dynamic tissue, is constantly changing by "remodeling." During this process, osteoblasts create new bone (bone deposition) and osteoclasts prepare bone for resorption (removal by absorption). Bone remodeling is not uniform throughout the skeleton, although it goes on continuously.

The 206 named bones in the human skeleton are divided into axial and appendicular skeletons. The skull, spinal (vertebral) column, and thorax (bony chest) comprise the axial skeleton. It forms the upright axis of the trunk and protects the brain, spinal cord, heart, and lungs. The appendicular skeleton consists of the bones in the arms and legs, as well as the shoulder and hip girdles that attach the limbs to the skeleton.

The spinal column deserves further discussion, since it is a significant structure affected by the aging process. It contains 26 vertebrae (33 in infants, but several fuse by adulthood) and extends from the skull to the pelvis, where it ends in the coccyx (the "tail bone"). The spinal cord runs through a central cavity and is protected by the vertebrae, which are separated from each other by intervertebral discs, cushion-like pads that are partially fluid-filled. Intervertebral discs act as shock absorbers and provide flexibility for the spine. The divisions of the spinal column are: (a) cervical, including 7 vertebrae that are somewhat thin and light, allowing for flexibility; (b) thoracic, including 12 vertebrae that are attachments for the ribs and heavier than the cervical vertebrae; (c) lumbar, including 5 vertebrae that are dense and heavy for weight-bearing and supporting the lower back; (d) sacrum, formed by 5 fused vertebrae that strengthen the pelvis; and (e) coccyx, formed by 3 or 4 fused vertebrae.

The functions of the skeletal system are:

1. Support for all soft body organs.
2. Protection of the brain, heart, and lungs.

3. Movement, in conjunction with muscles, acting as a leverage system to push, pull, and lift.
4. Storage for fat and minerals (calcium, phosphate, sodium, sulfur, magnesium, and copper). Stored minerals are released into the bloodstream and used by the body as needed. Mineral withdrawals and deposits occur almost constantly.
5. Blood cell formation, occurring within bone marrow (Marieb & Hoehn, 2007).

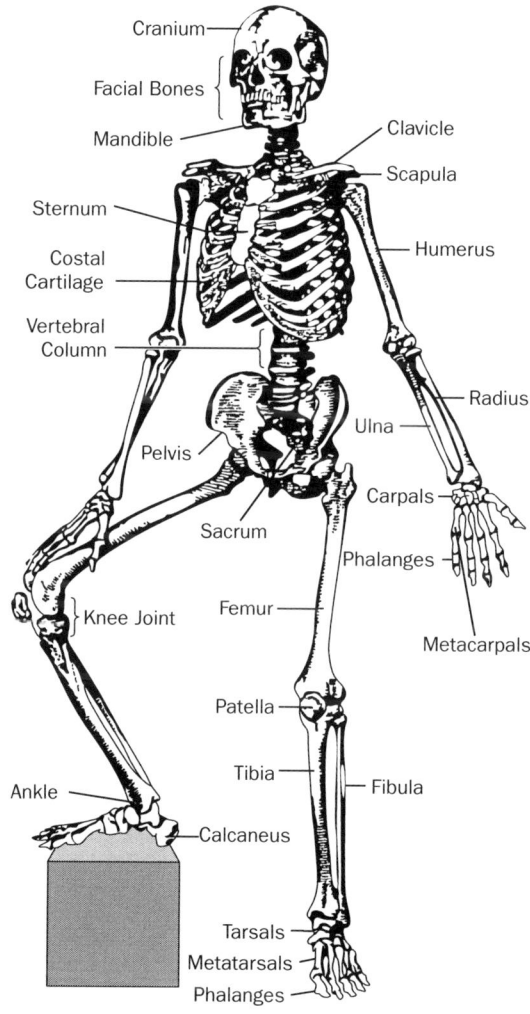

Figure 4.1. The skeleton

AGE-RELATED CHANGES IN THE SKELETAL SYSTEM

1. The primary, and probably most significant, age-related change in the skeletal system is the gradual loss of calcium from bone. Bone mass peaks at about age 35, after which there is a gradual loss of bone mass and bone density (osteopenia). Some of the factors influencing bone loss include genetics, smoking, excess consumption of alcohol, and hormonal factors (Linton, 2007). This is a nearly universal age-related change, irrespective of body size, race, or gender, although women tend to lose more bone mass than men (Meier, 1997; Mauk, 2006). If loss of bone mass becomes great enough to produce fractures, unremitting pain, or immobility, the process is considered pathological and is called osteoporosis. In aging, the balance between new bone formation and bone resorption is disturbed, and bone resorption begins to exceed bone formation. This results in a loss of both bone mass and bone density. Consequently, bone strength declines with age. Loss of bone mass varies both between and within individuals.
2. Aging affects the cartilage in the body's joints. Cartilage surfaces become rougher in joint areas receiving the greatest stress. This reduces flexibility and the cushioning effect of normal cartilage, allowing bones to rub against bones resulting in pain and restriction of joint movement. Hydration, or water content, in cartilage also decreases with age. Some of the change in cartilage may be attributed to wear-and-tear over the years, but since individuals who have led sedentary lives also experience these changes, there appears to be some internal process contributing to joint changes with age (Loeser & Delbono, 1999).
3. Normally, vertebrae are separated by intervertebral discs that both separate the vertebrae and act as shock absorbers in the vertebral column. Cartilage of the intervertebral discs changes with age by losing fluid and becoming stiffer or less compressible, restricting body flexibility. Lower back pain, common in older age, may reflect these age-related degenerative changes. Compression of spinal discs and loss of height in individual vertebrae result in some loss of overall height, so older adults are somewhat shorter than they were when younger.
4. Both tendons and ligaments lose strength with age and show some decrease in water content. These changes also contribute

to decreased strength and mobility in the skeletal system (Loeser & Delbono, 1999).

AGE-RELATED SKELETAL SYSTEM DISORDERS

Osteoporosis

The most common metabolic bone disease in older adults is characterized by a gradual, progressive change as the rate of bone resorption becomes greater than the rate of bone formation. This results in reduced bone mass. Although bone mass is reduced, the mineralization of bone does not change significantly. In other words, bones become more porous, fragile, and brittle, but the chemical composition of the bone remains normal. Reduced bone mass sufficient to cause fractures is called osteoporosis (Chestnut, 1994; Linton, 2007). Osteoporosis may be differentiated into primary and secondary osteoporosis.

Primary osteoporosis accounts for most cases of osteoporosis. The cause is usually not completely clear and no other disease state is present that could account for the osteoporosis. There are two types of primary osteoporosis. Type I, or postmenopausal, osteoporosis occurs between the ages of 51 and 75 and is largely responsible for vertebral fractures and fractures of the wrist. It primarily involves spongy, or cancellous, bone. Type II, or involutional, osteoporosis is a slow, age-related bone loss. It primarily occurs in those over 70, and often results in hip fractures and vertebral fractures. It primarily involves compact bone. Both Type I and Type II can be present simultaneously.

Secondary osteoporosis develops secondary to a number of factors or diseases that promote accelerated bone loss. It accounts for fewer than 5% of all cases of osteoporosis. Some possible causes of secondary osteoporosis are drugs (especially corticosteroids), diabetes, chronic renal failure, rheumatoid arthritis, chronic obstructive lung disease, osteomalacia, alcoholism, and immobilization.

Osteoporosis constitutes a major public health problem, especially for older women, and the costs of disability, dependency, and financial hardship are enormous. In the United States, osteoporosis accounts for 1 million hip fractures per year. Approximately 10 million Americans have osteoporosis, 8 million are women and 2 million are men. More than 44 million adults are at risk for this disease (Pharmacological Options for Osteoporosis, 2007). Fractures are the most serious problem associated with osteoporosis. Osteoporosis results in skeletal instability caused by increasingly porous bones that may not be capable of adequately supporting the body.

Fractures are common and are a leading cause of disability and serious restriction of mobility in the elderly. Early fractures typically involve weight-bearing vertebrae, especially those in the lower back. Compression fractures of the vertebrae often go undetected, as initially pain can be minimal. Even simple activities, such as bending, coughing, or sneezing, may cause vertebral fractures in osteoporotic bones. As small fractures cumulate in the spine, though, pain ranges from mild to severe. Over time, these small vertebral fractures undoubtedly contribute to poor posture, chronic back pain, and a shortened stature. Serious vertebral compression fractures cause severe pain and require immediate treatment. The first line of treatment for vertebral fractures usually involves hormone replacement therapy, bisphosphonates, calcitonin, and some degree of activity limitation. Surgical interventions may include vertebroplasty (injection of bone cement into the vertebral body) or kyphoplasty (using an inflatable balloon to expand the fractured vertebral body, removing the balloon, and then filling the cavity with cement). Reported pain relief rates are 70% to 92% with vertebroplasty and 90% with kyphoplasty (Linton, 2007). In older adults it is especially important to be attentive to preventing constipation, urinary retention, falls, and confusion during fracture treatment and in the recovery period.

Fractures of the wrist (Colle's fracture) usually occur when an individual puts a hand out to break a fall. Hip fractures are usually the result of a fall, but in a few cases the weakened joint may break spontaneously without any apparent trauma. When bones become too weak to withstand the force of gravity, they break and the person falls. Optimal recovery from a fractured hip requires appropriate and intense medical care and rehabilitation. According to Meier (1997), fractures of the hip affect twice as many women as men, and the rate in women quadruples with every decade past age 50. Statistics now indicate men also develop osteoporosis, although usually later in life than women. Men tend to have more bone mass than women, do not have comparable hormone depletion such as that which occurs at menopause, and also tend to fall less frequently. Nevertheless, Caucasian men do have a 25% likelihood of a fracture due to osteoporosis in their lifetimes, especially in their later years (Orwoll, 1997; Siddiqui, Shetty, & Duthie, 1999). One year mortality after hip fracture is nearly twice as high for men as it is for women. Factors contributing to osteoporosis in men include decreased testosterone levels, decreased calcium intake and absorption, and lack of regular weight-bearing exercise. Other risk factors identified for women also apply to men. The consequences of hip fractures for men and women can include hospitalization, surgery, nursing home placement, and permanently restricted mobility. Hip fractures are still associated with significant mortality rates.

Another serious consequence of osteoporosis involves postural or alignment problems frequently associated with aging. A "hump-backed" or flexed posture resulting from osteoporotic changes is called kyphosis; S-shaped curvature of the spine is called scoliosis; and sway-back posture is called lordosis. These are relatively common phenomena in older age. Kyphosis and scoliosis, especially, interfere with stability and balance, and may impede walking. A wide-stance or waddling gait is adopted as an attempt to change the center of gravity and offset misalignment created by bone and muscle changes. Kyphosis can also interfere with breathing and digestion.

Specific risk factors associated with the development of osteoporosis are: (a) age (the older, the greater the risk), as bone mass begins to decline after about age 30; (b) female, with women over age 50 having the greatest risk of developing osteoporosis; (c) Caucasian or Asian race; (d) low body weight and petite body build; (e) estrogen deficiency; (f) cigarette smoking; (g) heredity, with those having a parent or grandparent with osteoporosis at greater risk; (h) inadequate calcium and vitamin D intake; (i) alcoholism; (j) excessive intake of caffeine; (k) inactivity; (l) diet high in fat and protein; and (m) taking certain medications such as long term steroids.

Diagnosis of primary osteoporosis is difficult since it has no early symptoms and is not apparent until it is quite far advanced. Often, fractures are the first clear indication of osteoporosis. Other suspicious indicators are reduced height and kyphosis. There are currently no urine or blood tests to accurately diagnose osteoporosis, and standard X-rays do not show loss of bone density until at least 30% of bone mass has been lost. Diagnosis involves a thorough medical history, physical examination, selected laboratory studies to rule out other pathologies, and bone density tests. Dual energy X-ray absorptiometry (DEXA), which assesses bone density of the lower spine, wrist, and/or hip, is considered to be the most accurate procedure for indicating osteoporosis. Individuals who have hip or spine bone mineral density of 2.5 standard deviations or more below peak bone mass are considered to have osteoporosis, whereas those with bone density between

2.5 and 1.0 standard deviations below peak bone mass are considered to have osteopenia. Those diagnosed with osteopenia should be re-evaluated every two to five years. Those within 1.0 standard deviation of peak bone mass are considered to have normal bone density. Other procedures to evaluate bone density are single photon absorptiometry, CAT scan, and ultrasonographic techniques, but the DEXA procedure is currently considered to be the safest and most accurate. The National Osteoporosis Foundation recommends bone density testing for all women over age 65, and for those under age 65 who have one or more risk factors for osteoporosis. As osteoporosis increasingly is recognized as a significant health problem for older men, screening recommendations will be forthcoming for them. Newer guidelines are being proposed to include men 50 and older. These guidelines will utilize fracture-risk calculations from a computerized model (FRAX) to determine the likelihood of an osteoporotic fracture within 10 years. In addition to bone mineral density, it will include age, gender, fracture history, parental hip fracture history, oral steroid use, low BMI (body mass index), secondary osteoporosis, smoking, and alcohol intake. It is expected that DEXA machines will eventually report results in terms of FRAX indicators (Osteoporosis Diagnostic Guidelines Expanded, 2008).

Prevention is the best course. Understanding and modifying the various risk factors associated with osteoporosis (as early in life as possible) are necessary measures in reducing the chance of developing osteoporosis. Some risk factors are fixed and not subject to lifestyle modification, but those that can be modified should be. Education is necessary to encourage healthy lifestyle modifications. Currently, the two prevention and treatment strategies considered especially valuable are regular exercise and drug therapy.

Regular Exercise

Weight bearing exercises stimulate bone growth and are considered significant preventive measures for osteoporosis. Walking is one of the easiest and safest forms of exercise. Brisk walking or other moderate-intensity weight-bearing exercise for 30 to 45 minutes for at least 4 or 5 days a week is recommended, although even a shorter period of time over most days of the week is helpful. In addition, training with weights (resistance training) to strengthen and tone muscles and promote flexibility of the upper body contributes to better posture. Resistance training

The Musculoskeletal System

also reduces stress on the spinal column, which is a source of chronic back pain and body misalignment.

Drug Therapy

Controversy exists over the amount of calcium necessary and the form best utilized by the body, but adequate calcium intake is acknowledged as necessary to help prevent osteoporosis. Recommendations are for 1,200 to 1,500 mg/day for postmenopausal women not on estrogen replacement therapy, and 1,000 mg/day for premenopausal women. Dietary recommendations for men are 1,000 mg/day for younger men and 1,500 mg/day for men over 65. Calcium carbonate is the most widely used form of calcium, although in some individuals it may cause constipation, hyperacidity, and other gastrointestinal complaints. Calcium lactate, calcium gluconate, and calcium citrate are possible alternatives to calcium carbonate. Calcium is absorbed better if taken with food three to four times a day. A higher dose should be taken at bedtime. Vitamin D intake of at least 400 to 800 IU per day is essential for calcium supplementation to be effective, and many professionals are now recommending at least 800 to 1000 IU daily.

Hormone Therapy

The estrogen-progesterone combinations have been considered especially useful in preventing or treating excessive bone loss in post-menopausal women. This treatment remains controversial, however, because of possible increases in the risk of developing breast cancer, gallbladder disease, blood clots, stroke, and heart disease. Risks and benefits need to be carefully assessed by each individual in consultation with a primary health care practitioner. For those who choose not to take hormones, alternative choices include bisphosphonates, such as risedronate (Actonel), alendronate (Fosamax), and ibandronate (Boniva), which have been shown to slow bone loss and increase bone density and have now been approved by the FDA for both prevention and treatment of osteoporosis. Daily dosing schedules have had rather poor compliance, though, because one has to remain upright and not eat or drink for 30 to 60 minutes after taking the medication. Newer weekly or monthly oral doses are now approved, as are quarterly and yearly intravenous doses, which may make compliance easier. Unfortunately, researchers recently identified a rare side effect of these medicines. This side effect, osteonecrosis of the jaw (generalized death of bone tissue), must be considered when prescribing bisphosphonates (Levy & Armbruster, 2007).

Arthritis

Arthritis is a broad term referring to inflammation or degenerative changes in body joints, usually associated with the aging process. Joints, the junctions between bones, involve various types of articulating surfaces that protect bones and maintain smooth joint movements. The ends of bones at most joints are covered with cartilage and enclosed in a capsule. Synovial fluid lines the capsule and acts as a lubricant, which is necessary for smooth movement. Tendons and ligaments also help support and protect joints. Any or all of these structures can be involved in arthritic changes. The three most common types of arthritis are osteoarthritis, rheumatoid arthritis, and gout.

Osteoarthritis

Osteoarthritis, also referred to as OA or degenerative joint disease (DJD), is the most common form of arthritis and is one of the leading causes of disability in those over 65. It is virtually impossible to find anyone over age 60 without some osteoarthritis somewhere in his or her body. At least 20 million Americans have OA (Touhy, 2008). Age alone does not cause osteoarthritis, but age-related changes in cartilage predispose older adults to it. In addition to age, other factors presumed to be significant in the development of OA include obesity, trauma (wear and tear), diabetes, primary disorders of the joints, and genetic predisposition (Gorevic, 2004). OA primarily involves a progressive loss of articular cartilage that exposes the ends of the bones at the joint and allows the bones to rub together resulting in pain, stiffness, and joint instability. Bony growths or bone spurs may appear at joint surfaces and cause enlargement of the joint. Eventually the joint capsule thickens, contributing to restricted movement and joint instability. Symptoms are generally mild early in the disease, with intermittent joint pain, stiffness upon arising, and crepitation (creaking joints). As pain becomes more constant, limitation of movement and joint deformity occur, but inflammation is not usually present. Pain is relieved by rest and aggravated by movement or weight bearing. Eventually pain occurs at rest as well. Restriction of mobility due to joint pain increases stiffness, reduces muscle tone, and adds to weakness and joint instability.

Diagnosis includes a physical examination to detect limitation of motion, pain, tenderness, and deformity of joints. In addition, X-rays may reveal arthritic changes. The degree of arthritic change observed on X-rays does not necessarily correlate with symptoms described by the person. Some individuals with severe degenerative changes apparent on X-rays report few or mild symptoms. In addition, X-rays do not assess changes in cartilage damage; these changes are better assessed using MRI techniques (Linton, 2007).

Specific treatment options include physical therapy, exercise, rest, reduced stress on joints, dietary modifications, drug therapy, and various surgical procedures. Symptom relief depends on rest balanced with an appropriate exercise program, including physical and occupational therapy. Pain control is essential. Other significant components of treatment include exercise and physical therapy aimed at improving range of motion, strength training, increasing the individual's ability to carry out activities of daily living, and remaining independent (Krohn, 2007). Dietary modification often revolves around weight loss since obesity is a definite risk factor for osteoarthritis, especially in the knees. Weight reduction both reduces the risk of OA of the knees, and also generally reduces symptoms in those who already have OA. Drugs most commonly used for osteoarthritis are acetaminophen (usually the first choice) and the nonsteroidal anti-inflammatory drugs (NSAIDs). Side effects of these drugs over long term usage must be carefully monitored. For those with severe pain that is not responding to medications, corticosteroid or hyaluronic acid injections directly into the joint may be helpful, but these should be used infrequently. Other drugs, such as the previously popular COX-2 inhibitors, have been deemed inappropriate in most cases because of serious side effects. Newer drugs are constantly made available for the treatment of arthritis, but these should be carefully evaluated by both individuals and health care providers. Side effects of these medications are common and caution is necessary, especially for prolonged use. Bleeding may occur in the gastrointestinal (GI) tract, so these medications should never be taken on an empty stomach. Constant monitoring is essential.

Educating older adults concerning the advantages, disadvantages, and side effects of various medications that manage osteoarthritis is necessary, as is active involvement of the individual in the treatment program. Management is crucial as there is no cure for OA. If nonsurgical management of osteoarthritis is ineffective, surgical procedures may be indicated. Total joint replacement (arthroplasty) is an effective option if nonsurgical choices do not relieve severe pain and restriction of mobility. Joint replacement now has a 95% success rate in older adults (Linton, 2007). Partial joint replacement (especially in the knee) is another possibility that allows for faster recovery and rehabilitation. Significant advances have occurred in joint replacement surgery, and artificial joints are now expected to last 15 to 20 years or longer and allow for a higher level of activity than previously experienced. In addition, surgeons now have more options for less invasive surgery, which provides for fewer post-surgery complications, faster rehabilitation, and increased mobility.

Rheumatoid Arthritis

Rheumatoid arthritis (RA) is an autoimmune disorder in which the body's antibodies attack body tissues. In contrast to osteoarthritis, rheumatoid arthritis can involve the connective tissues of the entire body, however it is usually manifested in the joints. It is a systemic, chronic disease, with inflammation generally present. Its peak incidence is in people between 40 and 60, although it may appear for the first time in older age. Women are two or three times more likely to get RA than men, but men tend to be more severely affected (Linton, 2007). The etiology is still unknown, but genetic, immunological, and environmental factors are assumed to be significant in rheumatoid arthritis. In addition, exposure to a virus may possibly contribute to the onset of the disease.

In joints, the synovial membrane becomes inflamed and thickens; as the disease progresses, joint capsules and ligaments are stretched and destroyed. Tendons may shorten and move out of their usual position, producing deformity of the joints. Joints are usually involved symmetrically (i.e., the same joints on both sides of the body are involved). Hands and feet are most often affected, but the knee, hip, ankle, shoulder, and elbow can also be affected. Other symptoms include malaise, fatigue, low-grade fever, weight loss, and morning stiffness that lasts for more than one hour. When rheumatoid arthritis occurs for the first time in older age, it often has a sudden onset, but also tends to respond to treatment. Periods of remission are common.

Diagnosis is difficult as several diseases can masquerade as RA, but it generally involves a personal history and physical examination, plus the determination of an elevated erythrocyte (red blood cell) sedimentation rate (a laboratory test of speed at which erythrocytes settle) and the presence of a rheumatoid factor (an abnormal antibody) in the blood. Both of these tests may also indicate other disorders in addition to rheumatoid arthritis, so further evaluation may be required. Other tests include the C-reactive protein test, the antinuclear antibody test, and other specific blood tests. X-rays show some of the changes characteristic of rheumatoid arthritis, but MRIs, bone scans with isotopes, and DEXA scans provide more detailed information that is useful in assessing the progression of RA and the patient's response to treatment therapies.

Treatment is directed toward meeting three realistic goals: symptom relief, preserving joint function by learning to protect joints, and maintaining a reasonably normal lifestyle. Educating the individual and family, and actively involving them in the treatment regimen, is essential since rheumatoid arthritis is chronic, non-curable, and progressively disabling. Psychological support and pain management training are important in managing a long-term chronic disease. Every person with rheumatoid arthritis should engage in an appropriate program that balances exercise and rest. Neither excessive rest nor excessive exercise is therapeutic, and individuals must learn to monitor each of these therapies to prevent further deterioration from inactivity (disuse) and also to prevent exacerbation by excessive wear and tear on the affected joints. Controlling inflammation and relieving pain are obviously primary goals of treatment. Medicines used for RA include NSAIDs with special attention to side effects in older adults. If NSAIDs and physical therapies don't alleviate symptoms quickly, more potent anti-rheumatic drugs may be used since irreversible joint changes can occur within the first year of RA. Disease-modifying anti-rheumatic drugs (DMARDs) may be a more effective treatment, but may also have serious side effects. Gold salts, antimalarial drugs, immunosuppressants, and biological response modifiers (BRMs) are other possible treatment choices. All are potent medicines, have a variety of potentially serious side effects, and must be monitored closely. To further complicate the issue, combinations of these drug therapies are also frequently used. Corticosteroids are sometimes used as a bridging drug until another can be initiated, but long-term use is to be avoided when possible. If pharmacological interventions fail, surgical procedures, especially joint replacement, may be appropriate. Lifestyle modifications recommended for those with RA include heat; rest; weight reduction; regular, but appropriate, exercise; and special modifications in the home, such as utensils, door knobs, and drawer handles, designed for people with physical limitations. Some individuals opt for various complementary or alternative therapies such as acupuncture, homeopathy, selected nutritional supplements, and other approaches to help deal with the stresses of RA. Primary health care providers need to be notified when these options are being used in conjunction with more traditional treatments. Rheumatoid arthritis is a long-term, debilitating disease that is physically, psychologically, and socially difficult to manage. It requires extensive education about the disease, realistic expectations, and ongoing management options for patients and families.

Gout (Gouty Arthritis)

Gout is a disease of faulty metabolism in which there are deposits of uric acid crystals in the joints and an increased amount of uric acid in the blood. The increase in uric acid stems from an inherited defect in purine metabolism. Proteins in the body break down into purines (the end products of nucleoprotein digestion). Purine metabolism produces uric acid, which is usually excreted by the kidneys. Either increased production of uric acid or its faulty elimination cause excess amounts of uric acid to accumulate in the body. Excessive uric acid can form crystals in the joints called *tophi,* which produce inflammation of the joints. This inflammation results in an attack of gout. Attacks are sudden and pain is excruciating, usually lasting from five to eight days during which time the individual is incapacitated. Although the attacks last only for a limited time, repeated attacks usually damage the joints and lead to chronic gout. The joints may eventually become deformed and disabled. Although any joint may be affected, the big toe seems to be a prime site. Gout often occurs for the first time in middle age and is more common in men. Women rarely develop gout before menopause.

Diagnosis depends on the clinical presenting symptoms, a study of serum uric acid, urinary uric acid levels, and a study of joint synovial fluid as well as the material in the tophi. Treatment involves medications such as NSAIDs, colchicine, possible steroid injections into the joint, a diet free of purines, and drugs to lower the amount of uric acid in the blood. Aspirin is not recommended as it may increase uric acid levels. Currently, allopurinol is considered the treatment of choice for preventing further attacks, but it cannot be initiated during an acute flare-up as it could make the attacks worse (Linton, 2007). Individuals prone to gout attacks may need to take medications throughout their lives to reduce uric acid buildup in the blood. Secondary gout is not uncommon, and is associated with certain medical problems (e.g. leukemia or cirrhosis) and with other medications the individual may be taking. Diuretics in particular may cause attacks of gout. Other possible precipitating factors include being overweight; surgery; minor trauma; emotional upset; ingestion of certain foods, especially foods high in purines such as shellfish and organ meats; alcoholic beverages; and drugs (Fife, 1994; Meiner, 2006).

Osteomalacia

Osteomalacia, a metabolic bone disease, is characterized by demineralized bone leading to bone softening, deformity, fractures, and bone pain. This disease may be easily confused with osteoporosis, in which mineralization of bone is essentially normal, but bone mass is decreased. Symptomatology of both diseases is similar, but osteomalacia is not as common as osteoporosis in older adults. Since osteomalacia can be treated fairly easily, it is important to distinguish between these two bone pathologies. The primary cause of osteomalacia is vitamin D deficiency due to an inadequate diet (low in dairy products, fish, and fortified flour), lack of sunlight, liver disease, chronic kidney disease, phosphate deficiency (phosphate is essential to bone mineralization processes), and the use of some drugs (especially anticonvulsants). The classic symptom of osteomalacia is pain in skeletal areas (Linton, 2007). Other symptoms include muscle weakness, fractures, fatigue, and depression. Pain increases with movement.

The diagnosis depends on serum and urine laboratory studies. X-rays are of limited value in distinguishing between osteoporosis and osteomalacia until the disease is far advanced. Bone scans may distinguish between them, but not necessarily in the early stages, and a bone biopsy may be necessary to firmly establish the diagnosis. Treatment is based on the cause of osteomalacia. If it is caused by a vitamin D deficiency, vitamin D replacement and calcium are effective. If it is primarily due to phosphate deficiency it will respond to phosphate salts. If caused by liver or kidney disease, these diseases must be treated as well as the osteomalacia. Those on anticonvulsant medications over long periods of time may also need vitamin D and calcium replacement. Older adults in nursing homes, or those with extremely limited mobility, should be monitored for appropriate vitamin D levels since they are likely to be at high risk for the development of osteomalacia.

Paget's Disease

Paget's disease, a chronic metabolic bone disease, is characterized by excessive bone resorption and excessive formation of abnormal, extraordinarily vascular bone. The entire skeleton is usually not affected, but multiple localized sites may occur. Most commonly affected are the pelvis, spine, femur, tibia, and skull. It rarely occurs in those under 40, and is most often diagnosed in the 60s. Etiology is unknown, but it is likely there is a genetic influence which may be triggered by a slow virus or some environmental factor. Symptoms are usually minimal or nonexistent in the early stages of the disease. Often it is detected by X-ray or an elevated serum alkaline phosphatase level. Bone pain occurs later in the course of the disease and varies from mild to moderate. Pain is primarily associated with deformities of the skull and weight-bearing bones. Severe bone pain generally indicates coexisting arthritis, acute fracture, neurological impairment, or bone lesions. Enlarged skull structures can result in headache, vertigo, tinnitus, and hearing loss (Meier, 1997; Linton, 2007). Bony enlargements at the base of the skull can cause slurred speech, incontinence, visual difficulties, and problems in swallowing if the enlarged bones press on areas controlling these activities. If lumbar and thoracic vertebrae are enlarged, spinal nerves may be pinched or pressured. One of the most serious complications of Paget's disease is malignant bone tumors, which are difficult to detect in the early stages.

Diagnosis depends on finding elevated levels of serum alkaline phosphatase in the blood tests, urine studies, physical examinations, MRIs, and isotope bone scans. Treatment is indicated when pain, bone deformities, neurological complications, and/or medical complications are present. The most effective drug therapies include bisphosphonates, which have replaced calcitonin as the treatment of choice (Linton, 2007). Calcitonin may be given if a person cannot tolerate bisphosphonates (Walsh, 2007). NSAIDs are used to relieve pain and to reduce inflammation. Surgical interventions may be necessary if there are nerve compressions or fractures.

THE MUSCLES

Components and Functions

The three specific types of muscles in the human body are differentiated on the basis of histological (microscopic study of tissues) structure: skeletal, smooth, and cardiac.

Skeletal Muscle

Skeletal muscle, also referred to as striated muscle because of its striped appearance, is attached to and covers the bony skeleton. Some skeletal muscles are attached directly to bones, whereas a band of dense, fibrous tissue (tendon) connects other skeletal muscles to bones. In addition, striated muscle is also found in the tongue, soft palate, scalp, pharynx, upper part of the esophagus, and in extrinsic eye muscles. Skeletal muscles are the true voluntary muscles because they are the only type of muscle normally under conscious control. Mobility of the body depends on skeletal muscles. These muscles are able to contract rapidly and vigorously, but they fatigue easily and need to rest after even short periods of intense effort. Also, muscles must be exercised to maintain their strength and function. Exercising muscles increases the size of individual muscle fibers and promotes strength and endurance. Conversely, disuse results in decreased size of muscles (atrophy) and loss of strength. Muscle strength peaks between 20 and 30 years of age; there is a gradual decline thereafter, however, the rate of decline in strength in the later years may be slowed by remaining physically fit (Marieb & Hoehn, 2007). Muscle atrophy tends to occur more rapidly in older age, so it is imperative for older adults to maintain strength and mobility with appropriate and regular exercise.

Skeletal muscles perform four important functions:

1. *Movement.* Essentially all movements of the body involve muscles. Muscles contract and relax to produce movement. A muscle that causes a specific motion is called the prime mover (agonist), and those assisting the agonist are called the synergists. Muscles causing movement opposite that of the agonist are called antagonists. The antagonist has to relax to allow the agonist to contract and produce movement (Smeltzer & Bare, 1992). For example, bending the arm at the elbow to touch the face involves contracting the biceps muscle and relaxing the triceps muscles opposite the biceps. Muscles act on bones to create an efficient leverage system for pushing, pulling, and lifting. All body movement involves interrelationships between muscles, the bony skeleton, and the nervous system.
2. *Posture.* Skeletal muscles are crucial for maintaining posture against the force of gravity. Although we give little thought to this, skeletal muscles are constantly making necessary adjustments for us to maintain an erect or seated posture. Muscle tone (tonus) is also maintained constantly by some degree of muscle contraction in certain muscle fibers to keep muscles in a state of readiness to respond to contraction stimuli. Muscles with less

than normal tonus are flaccid, while muscles with greater than normal tonus are spastic.
3. *Stabilizing joints.* As muscles pull on bones for movement, they stabilize and strengthen joints.
4. *Heat production.* The fourth function of muscles is heat production. Body heat is a byproduct of muscle metabolism and contraction, and is essential in maintaining normal body temperature.

Skeletal muscle tissue has four special characteristics:

(a) *Excitability,* the ability to respond to stimulation. The usual stimulus for muscle action is chemical, as when a neurotransmitter is released from a nerve cell. The response is the transformation of chemical energy into mechanical energy.

(b) *Contractility,* the ability to contract and become shorter when an appropriate stimulus is received.

(c) *Extensibility,* the ability to lengthen (stretch). Muscle fibers shorten when contracting and lengthen when relaxing.

(d) *Elasticity,* the ability to regain its original shape after having been stretched or contracted.

Smooth Muscle

Smooth muscle, so named because of its appearance, is found primarily in the walls of the digestive tract, trachea (windpipe), bronchi leading to the lungs, urinary bladder, gallbladder, ducts of the urinary and genital organs, walls of the blood vessels, spleen, iris of the eye, and hair follicles of the skin. The action of smooth muscle is typically slow, sustained, and often rhythmical. It is mostly under the control of the autonomic nervous system and usually acts without conscious thought directed to its activity. Thus it is not necessary to will or command the smooth muscle of the digestive tract to begin digesting food. Digestion occurs without conscious attention, but thoughts and emotions do influence the process. For example, some body processes involving smooth muscles previously thought to be involuntary activities, such as digestion, blood pressure, and heart rate, can be brought under at least partial voluntary control by learning conditioning and biofeedback techniques. These interventions have been helpful in managing health problems such as chronic hypertension and muscle spasms. Consequently, the older, clear distinction between voluntary and involuntary muscles has to be qualified somewhat in light of ongoing behavioral research and clinical applications.

Cardiac Muscle

Cardiac muscle is a special kind of muscle tissue found only in the heart. It has its own pacemaker system (a group of cells generating impulses to other areas of the heart), but additional stimulation is provided by the autonomic nervous system. Action is primarily (but not exclusively) involuntary, automatic, and rhythmic.

In summary, muscles are complex in both structure and function, and are among the most remarkable of all body tissues. Although the distinction between voluntary and involuntary muscle action is not always clear, muscle activities primarily under voluntary control include: (a) the maintenance of posture; and (b) the majority of visible movements such as facial expression, locomotion, chewing, and the manipulation of objects. Muscle activities under involuntary control include: (a) propulsion of material through the body (food and blood, for example); (b) expulsion of stored substances (bile from the gallbladder, urine from the bladder, and feces from the anus, although the latter two processes can also be under voluntary control); (c) regulation of the size of some body openings (such as the anus and urethral openings); (d) regulation of the diameter of some tubes (as, for example, the size of blood vessels and bronchioles).

Specific Age-Related Changes in Muscles

1. Muscle strength tends to decline with age due partially to loss of motor units and muscle fibers (Bruce, 1998). Nevertheless, a large body of evidence indicates that regular, appropriate exercise can slow loss of muscle strength and also increase strength, even in very old age. Resistance training is most beneficial (Mauk, 2006).
2. There is some muscle atrophy with age, although how much is due to the aging process and how much to disuse is not clear.
3. The decrease in muscle mass and in contractile force or weakness frequently noted in older adults is called sarcopenia. Sarcopenia increases fatigue, frailty, disabilities, is a major risk factor for falling, and makes activities of daily living more difficult, Therefore it compromises independence in many older adults.

SPECIFIC AGE-RELATED DISORDERS IN MUSCLES

Muscle Cramps

Muscle cramping, or sustained contraction of an entire muscle lasting anywhere from a few seconds to several hours, increases with age. The muscle feels tight and painful. In older adults, muscle cramps frequently occur at night, especially after activity. Cramps commonly affect the thigh, calf, foot, hip, or hand. They result from peripheral vascular insufficiency and can be related to low blood sugar levels, dehydration, irritability of spinal cord neurons, and electrolyte imbalances (especially sodium and calcium). Stretching the muscles prior to sleeping and soaking in a hot tub may be helpful in relieving severe cramping (Meiner, 2006).

Myasthenia Gravis

Myasthenia gravis, a progressive, chronic, acquired autoimmune disease, involves a defect in impulses transmitted from nerves to muscle cells. Antibodies attack and destroy acetylcholine receptors necessary for muscle contraction. Clinically, it is characterized by an unusual susceptibility of muscles to fatigue. One peak period of onset is between 20 and 40, and at this age more females than males are affected. Another peak period of onset is between 50 and 70, with more men developing the disease. Symptoms often first occur in the eyes, the bulbar muscles (those involved in chewing, swallowing, and talking), or the limbs. Ptosis (sagging) of the eyelids is a common early sign of myasthenia gravis. As the disease progresses, muscles of the face weaken and speech may be difficult to understand. Fluctuations in the progress of this disease occur unpredictably.

Diagnosis involves observation of signs of muscle weakness and testing for muscle strength. A CT scan or MRI provides information on possible tumors (particularly of the thymus gland), and blood tests assess other possible pathological states or other autoimmune disorders. Treatment is complex. Anticholinesterase therapy is a major form of first-line treatment, but problems include the possibility of overdosing and the variability of medication effects. When this form of treatment is not effective, immunosuppressive treatment is usually the next choice. Caution is advised because of the high incidence of undesirable side effects in older adults. Many drugs are contraindicated or must be used cautiously.

Polymyalgia Rheumatica

Polymyalgia rheumatica (PMR) is a rheumatic syndrome occurring most frequently in women over age 50. It is characterized by aching and stiffness in muscles of the neck, upper arms, shoulder girdle, and pelvic girdle. Frequently, polymyalgia rheumatica is accompanied by temporal arteritis (also known as giant cell arteritis), which is an inflammation of arteries, especially the arteries serving the temporal area of the brain. Major symptoms of this form of arteritis are headaches, changes in vision, and pain in the jaw. Giant cell arteritis may result in spontaneous blindness. Etiology of both PMR and temporal arteritis is unclear, although genetic and environmental factors are suspected. Both of these conditions are generally self-limiting, but still may last from months to several years. Treatment is necessary, though, to control pain and to prevent blindness.

Diagnosis depends on physical examination and laboratory tests, especially a test of erythrocyte sedimentation rate. A temporal artery biopsy may be necessary to confirm temporal arteritis. Treatment with corticosteroids produces a dramatic and immediate response, but early diagnosis is essential for treatment to be most effective. NSAIDs may be used for pain management.

Bursitis

Bursitis is a soft tissue disorder. Bursae are sacs containing a small amount of fluid. They are located in the joints where tendons or muscles pass over bones. Infection, calcium deposits, overuse, or trauma cause bursae to become inflamed and the fluid in them to increase, causing pain upon movement of the joint. The most commonly affected sites are the shoulder and the elbow. Repetitive movements are a definite risk factor for bursitis.

Diagnosis involves a physical examination and an analysis of daily activities. In addition, X-rays, MRIs, or ultrasounds may be used to assess tissue injuries. Treatment includes rest, ice, and pain medications as necessary. Gentle stretching and range of motion exercises prevent stiffness. In severe situations, extra fluid may be aspirated from the bursa. To prevent reoccurrences, daily range of motion exercises, modified activities that do not repeatedly strain muscles or joints, and protecting joints from excessive pressure are recommended.

SUMMARY

Aging in muscles and bones has a significant effect on the efficiency of a number of other body organs or organ systems.

1. Sharpness of vision decreases with age, partially because of weakening of the small muscles attached to the lens.
2. Skeletal and muscular changes associated with age affect the respiratory system when skeletal kyphosis (humpback) reduces the overall volume of the lungs, while loss of muscle strength affects efficiency of breathing. Age-related changes in both bone and muscle contribute to reduced reserve capacity in the respiratory system.
3. Alterations in the musculature of the gastrointestinal tract and the urinary system produce changes in the ability to digest food and to regulate defecation and urination. The embarrassment of partial or complete incontinence often has a severely deleterious effect on self-confidence and self-esteem in older age.
4. Muscles are one site of glycogen storage. Reduction in muscle mass results in reduced capacity to store glycogen, which is derived from carbohydrates and released when necessary to furnish quick energy in emergency situations. Thus, older adults may be expected to react more slowly to emergencies or fast-paced situations.

Pacing

As we age, physical activities need to be paced more carefully to compensate for slower movements and decreased strength and stamina. The concept of pacing suggests that each individual should perform in his or her own way and in his or her own time frame. Attention to individual pacing schedules becomes much more important from middle age on as an effective way to cope with age-related changes. Older adults, family members, caregivers, and health care professionals must all be more attentive to the need for pacing most behaviors and activities. Pacing can make the difference between competent performance and disorganized, inept efforts that may cause frustration for all involved.

Environmental Modifications

Whenever one is planning programs and activities for older age groups, it is especially important to allow for periodic "stretch" breaks if participants have been sitting, or rest breaks if participants have been active. Sitting for long periods of time can result in painful joint stiffness, which lessens concentration on the activity or program.

In the home, furniture should accommodate the older person's less flexible muscular and skeletal systems. For example, low, overstuffed chairs without arms make it difficult to rise and at the same time maintain balance. Protruding furniture legs increase the probability of accidents, as do scatter rugs and waxed floors. Lighting must be adequate. In general, the home should be arranged so that accident hazards are reduced and safety devices increased. Such modifications can increase the competence of older persons and prolong independence (see Appendix A). Maintaining physical fitness throughout older age is essential to compensate for age-related changes in the musculoskeletal system. Aerobic exercise, strength building, and flexibility exercises are all absolutely necessary to preserve mobility and independence.

REFERENCES

Bruce, S. (1998). Muscle strength. In R. C. Tallis, H. M. Fillit, & J. C. Brocklehurst (Eds.), *Geriatric medicine and gerontology* (5th ed., pp. 1107–1114). London: Churchill Livingstone.

Chestnut, C. H. (1994). Osteoporosis. In W. R. Hazzard, E. L. Bierman, J. P. Blass, W. H. Ettinger, & J. B. Halter (Eds.), *Principles of geriatric medicine and gerontology* (3rd ed., pp. 897–910). New York: McGraw-Hill.

Fife, R. S. (1994). Osteoarthritis. In W. R. Hazzard, E. L. Bierman, J. P. Blass, W. H. Ettinger, & J. B. Halter (Eds.), *Principles of geriatric medicine and gerontology* (3rd ed., pp. 981–986). New York: McGraw-Hill.

Gorevic, P. D. (2004). Osteoarthritis–A review of musculoskeletal aging and treatment issues in geriatric patients. *Geriatrics, 59,* 29–32.

Krohn, K. (2007, Sept./Oct.). Combating knee pain. *Healthy Aging,* 37–40.

Levy, R., & Armbruster, M. A. (2007, Sept./Oct.). Keeping bones strong. *Healthy Aging,* 45–48.

Linton, A. D. (2007) Musculoskeletal system. In A. D. Linton, & H.W. Lach (Eds.), *Matteson & McConnell's gerontological nursing* (3rd ed., pp. 259–312). St. Louis: Saunders Elsevier.

Loeser, R. F., & Delbono, O. (1999). Aging and the musculoskeletal system. In W. R. Hazzard, J. P. Blass, W. H. Ettinger, J. B. Halter, & J. G. Ouslander (Eds.), *Principles of geriatric medicine and gerontology* (4th ed., pp. 1097–1111). New York: McGraw-Hill.

Marieb, E. N., & Hoehn, K. (2007). *Human anatomy and physiology* (7th ed.). San Francisco: Pearson Benjamin Cummings.

Mauk, K. (2006). *Gerontological nursing.* Boston: Jones & Bartlett.

Meier, D.E. (1997). Osteoporosis and other disorders of skeletal aging. In C. K. Cassel, H. J. Cohen, E. B. Larson, D. E. Meier, N. M. Resnick, L. A. Rubenstein, & L. B. Sorensen (Eds.), *Geriatric medicine* (3rd ed., pp. 411–432). New York: Springer-Verlag.

Meiner, S.E. (2006). Musculoskeletal function. In S.E. Meiner, & A.G. Lueckenotte (Eds.), *Gerontologic nursing* (3rd ed., pp. 596–629). St. Louis: Mosby Elsevier.

Orwoll, E. (1997). Osteoporosis in men. *Osteoporosis Report, 15,* 1–2.

Osteoporosis diagnostic guidelines expanded. (2008, April). *The Clinical Advisor, 11,* 16.

Pharmacological options for osteoporosis (2007, August). *Partners in Healthcare Education,* S3–S14.

Siddiqui, N. A., Shetty, K. R., & Duthie, E. H. (1999). Osteoporosis in older men: Discovering when and how to treat it. *Geriatrics, 54,* 20–37.

Smeltzer, S.C., & Bare, B.G. (1992). *Brunner & Suddarth's textbook of medical-surgical nursing* (7th ed.). Philadelphia: J.B. Lippincott.

Touhy, T.A. (2008). Mobility. In P. Ebersole, P. Hess, T. A. Touhy, K. Jett, & A. S. Luggen (Eds.), *Toward healthy aging* (7th ed., pp. 370–411). St. Louis: Mosby Elsevier.

Walsh, C.R. (2007). Musculoskeletal problems. In S. L. Lewis, M. M. Heitkemper, S. R. Dirksen, P. G. O'Brien, & L. Bucher (Eds.), *Medical-surgical nursing* (7th ed., pp. 1668–1692). St. Louis: Mosby Elsevier.

7 The Sensory Systems

All knowledge of the world in which we live comes to us through our sensory systems. To survive, we must constantly be aware of the environment and changes taking place within it. We must also be able to interpret incoming information, integrate it with knowledge about our body state at the moment, and act upon it adaptively. Adaptive behavior depends upon the integrity of the receptor-nervous system-effector system. Inaccurate or partial information received in the nervous system results in distorted or inappropriate behavior. Such behavior is particularly significant in older persons attempting to maintain independence and control in the face of the various decline factors and cumulating losses associated with advancing age. In older age, both the amount and quality of sensory input are vital factors in adaptive and adjustive behavior. Various research and clinical data suggest that humans need both an adequate amount and an adequate variety of stimulation in order to remain mentally intact and in contact with the real world. The behavioral implications of sensory deprivation resulting from the aging process are complex and intriguing.

Sensory systems of major concern in the study of aging are vision (sight), audition (hearing), gustation (taste), olfaction (smell), tactile (touch), vestibular (balance), and kinesthetic ("muscle sense"). Each contributes a specific type of information necessary for continuing adaptation and adjustment. Sensory changes usually begin in the 40s and 50s with a gradual reduction in acuity or sharpness of discrimination, but they do not appreciably limit behavior until about the 70s or 80s. For example, it is common to observe a 40-year-old person holding a newspaper at arm's length due to increasing farsightedness in middle age, but age-related poor vision probably will not curtail his or her driving until many years later. Having to hold a paper at arm's length may be a nuisance, but it does not limit behavior or change lifestyle in the way driving restriction does. Lacking personal transportation in our mobile society has far-reaching psychological and social consequences for older persons. The best programs and services will be of little use if lack of transportation makes them inaccessible, as is often the case among the elderly. Certainly, not being able to comfortably and safely negotiate one's day-to-day environment limits independence, self-sufficiency, and one's sense of personal competence.

Measuring the decrease in functioning of a given sensory system does not enable one to predict an older person's unique behavioral capabilities or limitations that may be associated with the particular sensory loss. First, there is significant variation among individuals in the rate of aging. Second, the amount of loss is highly variable from one organ system to another within a given individual. Third, humans have an amazing ability to adapt and compensate for gradual changes. For some, compensation and adaptation to a large sensory loss may be so effective that activities of daily living (ADL) are only minimally affected, but for others, a minimal sensory loss will produce major changes in lifestyle and possibly even result in the individual becoming housebound or a functional invalid. Utilizing more effective ways to assist people in adapting and compensating efficiently to gradual age-related changes would probably eliminate a number of common problems besetting many older adults as well as prolong their personal independence and self-maintenance. Fourth, some sensory systems are obviously more important in everyday functioning than others. We live primarily in a visual and auditory world and are very dependent on the integrity of our sight and hearing in dealing with day-to-day needs. Loss of smell, for instance, does not handicap a person nearly as much as loss of vision.

One generalization that can safely be made about sensory changes and age is that as we age, it takes stronger stimuli to activate sensory receptors; lights need to be brighter, sounds louder, and smells stronger for the aging person to obtain the quality and quantity of information from the environment needed for effective, adaptive action. This fact has enormous practical implications for creatively improving and modifying living and/or working environments to make them more supportive and appropriate for older individuals.

VISION

The main structures of the eye are:

1. Sclera. The sclera is the outer layer of the eyeball, which is the "white" of the eye. It protects and shapes the eyeball.
2. Cornea. The cornea is the transparent avascular (without blood vessels) surface of the eyeball through which light rays enter the eye. The primary function of the cornea is to bend (refract) light rays so they will come to a focal point directly on the retina for maximal stimulation of visual receptors. It is the most exposed part of the eye and therefore most vulnerable to damage.
3. Anterior and Posterior Chambers. The anterior chamber is the space between the cornea and the iris. The posterior chamber is between the iris and the lens. Both are filled with aqueous humor, a clear liquid that transports nutrients and waste products to and from the lens and cornea. Aqueous humor is continually produced and drained away. Usually the production and drainage are equal, and a constant intraocular pressure is maintained; however, if the drainage of aqueous humor is blocked, intraocular pressure in the eye increases, causing compression of both the retina and the optic nerve and possibly resulting in glaucoma.
4. Iris. The iris is a thin, pigmented, circular, muscular sphincter suspended between the cornea and the lens. The opening at the center is the pupil. The amount of pigment in the iris gives color to the eye, and the function of the iris is to regulate the amount of light entering the eye through dilation (opening) and constriction (closing) actions that change the pupil size. When illumination is low or dim, the pupil opening becomes large, or dilated, allowing a maximum amount of light to stimulate visual receptors. In bright light, pupils constrict and the opening becomes smaller so receptors will be stimulated but not damaged by intense light rays.
5. Lens. The transparent, flexible, avascular crystalline lens helps to focus light rays so they converge, or come to a focal point, precisely on the part of the retinal surface producing the sharpest vision at different viewing distances. The lens is enclosed in a

capsule and arranged in concentric layers that continue to grow by adding layers throughout life. The relatively flexible lens, suspended in place behind the iris by ligaments and ciliary muscles, can flatten or bulge to change its shape as necessary for sharp vision. In distance vision the ciliary muscles relax and the lens flattens; in near or close vision ciliary muscles contract, making the lens bulge to focus light rays from a near object so they fall on the retina correctly. This process is called visual accommodation. Changing lens shape to bring converging light rays to a focus directly on the retinal surface allows for very sharp and precise vision at both near and far distances. In some people, the shape of the eyeball, the cornea, and/or the lens brings light rays to a focus at a point behind the retinal surface, resulting in hyperopia (farsightedness). Similarly, the shape of either the eyeball, cornea, and/or lens may produce myopia (nearsightedness) when light rays come to a focus at a point in front of the retinal surface rather than directly on it. Astigmatism, or irregularities in the curvature of the cornea or lens, is another common visual problem; it causes blurred or indistinct visual images. Hyperopia, myopia, and astigmatism can usually be corrected by prescription eyeglasses, contact lens, or various surgical procedures. Surgical options commonly used are laser surgeries or implants.

6. Vitreous humor. This is a clear, gel-like material contained in the area behind the lens and in front of the retina of the eye. The vitreous humor helps to maintain the shape of the eyeball, contributes to intraocular pressure, and transmits light.

7. Retina. The retina, consisting of several distinct layers of cells, is photosensitive tissue at the back of the eye. Visual receptors (rods and cones) and nerve pathways are contained in the retina. Seventy percent of all sensory receptors in the body are in the eyes (Marieb & Hoehn, 2007). Both rods and cones manufacture pigments, which are changed by light rays and result in the initiation of a nerve impulse. Rods mediate dim light, or night vision, and peripheral vision, whereas cones are responsible for day vision and color vision. Rods and cones are distributed differentially on the retinal surface—cones are densely clustered at the back of the retina and rods are located predominantly along the sides of the retina. Thus, to see an object most distinctly at night or under very low illumination, look slightly off to the side of the object rather than directly at it. This positioning stimulates

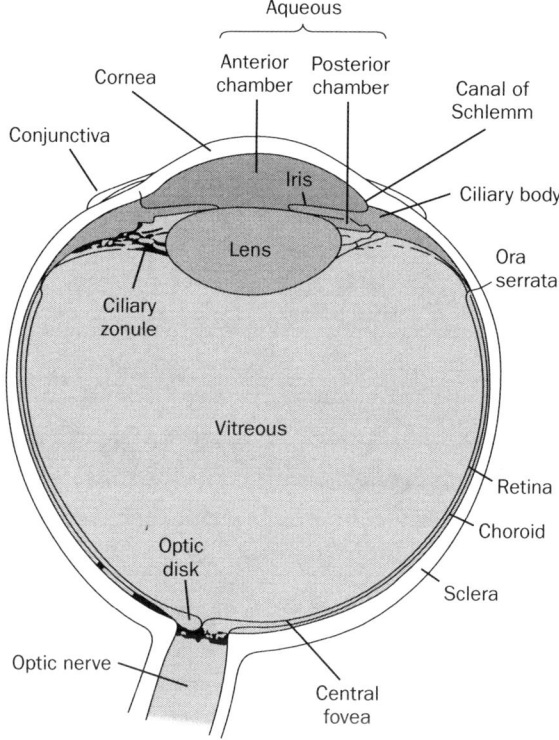

Figure 7.1. Structure of the eye

more rods than cones. The human retina is estimated to contain about 125 million rods and 6 million cones. Approximately 50,000 cones are concentrated in the macula, the area of sharpest and most distinct vision. In the center of the macula is a small area called the fovea.

8. Optic nerve. The optic disc, a blind spot with no sensory receptors, is at the back of the eyeball where the optic nerve leaves the eye. The optic nerve contains over a million nerve fibers.

AGE-RELATED CHANGES IN VISION

Cornea

The cornea becomes thicker and less curved with age. This affects its refractive ability and causes older adults to be more prone to astigmatism.

112 Physical Change & Aging

Frequently, in those over age 60 a gray ring, arcus senilis, forms around the outer edge of the cornea, but this does not affect vision appreciably.

Anterior Chamber

As the lens thickens with age, the anterior chamber decreases in size. Sometimes the growth of the lens puts pressure on the Canal of Schlemm (the channel through which aqueous humor drains from the eye) at the junction of the iris and cornea. The resulting increase in intraocular pressure can lead to glaucoma.

Iris

Eye color is determined by the pigmentation of the iris. With age, eye color fades somewhat and older people's eyes may not appear as lustrous as those of younger individuals.

Pupil

The pupil is the aperture, or opening, in the iris. With age, pupil diameter decreases, and the amount of light reaching the visual receptors by age 70 may be only a third of the amount reaching a younger person's eye. This reduction in pupil size is called miosis and results from age-related changes in the smooth muscle of the iris.

Lens

The lens has two extremely important functions in vision—refraction and accommodation. Refraction requires a crystalline clear lens, whereas accommodation requires the lens to be elastic and able to change shape. Both of these processes are affected by aging. The lens continues to grow with age by adding layers so that between the ages of 20 and 80 the width of the lens increases by approximately 50% (Meisami, 1988). As a result, the lens becomes thicker, denser, and less elastic. As the lens becomes more dense or cloudy (more opaque), it also becomes more yellow, impairing refractive ability.

Yellowing of the lens ("yellow filter effect") eventually produces changes in color vision, although many older adults remain unaware that color discrimination has changed. Older persons with distorted color perception are often able to discriminate between bright colors, such as reds and yellows, better than between darker colors, such as blues and greens. Color coding is one effective way to utilize color perception information. For example, painting restroom doors one bright color and dining room doors another color can likely increase mobility and social interaction among nursing home residents. Distinct color coding improves space and place orientation, and residents will be more inclined to move about. Color coding can be effective in many other situations, such as public buildings, transportation systems, or in housing areas, to maximize legibility and effectiveness of visual messages. Color contrast also aids in depth perception (the ability to judge distances). Since color perception changes are often subtle, behavioral changes related to deficient color perception may be misinterpreted. For instance, people may assume that an older person who is not able to discriminate medications by color is just careless or not paying attention when medication errors occur. Similarly, mismatched or dirty clothing may be interpreted as lack of interest in self-care, or even as early stages of dementia, when in reality the older person simply cannot discriminate colors accurately.

If the lens becomes increasingly cloudy or opaque, a cataract results. Cataracts are the most common disability of the aging eye and will be discussed under age-related disorders of the eye. As the lens becomes less elastic, larger, and more dense, visual accommodation is affected. Farsightedness increases with age and near-vision tasks become more difficult, an age-related change called presbyopia. Most adults in their 40s and 50s need corrective lenses for reading or other near-vision activities. Although decreased elasticity of the lens is the major reason for presbyopia, lessened tone in the suspensory ligaments and ciliary muscles holding the lens in place also contributes to a decline in visual accommodation.

Vitreous Humor

The vitreous humor becomes less gel-like and more liquid-like with age. It also becomes less transparent and causes light rays to scatter as they pass through the vitreous humor to the retina. This leads to less distinct vision. Older adults are frequently aware of brief flashes of light and/or of opacities in the eyes called "floaters." Floaters are due to changes in the vitreous humor and are generally loose cells and tissues casting shadows on the retina. Floaters are at times annoying, but are not usually dangerous.

Retina

Age-related changes in the retina include: (a) blood vessels and capillaries narrowing with the potential to atrophy; (b) some loss of rods and cones; and (c) a decline in light and dark adaptation processes as changes occur in the chemical sensitivity of the rods and cones.

Specific Implications of Age-Related Visual Changes

Age-related changes in the visual system have numerous significant implications for behavior.

1. Decreased visual acuity. The decreased sharpness of vision occurs because of: (a) changes in the refraction of light rays by the cornea and lens; (b) decreased accommodation ability; (c) less light admitted to the eyes due to smaller pupils; and (d) reduced numbers of visual receptors (rods and cones). Increasing the illumination, eliminating glare, and using larger print materials help to offset the behavioral impact of age-related lessened visual acuity.
2. Light and dark adaptation. There is a decrease in light and dark adaptation processes with age. Dark adaptation is the process by which the eyes become maximally sensitive to the dark after having been in the light; light adaptation is the converse, when eyes become maximally sensitive to the light after having been in the dark. A good example of these processes is the experience of walking out of bright sunlight into a dark movie theatre. Initially, it is impossible to see anything, but after a few minutes the eyes become sensitive to the dark (they become dark-adapted) so that empty seats can be identified and even individuals can be recognized. Dark adaptation is a chemical and neural process that takes time for completion. Reasonable sensitivity is usually attained in two to four minutes, although the chemical process is not complete for about 20 minutes. Conversely, when coming out of the dark theatre into the light, the brightness is very uncomfortable for a few minutes before the eyes become light-adapted. Dark and light adaptation are both mediated by photosensitive pigments contained in the rods and cones that are bleached out and restored according to prevailing levels of illumination.
3. Visual threshold. There is a higher visual threshold of sensitivity with age; more light is required to adequately stimulate visual

receptors. Visual threshold refers to the minimum amount of light that will stimulate visual receptors and trigger a nerve impulse to the brain, thereby registering visual information in the highest cortical centers of the nervous system. A higher threshold means greater illumination is needed to obtain the maximum amount of visual information from the environment, a fact important in designing optimal living and working situations for middle-aged and older persons.

4. Increased sensitivity to glare. Exposure to glare is more difficult for older adults because of age-related changes in the cornea, lens, and vitreous humor. Light is scattered throughout the eyeball rather than being focused at a precise point on the retinal surface and thus interferes with sharp vision. Common sources of glare include bright sunlight, exposed light bulbs, and light reflected off white, shiny surfaces. Even bright and shiny walls and floors can produce disturbing glare.

5. Peripheral vision. A significant loss of peripheral vision is common in aging and may influence both physical activity and social interactions. Older adults may be more likely to spill food or drinks placed in their visual periphery or not see objects out of their range of vision. Similarly, they may be unable to see people who are outside their range of vision. Loss of peripheral vision also has implications for driving (Linton, 2007).

General Implications of Age-Related Visual Changes

Behavioral implications of changes in vision are primarily associated with older adults' decreasing efficiency in responding to the visual world as well as with accident prevention. For instance, driving at night and coping with the glaring headlights of oncoming cars may be hazardous for most older people due to slower dark and light adaptation and lessened visual acuity. For the same reasons, moving from lighter to darker areas in the home (or vice versa) increases the possibility of accidents.

The visual system is without question one of the most important links to the world in which we live. A variety of gradual changes take place with aging in this very complex sensory system, and awareness of these changes should provide greater motivation for preventive care. Regular eye examinations, proper lighting, and avoidance of excessive eye strain are important in preserving vision. There are effective ways to compensate for age-related visual changes and thereby reduce behavioral limitations associated with visual impairments. This should be a significant area of interest both to the gerontologist and to older persons because it has enormous practical applications for the maintenance of activities of daily living and for the enjoyment of life.

AGE-RELATED DISORDERS OF THE VISUAL SYSTEM

Cataract

A cataract is a cloudy or opaque lens that impairs vision by interfering with light rays passing through the lens. Cataracts are the most common age-related disorder of the aging eye and affect approximately 70% of those over age 70. The exact causes of cataracts associated with aging are not yet clearly identified, but it appears that metabolic changes in the proteins of the lens are significant in cataract formation. Other risk factors are high blood pressure, diabetes, prolonged use of corticosteroid drugs, excessive exposure to sunlight, excessive use of alcohol, and, possibly, family history of cataracts.

Early symptoms of cataracts include myopia (nearsightedess) and sensitivity to glare as the refractive power of the lens increases when opacities develop. This increase in refractive power temporarily compensates for presbyopia, and some 60 to 70 year-old people can read again without glasses ("second sight"). Nevertheless, as lens changes progress, vision becomes increasingly impaired, making reading difficult even with glasses. Other classic symptoms experienced eventually are halos around objects, blurred vision, and decreased light and color perception (Touhy, 2008). At one time, older adults were advised to wait until cataracts were "ripe" before having surgery to remove them, but now they are encouraged to have cataracts removed whenever visual acuity changes interfere with their lifestyle. Opacity of the lens can be seen in an opthalmoscopic examination. Verbal complaints about reduced vision help determine how much the individual is affected by the cataract.

Surgery to remove the lens is the treatment of choice for cataracts. The success rate for cataract surgery is over 90% (Houde & Huff, 2003). When the lens is removed, there must be some way to make up for its loss. Options are: (a) thick prescription eyeglasses can magnify objects by about 25% but interfere with peripheral vision; (b) contact lenses, which provide more peripheral vision than eyeglasses and don't magnify objects as much but are difficult to manipulate, especially for those with arthritic hands or coordination difficulties; (c) intraocular lens, a plastic lens permanently implanted in the eye that provides good central and peripheral vision and does not magnify objects significantly. Most cataract surgery is now performed under regional or local anesthesia and often in an outpatient setting.

Glaucoma

Glaucoma, one of the major causes of blindness, is particularly dangerous because it progresses slowly and often does not present noticeable symptoms. Approximately three million Americans have glaucoma and about 120,000 are blind because of it. Age is the most important predictor of glaucoma, with older women affected about twice as often as men. Other contributing factors are family history of glaucoma, diabetes, and possibly long term use of some medications with anticholinergic effects (Touhy, 2008). Glaucoma occurs when there is an increase in intraocular pressure in the eye. Intraocular pressure is normal when the amount of intraocular fluid (aqueous humor) produced is equal to the amount drained from the eye. When intraocular fluid does not drain as quickly as more is formed, pressure within the eye increases. Increased intraocular pressure, if untreated, damages both the retina and the optic nerve, resulting in irreversible blindness. Glaucoma is classified as primary or secondary. In secondary glaucoma a pathological process blocks the outflow channels through which aqueous humor drains from the eye. Possible causes are congenital glaucoma, inflammation, diabetes, and tumors. Treatment of secondary glaucoma is difficult and oriented toward removal or control of whatever prevents the outflow of the aqueous humor.

Primary glaucoma can be primary open-angle (POAG) or primary angle-closure (PACG). Angle-closure glaucoma is relatively rare and accounts for only 5% to 10% of all glaucomas. Individuals with an anatomically shallow anterior chamber of the eye may develop angle-closure glaucoma as the lens grows and thickens with age, further reducing the size of the chamber and blocking the outflow of fluid. An acute situation then develops, with eye pain, clouded vision, nausea, and vomiting. Prompt treatment is necessary if blindness is to be averted. Laser surgery is often very successful, but some may require medications afterward for long-term control of intraocular pressure (Kalina, 1999; Miller, 2009). Approximately 90% of all primary glaucomas are open-angle. The outflow of aqueous humor gradually becomes impaired as degenerative changes occur in the eye. Symptoms are not usually apparent, and much damage may be done before the condition is ever diagnosed. This type of glaucoma is not curable, but can usually be controlled with both topical and systemic medications to help constrict the pupil and increase the outflow of fluid from the eye. Medications may also be prescribed to inhibit aqueous humor production. If medications fail, laser treatment and/or surgery are indicated to establish an alternate pathway for aqueous humor circulation. Since glaucoma is usually symptomless, individuals over age 40 should have periodic eye examinations that include glaucoma testing. Diagnosis of glaucoma is no longer based on measures of intraocular pressure alone but includes an examination of the optic disc for cupping (atrophy) and visual field evaluations.

Diabetic Retinopathy

Diabetic retinopathy is a serious visual problem associated with diabetes and is a leading cause of adult blindness (Kupfer, 1990; Brant, 1999; Touhy, 2008). Prevalence increases with the length of time a person has diabetes and nearly all diabetics will have some retinopathy after 20 years of diabetes. Essentially, retinal blood vessels develop small aneurysms, which result in retinal hemorrhages. Recurring hemorrhages block light from reaching visual receptors and also damage the receptors themselves. Initially, the macula area is most affected, but in time damage occurs over a wider area of the retina.

Symptoms usually do not appear until at least three to five years after the onset of diabetes. Early symptoms are subtle, such as cloudy vision or seeing a shower of spots. Symptoms increase with recurring hemorrhages, retinal detachment, or secondary glaucoma. Early diagnosis is of paramount importance, as laser photocoagulation is extremely effective in preventing or slowing visual loss, especially in the early stages of diabetic retinopathy.

Age-Related Macular Degeneration (AMD)

Age-related macular degeneration is a leading cause of legal blindness in older adults. Types of age-related macular degeneration include dry (nonexudative) and wet (exudative). Approximately 90% of all cases are of the dry form, in which cells of the macula start to atrophy leading to slow, but progressive, loss of vision. Only 10% to 15% of those with the dry form will develop the wet form, and those are usually people not under treatment for AMD. The wet form is more severe, and if untreated the majority of people become functionally blind. Abnormal blood vessels grow beneath the retina and may leak, causing irreversible damage. The macula is the retinal area most densely populated by cones and is responsible for sharp vision. Decreased blood supply to the macula and fovea damages receptors, resulting in central vision loss, usually bilaterally, although peripheral vision is not adversely affected. As central vision declines, tasks involving discrimination of detail or high visual acuity (such as reading or driving) become difficult or impossible. Complete blindness does not occur because peripheral vision remains reasonably intact. Aging is not the only causal factor in macular degeneration; genetics, smoking, cardiovascular disease, and long term sunlight exposure are also assumed to be significant. Nutrition is likely a factor in the progression of AMD and vitamin C, vitamin E, beta-carotene, zinc, and green leafy vegetables may be helpful in preventing and slowing the disease (Smith & Neely, 2007).

Symptoms include evidence of central vision distortion, such as objects appearing larger or smaller or straight lines appearing bent, and there is usually other evidence of loss of central vision acuity. Ophthalmoscopy is the primary diagnostic procedure. Drusen, yellowish extracellular deposits, occur in the early stages of the dry form. Fluorescein IV angiography and photography are also helpful in determining the extent and type of AMD. Treatment reduces the risk of further vision loss and may involve laser photocoagulation, pharmacological control of inflammatory conditions, photodynamic therapy, and use of low-vision aids if laser and pharmacological interventions do not help. New treatment procedures are constantly being developed.

AUDITION (HEARING)

Hearing is crucial because most of the time we relate to each other primarily through verbal communication. Hearing loss is thought by many to be the most devastating sensory handicap of all, frequently resulting in withdrawal from interactions with family, friends, and society in general. Paranoid ideas and behavior, suspicion, isolation, and loss of contact with reality are phenomena reported to occur in certain individuals as a result of becoming hearing-impaired or deaf (Crews & Campbell, 2004; Smith & Neely, 2007). Increasing evidence, however, indicates that people do not necessarily demonstrate such personality changes as a direct result of deafness or hearing impairment, but if these attributes already exist in one's personality, hearing impairment may well exacerbate or intensify them.

The basic structures of the auditory system are:

Outer Ear

The outer ear is composed of the pinna, or auricle, and the auditory canal. The pinna, the external part of the ear, is useful in directing sounds into the ear. The auditory canal is a short passageway through which sound travels to reach the middle and inner ear. The auditory canal, containing hairs and glands that produce cerumen (ear wax), terminates at the eardrum (tympanic membrane).

Middle Ear

The middle ear has substantial functional significance for hearing because the mechanical transmission of sound takes place there. The eardrum, or tympanic membrane, separates the outer ear from the middle ear. Pharyngotympanic tubes (formerly called Eustachian tubes) open into the middle ear from the throat and are important in equalizing pressures between the outside and inside of the head. When extreme pressure differences exist between the outer and middle ear, pain results, and the eardrum may rupture unless pressures are equalized. For example, ears "pop" at high altitudes or when scuba diving as pressures become equalized.

Structures of importance in the middle ear are three small bones (malleus, incus, and stapes) called the ossicles that transmit sound vibrations from the eardrum through the middle ear to the oval window, a membrane separating the middle ear from the inner ear. Another membrane, the round window, is situated below the oval window. The ossicles are the three smallest bones in the body and are named for their shapes: the malleus (hammer), the incus (anvil), and the stapes (stirrup). The "handle" of the malleus fits against the eardrum, and the base of the stapes fits against the oval window. The incus articulates with the malleus and the stapes. When the eardrum is vibrated by sound waves, the ossicles transmit the vibrations to the oval window, which in turn sets fluids in the inner ear in motion, thus stimulating auditory receptors. Two small muscles attach to the malleus and the stapes, and when unusually loud sounds occur, these muscles pull the ossicles away from the membranes they contact. This is called the tympanic reflex, and it helps protect the auditory receptors from extremely loud sounds; however, the reflex has a lag time long enough to be fairly ineffective in protecting against extremely sudden, very loud noises.

Inner Ear

The inner ear, located in the temporal bone, is highly complicated and contains structures for both hearing and equilibrium. It contains: (a) the bony (osseous) labyrinth, which consists of the vestibule, cochlea, semicircular canals, and a system of channels through bone; and (b) the membranous labyrinth, which consists of interconnecting membranous ducts in the bony labyrinth. Two fluids, perilymph and endolymph, are contained in the labyrinths to conduct sound vibrations and respond to changes in body position and acceleration. The cochlea, contained in the bony labyrinth, is a spiral bony chamber containing the auditory receptors. The cochlea contains the spiral organ of Corti in which hair cells, the actual receptors for hearing, are found. The spiral organ of Corti rests on top of the basilar membrane.

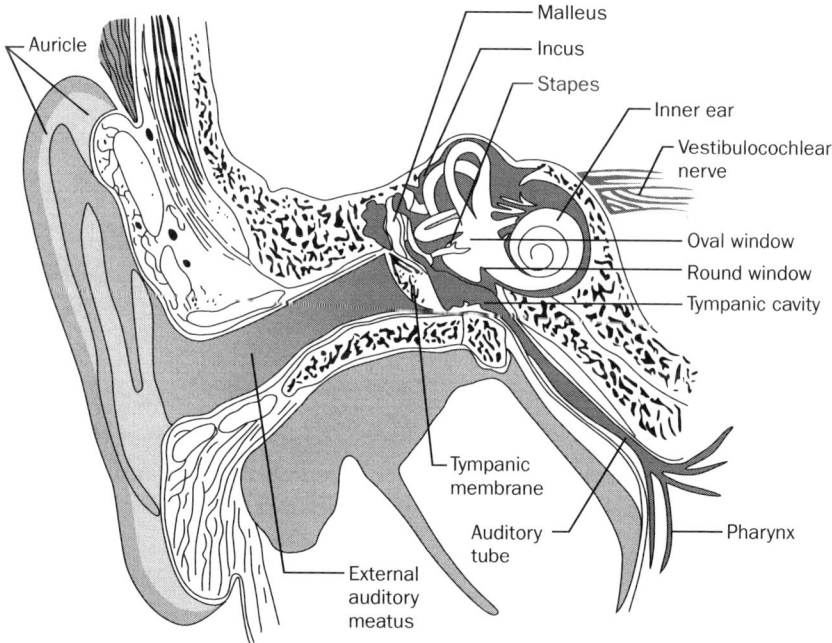

Figure 7.2. The ear

Sound waves enter the outer ear and initiate a vibration of the eardrum that causes the ossicles in the middle ear to transmit the sound vibration to the oval window. This movement, or vibration, passes through the oval window creating a vibration of fluid in the cochlea of the inner ear. In response to a wave of sound pressure, the basilar membrane moves up and down, stimulating the hair cells of the spiral organ of Corti and initiating nerve impulses. Nerve impulses are sent from the ears via the auditory nerve to the auditory center of the brain (located in the temporal lobe of the cerebrum). High-frequency sounds vibrate hair cells on the basal part of the basilar membrane (near the oval window), mid-frequency sounds vibrate hair cells on the middle part of the membrane, and low-frequency sounds vibrate hair cells primarily near the cochlear apex of the membrane. Below the oval window another membrane, called the round window, serves to dampen sound waves in the inner ear and restores the system to equilibrium in preparation for the next stimulus entering the ear. The auditory nerve contains from 24,000 to 28,000 fibers, and the range of human hearing is approximately 20 to 20,000 cycles per second. The human ear is thus a very sensitive organ, but if it were more sensitive it would be less efficient. For example, a movement of the eardrum of less than one tenth the diameter of a hydrogen atom can result in an auditory sensation. If the ear were more sensitive it would respond to the movement of air molecules, and the resulting roaring sounds would all but mask other auditory stimuli.

AGE-RELATED CHANGES IN HEARING

Subtle changes in hearing usually begin in the 40s and gradually progress with age. An estimated 28 million people in the United States have hearing loss, with approximately 40% to 50% of those over 75 experiencing a hearing loss (Linton, 2007). In our culture, men tend to show hearing loss earlier than women, partly because men have generally been exposed to more prolonged, high-level occupational noise than women, and environmental noise factors have a definite impact on auditory integrity. Hearing impairments are generally classified as conductive, sensorineural, central, or mixed. Conductive impairments result from anything interfering with the transmission of sound through the outer or middle ear so that sound stimuli do not reach the inner ear and auditory receptors. Impacted ear wax, arthritic changes in the ossicles, otosclerosis, or stiffening of the tympanic membrane or oval window membrane are possible reasons for conductive hearing impairments. Sensorineural impairments result from disorders of the inner ear (especially loss of hair cells with age) that affect the transmission of sound to the auditory receptors and/or through the auditory pathways. Presbycusis is the most common form of sensorineural hearing impairment or loss in older adults, with drug toxicity another common cause. Many drugs commonly used by older adults, such as antibiotics, aspirin, NSAIDs, and diuretics, have potential side effects affecting hearing (ototoxicity). Usually ototoxicity will be reversed with discontinuation of the particular drug. Central hearing loss results from lesions in the central auditory pathways. Mixed hearing impairment involves both conductive and sensorineural hearing loss.

There are several specific changes in hearing that are associated with the aging process:

1. In the outer ear, the pinna loses some flexibility and becomes a bit longer and wider. Hairs in the external ear canal tend to become stiffer. This, combined with the drying and thinning of tissues in the external ear canal, contributes to a likelihood of cerumen (ear wax) accumulation with age. Cerumen produced in the later years is of thicker consistency (dryer) and is not always easily removed. Accumulation of cerumen in the external ear canal can occlude the auditory canal and is responsible for a substantial amount of conductive hearing impairment (Mahoney, 1993). This can be avoided by keeping the ears free of excessive ear wax build-up. When ear wax accumulates, it should be removed only by a professional because it is not a safe do-it-yourself project; perforation of the eardrum resulting in serious hearing impairment is not uncommon.
2. Aging changes in the middle ear involve lessened flexibility of the tympanic membrane, the oval window membrane, and the round window membrane; an increased possibility of stiffness (calcification) of the ossicles; and likely decreased efficiency of the acoustic reflex. Changes in the membranes of the middle ear and the ossicles somewhat impair the transmission of sound vibrations, but normally do not impair hearing significantly.
3. Age-related changes in the inner ear are primarily presbycusis. With age, auditory loss generally affects perception of high frequencies first. Later, age-related changes may involve middle- and low-frequency ranges as well. Four types of presbycusis

have been identified. The most common form is sensory presbycusis, which involves degeneration in the spiral organ of Corti in the cochlea. The other forms involve loss of cochlear and higher auditory pathway neurons (neural presbycusis), atrophy of fibrous vascular cochlear tissue (strial or metabolic presbycusis), and degenerative change in the basilar membrane of the cochlea (mechanical or cochlear presbycusis). Presbycusis has many important influences on behavior because it especially affects the ability to understand speech. Individuals can hear sounds, but are not able to discriminate words or comprehend what is being said.

Implications of Age-Related Hearing Impairments

Hearing impairments are not life-threatening and do not result in actual physical disability, but they are disabling because they can seriously disrupt quality of life. Few people appreciate the extent to which hearing impairments affect all aspects of daily life. Age-related hearing impairment usually occurs gradually, affecting the ability to respond appropriately to auditory signals of danger, but even more importantly, impairing the ability to understand what is said and to communicate.

Presbycusis interferes substantially with the perception of high-frequency sounds. In the English language, the sounds of consonants have a higher frequency than vowels. Consonants enable us to differentiate one word from another. For example, the words bear, care, and wear can only be differentiated by consonants. To the individual with presbycusis, these words may all sound alike. Therefore, those with presbycusis hear part of a word or sentence and either have to ask to have it repeated or else guess what was said. Being asked to repeat words or sentences too often almost always produces impatience or irritability in others and frustration for both speaker and listener. When words or sentences are misinterpreted or misunderstood and are responded to inappropriately, those attempting to communicate with the hearing-impaired person often react emotionally and with impatience.

Too often older hearing-impaired individuals are treated as though they are mentally incompetent or in the early stages of dementia. To further complicate the situation, since hearing impairments are not as obvious as visual impairments, a hearing impairment is often not noticed until communication problems arise. In addition, many older adults are extremely sensitive about being hearing impaired and will deny the problem exists. Because hearing loss is an invisible handicap, other people find it difficult to remember the impairment exists and become insensitive to the impact it has on the person affected. Rees, Duckett and Milczuk (1994, p.458) state that: "Misunderstanding, mistrust, and lack of sympathy for the hearing impaired seem to be built into our cultural heritage. These attitudes are certainly quite different from our perceptions about and treatment of blindness."

As indicated earlier, certain personality changes have been reported to occur in some, but not all, older individuals with hearing loss. There is widespread variation in the psychosocial effects of hearing impairment in older adults, and each person should be assessed for his or her idiosyncratic reactions to this sensory handicap (Kart, Metress, & Metress, 1992). The following suggestions are helpful in communicating with someone who is hearing impaired:

(a) Face the person so you can be seen clearly.

(b) Speak slowly and enunciate carefully.

(c) Lower the pitch of your voice. This is especially important for women, who usually have higher-pitched voices than men.

(d) Do not shout, as this makes the voice pitch even higher and is embarrassing to the hearing impaired person.

(e) Use touch as an adjunct to communication if appropriate.

(f) Remember that it takes a lot of motivation, concentration, and energy for the hearing impaired to function well in communication situations. If the person doesn't feel well or doesn't have the energy to expend, he or she will not hear as well as at other, more optimal times.

Assessment of hearing impairments should include an examination by an otologist or otolaryngologist to assess any medical condition contributing to hearing loss and a complete audiologic evaluation by an audiologist. Audiologic rehabilitation options include assistive listening devices such as amplified telephones, hearing aids, speech reading, and educational/counseling programs. Most hearing impaired persons can now be helped with some type of hearing aid, but only a qualified professional can match the specific impairment to the most appropriate type of hearing aid. Hearing aid technology has progressed enormously in the past few years, and many options, such as programmed and digital aids, are now available. For those who are profoundly deaf, cochlear implants are becoming more common for older adults. Human voices will sound tinny and not of normal quality, but for the profoundly deaf, even these sounds may be helpful. Education, counseling, and referrals to rehabilitation options such as speech reading are also part of an appropriate hearing rehabilitation program. A number of older adults do not wear their hearing aids after purchase because they do not get adequate follow-up and education about expectations, use, and care of these instruments. There are many choices and options available to deal with hearing losses, and older adults need to be encouraged to pursue these to improve their quality of life.

AGE-RELATED DISORDERS OF HEARING

Tinnitus

Tinnitus is the perception of sounds in one or both ears in the absence of an auditory stimulus. Eighty-five percent of those with hearing or ear problems experience tinnitus, and it is more common in older adults. Sounds are described as a ringing, buzzing, whistling, or roaring in the ears. Tinnitus sounds are most often subjective (only the affected person hears them), but they may also be objective (the examiner is able to hear the sounds), although this form of tinnitus is rare. Causes may be local (impacted ear wax, infections of the external or middle ear, or conductive hearing losses), or systemic (meningitis, drug-induced ototoxicity, hypertension, or cardiovascular diseases). More than 200 prescription or nonprescription drugs include tinnitus as a possible side effect (Touhy, 2008). A thorough medical evaluation is needed to determine the specific causes of tinnitus.

Once it is clear that tinnitus is chronic and not caused by a surgically correctable medical problem, a long-term program of management can be established. According to Ross, Echevarria, & Robinson (1991), major components of a management plan include:

1. Treating related problems that are correctable. For instance, have the individual avoid loud or continuous noises.
2. Avoiding irritants that may aggravate or perpetuate tinnitus. Examples are alcohol, caffeine, chocolate, tea, some anti-inflammatory drugs, aspirin, and quinine.

3. Reassuring the older adult that tinnitus is not life-threatening, but a symptom that can be managed. Remember that fatigue, worry, and high stress worsen the annoyance.
4. Teaching individuals with tinnitus how to manage it by using various noise-masking techniques. Radios and other masking noises may help distract from tinnitus sounds. A proper hearing aid sometimes helps in reducing tinnitus.
5. Teaching biofeedback, relaxation training, and stress management to improve coping strategies.
6. Referring to self-help and support groups for additional information and strategies aiding in more effective management.
7. Medications may be of help in certain situations.

Otosclerosis

Otosclerosis refers to a form of bilateral progressive hearing impairment caused by abnormal bone formation that occurs primarily at the oval window and eventually immobilizes the stapes. Sound transmission into the inner ear is prevented if the stapes is unable to transmit the sound. The cause of otosclerosis is unknown, but heredity is a factor. Treatment may require drug therapy with sodium fluoride, vitamin D and calcium carbonate supplements, surgery involving partial removal of the stapes (stapedectomy), or complete removal of the stapes with an implant to replace it (fenestration). A well-fitted hearing aid can be of substantial help as well (Smith & Neely, 2007).

VESTIBULAR SYSTEM

The vestibular system is significant for mobility and accident prevention. Receptors providing information on the body's orientation in space are located in the inner ear within the bony labyrinth close to the cochlea. The structures of the vestibular system include two compartments, the utricle and the saccule, plus three tubes (semicircular canals) filled with fluid. The utricle and saccule contain receptors (hair cells) responsive to changes in the position of the head with respect to gravity. Such movements stimulate the hair cell receptors and initiate nerve impulses that travel the vestibular nerve to the brain. The semicircular canals, placed at right angles to each other, each contain fluid as well as an enlargement (ampulla) at one end containing hair cell receptors. Changes in the rate of motion of the head stimulate hair cells in the ampullae and initiate nerve impulses.

AGE-RELATED CHANGES IN THE VESTIBULAR SYSTEM

The bony labyrinth undergoes degenerative changes similar to those in the cochlea as discussed under age-related changes in the inner ear.

1. Sensory receptors (hair cells) decrease in number, and peripheral neural fibers are reduced (Mhoon, 1997).
2. Body sway increases and may be partially responsible for general postural unsteadiness (especially falls) experienced by many older people. Equilibrium and balance become impaired, especially when fast movement is required. Older adults generally adapt by moving slowly and walking with a wide-stance (feet-apart) gait to provide greater stability. Pacing one's speed of movement becomes much more important in old age, not only for conserving energy but also for safety.

AGE-RELATED DISORDERS OF THE VESTIBULAR SYSTEM

Disturbances of the vestibular system are frequently implicated in dizziness, vertigo, and other equilibrium problems affecting older adults. Dizziness, a complaint of many older adults, is not easy for the professional to interpret. According to Ross and Robinson (1984), four types of complaints are labeled dizziness:

1. Dysequilibrium, or imbalance, characterized by difficulties in walking. Those with Parkinson's disease or Alzheimer's are illustrative of dysequilibrium problems.
2. Faintness, or a feeling of impending loss of consciousness. This type of dizziness is usually caused by circulatory insufficiency. Systemic disorders such as anemias, thyroid disease, hypoglycemia, and medical problems that lessen oxygenation in the brain contribute to faintness.
3. Vague, non-specific lightheadedness. Although usually imprecisely described by those affected, three likely causes are multiple

sensory deficits, anxiety with hyperventilation, and chronic systemic disease.
4. Vertigo, a sensation of rotating in space or spinning. The illusion that one is moving, or one's surroundings are moving, differentiates vertigo from other types of dizziness. Dizziness most often results when several sensory modalities bring contradictory sensory information to the brain. Thus, dizziness often has multiple causes and involves several dysfunctioning systems of the body. Diagnosis of various causal factors is difficult but necessary for effective treatment.

Ménière's Disease

Ménière's disease, an inner ear disturbance, results from a dysfunction of the bony labyrinth. Its specific cause is not known. Symptoms characteristic of the disorder include vertigo with nausea and vomiting, tinnitus, neurosensory hearing loss, and/or a sensation of pressure within the ears. Vertigo attacks occur suddenly and may last for several hours. In the early stages of the disease, weeks or months pass between attacks, but as the disorder progresses, attacks can occur every two or three days. Usually, only one ear is involved.

Diagnostic evaluation may include audiogram, head scan, allergy evaluation, glucose tolerance test, and specific techniques to assess labyrinthine function. Treatment goals are to eliminate the vertigo and stabilize hearing. Treatment approaches include medical, surgical, rehabilitative, and dietary strategies depending on the underlying primary cause. Thus, treatment of vestibular disorders involves alleviating symptoms and correcting underlying causes if they can be accurately identified. Medication choices depend on the individual's tolerance for a particular drug, the efficacy of the drug, and its safety for long-term use. Medications used to treat vertigo often have side effects that are disturbing to older adults. Surgery may be necessary to treat uncontrolled vertigo.

Balancing the body under the influence of gravity, maintaining equilibrium under a variety of movement conditions, and engaging in coordinated, controlled psychomotor activities all involve the interplay of many intricate mechanisms influenced by the aging process. Falls and other accidents tend to increase with age as these controlling and integrative aspects of movement, balance, and equilibrium decline in efficiency.

TASTE (GUSTATION)

Receptors for taste are located in taste buds, primarily on the tongue, with each taste bud having 15 to 20 or more sensory cells. These cells replace themselves constantly, but replacement may be slower in older people. Receptors specific to four different taste sensations have previously been identified with different locations: sweet and salt receptors mostly at the tip of the tongue, sour receptors along the sides of the tongue, and bitter receptors toward the back of the tongue. This specificity is now in question, and it is possible that all taste buds may respond to a taste stimulus (Duffy & Chapo, 2006). Taste is one of the chemical senses because substances must be in solution to be tasted; insoluble materials have no taste. The blending of substances produces a variety of taste sensations that contribute to enjoyable eating.

AGE-RELATED CHANGES IN TASTE

Research on age-related changes in both taste and smell is difficult because these senses are so interrelated. Older persons may notice a decrease in the sense of taste around age 60 and especially after age 70 (Linton, 2007). The behavioral significance of changes in taste for eating has not been established. Taste has always been considered to be a relatively minor sensory modality, and its age-related changes occur gradually. Individuals, then, may not be as consciously aware of changes in taste as they are of changes in vision or hearing. Many older adults do complain that foods taste bland, and they regularly pour on salt, sauces, sugar, or spices to enhance flavor. If, with age, foods begin to taste bland, this may be partly due to changes in taste receptors and partly to other factors contributing to the enjoyment of food. For example, ill-fitting dentures can modify eating patterns; eating alone is a situation often not conducive to preparation of nutritionally balanced meals; and loss of appetite occurs with inactivity. In addition, certain medications may alter taste sensations, and older adults commonly use many medications. Medications that decrease the ability to taste may therefore contribute to nutritional difficulties in older age. An adequate diet is important, especially in older age, and continuing research and education are needed in this area. Nutrition has far-reaching implications for health and vitality in older age.

SMELL (OLFACTION)

Specific receptors for the sense of smell are located in the nasal passages. Various kinds of receptors have been identified, but research is difficult and results sometimes contradictory.

AGE-RELATED CHANGES IN SMELL

Smell appears to be more affected by age than is taste (Duffy & Chapo, 2006). As in taste, olfactory receptors are constantly being replaced, but not all receptors may be replaced in older age. Also, environmental factors such as smoking affect olfactory sensitivity and make specific age-related changes difficult to differentiate. There is a higher threshold of smell sensitivity with age, suggesting that odor identification seems to be less efficient, and that odors need to be stronger and more intense to be perceived and differentiated by older adults. For example, ethyl mercaptan is an odorous substance once added to propane to enable natural gas consumers to be aware of leaks, but older adults were found to have more difficulty identifying this substance than younger people, which posed a serious safety hazard for older persons.

Smell, like taste, is considered a relatively minor sensory modality compared to vision and hearing. Doty (1990) suggests several reasons for lack of attention to smell in both research and applied settings. First, disturbances in the sense of smell are less obvious and have less influence on everyday activities than do the major sensory modalities. Second, this system is considered to be primitive and not as useful to humans. Third, easy-to-use assessments of olfactory functioning are not readily available. Fourth, olfaction is taken for granted and its significance is not appreciated until disturbances or losses occur.

Changes occurring in the sense of smell have behavioral implications for the proper ingestion of food, for safety, and for personal hygiene. The smell of escaping gas fumes from a stove or heater, electrical wires burning, or spoiled foods are important cues for personal safety. Taste and smell are related senses, and both contribute substantially to the pleasure of eating. Personal cleanliness is important in our society. Older adults with reduced olfactory perception may not be aware of unpleasant body odors or other aspects of personal hygiene. Some older adults use such large amounts of perfume or cologne that it is offensive to those around them, but they are unaware of this reaction.

AGE-RELATED DISORDERS IN TASTE AND SMELL

Pathologies do exist, but diseases in these systems are idiosyncratic and vary greatly from one person to another; no one disorder is particularly associated with aging. The most common causes of loss of smell (and probably taste) are upper respiratory infection, head traumas, and nasal/sinus disease. Olfactory distortions or losses have also been associated with Alzheimer's disease, Parkinson's disease, and Huntington's disease.

SKIN (CUTANEOUS) SENSES

The skin senses are touch, pressure, heat, cold, and pain. Each sense has specific receptors. As with other sensory receptors, differential distribution of cutaneous receptors is found throughout the body. The fingertips, for example, are more sensitive to touch and pressure than is the forearm.

AGE-RELATED CHANGES IN THE SKIN SENSES

Research on age-related changes in the skin senses is sparse. Evidence suggests that changes take place gradually, involving some loss of receptors with age and higher thresholds of stimulation in remaining receptors. Behavioral implications of age-related changes in the skin senses primarily concern personal safety. Burns are likely to occur if an older person does not accurately perceive temperatures. When touch receptors on the soles of the feet do not function effectively, falls occur before the individual even realizes the foot is not on a solid surface. Certain social behaviors may be affected adversely, as when, for example, it is difficult to know how much pressure to exert when holding a glass or fork without dropping it. Some older adults become overly sensitive about such perceived clumsiness and avoid public or social situations. Touch sensitivity changes can exert subtle influences on various aspects of behavior because touch is necessary to orient ourselves to many aspects of the daily environment and to prevent accidents.

Another significant aspect of touch that is often neglected in discussions of sensory changes and age is touch as a mode of communication. The use of touch conveys various messages (Vortherms, 1991). Appropriate use of affective ("caring") touch improves communication with older adults, whether they are oriented or confused. How touch is perceived, though, depends on cultural and family experiences, gender differences, location of touch, and basic personality preferences. Professionals must be sensitive to the complex dynamics involved in touch because it can serve as a powerful adjunct to verbal communication with older adults.

THE IMPORTANCE OF SENSORY CHANGES IN AGING

Sensory changes with age are some of the most crucial, and possibly the most underrated, changes associated with the entire aging process. Perhaps this is because these changes usually occur gradually and are not as dramatic as handicaps that occur suddenly through an accident or health crisis. Perhaps our lack of active concern in this area arises from the "error of familiarity," as most people are at least vaguely aware that sensory changes take place with age but do not dwell on the possible implications of such changes. Perhaps we tend to write these changes off with a "what can you expect from old age?" attitude. Whatever the reasons, most people interested and involved in the study of the aging process do not give sensory changes and their cumulating impact on behavior the significance they deserve.

Changes in each of these systems interfere with a person's ability to gather pertinent information about the environment that is essential to a high quality of life and even to the maintenance of life itself. Is it not reasonable, then, that as sensory changes gradually occur, the organism also experiences gradual sensory deprivation that may lead to social isolation as the individual becomes less mobile, increasingly housebound, or more difficult to engage in communication? The next stage might well be "functional senility," a state in which the person generates his or her own world of fantasy or lives in the past because the real world is not interesting enough to provide the variety of stimulation needed to keep psychologically intact. Continued stimulation of sensory modalities is very necessary to maintain adequate functioning in older age. Preventive care and early intervention are extremely important in retaining sensory efficiency in the later years.

REFERENCES

Brant, B. B. (1999). Sensory disorders. In J. T. Stone, J. F. Wyman, & S. A. Salisbury (Eds.), *Clinical gerontological nursing* (2nd ed., pp. 515–533). Philadelphia: W.B. Saunders.

Crews, J. E., & Campbell, V. A. (2004). Vision impairment and hearing loss among community-dwelling older Americans: Implications for health and functioning. *American Journal of Public Health, 94,* 823–829.
Doty, R. L. (1990). Olfaction. In F. Boller, & J. Grafman (Eds.), *Handbook of neuropsychology* (pp. 211–226). Amsterdam: Elsevier.
Duffy, V. B., & Chapo, A. K. (2006). Smell, taste, and somatosensation in the elderly. In R. Chernoff (Ed.), *Geriatric nutrition* (3rd ed., pp. 115–162). Boston: Jones & Bartlett.
Houde, S. C., & Huff, M. A. (2003). Age-related vision loss in older adults. *Journal of Gerontological Nursing, 29,* 25–27.
Kalina, R. E. (1999). Aging and visual function. In W. R. Hazzard, J. P. Blass, W. H. Ettinger, J. B. Halter, & J. G. Ouslander (Eds.), *Principles of geriatric medicine and gerontology* (4th ed., pp. 603–616). New York: McGraw-Hill.
Kart, C. S., Metress, E. K., & Metress, S. P. (1992). *Human aging and chronic disease.* Boston: Jones & Bartlett.
Kupfer, C. (1990). Ophthalmologic disorders. In W. B. Abrams, & R. Berkow (Eds.), *Merck manual of geriatrics* (pp. 1055–1081). Rahway, NJ: Merck Sharp & Dohme Research Laboratories.
Linton, A.D. (2007). Age-related changes in the special senses. In A.D. Linton, & H.W. Lach (Eds.), *Matteson & McConnell's gerontological nursing* (3rd ed., pp. 600–627). St. Louis: Saunders Elsevier.
Mahoney, D.F. (1993). Cerumen impaction: Prevalence and detection in nursing homes. *Journal of Gerontological Nursing, 19,* 23–30.
Marieb, E.N., & Hoehn, K. (2007). *Human anatomy and physiology* (7th ed.). San Francisco: Pearson Benjamin Cummings.
Meisami, F. (1988). Aging of the nervous system: Sensory changes. In P. S. Timiras (Ed.), *Physiological basis of geriatrics* (pp. 156–178). New York: Macmillan.
Mhoon, E. (1997). Otologic changes and disorders. In C. K. Cassel, H. J. Cohen, E. B. Larson, D. E. Meier, N. M. Resnick, L. Z. Rubenstein, & L. B. Sorensen (Eds.), *Geriatric medicine* (3rd ed., pp. 699–716). New York: Springer-Verlag.
Miller, C. A. (2009). *Nursing for wellness in older adults* (5th ed.). Philadelphia: Wolters Kluwer/Lippincott Williams & Wilkins.
Rees, T. S., Duckett, L. G., & Milczuk, H. A. (1994). Auditory and vestibular dysfunction. In W. R. Hazzard, E. L. Bierman, J. P .Blass, W. H. Ettinger, & J.B. Halter (Eds.), *Principles of geriatric medicine and gerontology* (3rd ed., pp. 457–472). New York: McGraw-Hill.
Ross, V., Echevarria, K., & Robinson, B. (1991). Geriatric tinnitus: Causes, clinical treatment, and prevention. *Gerontological Nursing, 17,* 6–11.
Ross, V., & Robinson, B. (1984). Dizziness: Causes, prevention, and management. *Geriatric Nursing, Sept/Oct5*(7), 289–304.
Smith, S. C., & Neely, S. (2007). Visual and auditory problems. In. S. L. Lewis, M. M. Heitkemper, S. R. Dirksen, P. G. O'Brien, & L. Bucher (Eds.), *Medical surgical nursing* (7th ed., pp. 416–448). St. Louis: Elsevier.
Touhy, T.A. (2008). Sensory function. In P. Ebersole, P. Hess, T. A. Touhy, K. Jett, & A. S. Luggen (Eds.), *Toward healthy aging* (7th ed., pp. 338–369). St. Louis: Mosby Elsevier.
Vortherms, R.C. (1991). Clinically improving communication through touch. *Journal of Gerontological Nursing, 17,* 6–10.

8 The Cardiovascular System

Death from heart disease remains the primary cause of death and second cause of disability among older adults. Elders undergo most of the cardiovascular-related medical procedures and make up 65% of hospitalizations for cardiovascular disorders although they represent only 13% of the population (Rich, 2004; Jett, 2008).

Health problems in the cardiovascular system resulting from age-related changes and disease are often preventable. Primary modes of preventions include eating a healthy diet and exercising regularly. Data indicate a consistent exercise program changes both heart functioning and heart size and lowers blood pressure levels. Maintaining weight within a normal range and effective management of existing health problems can also do much to decrease the likelihood of heart disease.

Risk factors for cardiovascular disease include those not modifiable by lifestyle changes and those that can be modified, or changed. Non-modifiable risk factors include family history, gender (men are more likely to have cardiovascular disease than women), and age. Risk factors that can be modified by lifestyle changes include hypertension, diabetes, high cholesterol levels, obesity, alcohol use, smoking, a diet high in animal fats and calories, and a sedentary lifestyle (Jett, 2008). Personality characteristics also influence the development of heart disease. Stress, a significant factor in heart disease, may be modified by the use of relaxation techniques, lifestyle changes, and psychosocial therapies (Lakatta, 1999).

ANATOMY AND PHYSIOLOGY OF THE CARDIOVASCULAR SYSTEM

The cardiovascular system serves as a pump that moves arterial blood containing nutrients and oxygen through the arteries to the cells of the body where metabolism takes place. Waste products from cellular metabolic processes are then returned through the veins to be excreted by the excretory organs.

The Blood

Blood is a sticky, opaque fluid that accounts for about 8% of total body weight. Males have about five or six liters of blood in their bodies, whereas females have four or five liters. (Marieb & Hoehn, 2007). The blood is composed of:

1. Red blood cells (erythrocytes), which carry oxygen to all the cells of the body
2. White blood cells (leukocytes), which protect the body from attack by viruses, bacteria, toxins, parasites, and tumor cells
3. Platelets (thrombocytes), which are essential for blood clotting
4. Plasma, the fluid component of the blood in which solute (substances dissolved in a solution) and elements are suspended and circulated

Functions of the Blood

Blood, the major medium for the transportation of fluids throughout the body, has four significant functions in the maintenance of life and health. These functions are:

1. Respiratory. Blood distributes oxygen from the lungs to the tissues of the body for cell use, and takes carbon dioxide from the body tissues back to the lungs where it is expelled.
2. Nutritive. Blood transports food substances such as glucose, fat, and amino acids from storage places (e.g. the liver and intestines)

to body tissues where these materials are needed to produce energy and to maintain life.
3. Excretory. Blood moves waste products from body cells to the excretory organs.
4. Regulatory. Blood controls body equilibrium (homeostasis). Specifically, it distributes hormones, maintains water balance, and regulates temperature. For example, excess heat generated in the body is transported continuously by the blood to the lungs and to body surfaces where it is dissipated.

The Lymphatic System

The lymphatic system is composed of:

1. Lymph, a fluid originating in tissue spaces throughout the body
2. A one-way system of lymph vessels transporting lymph from tissue spaces to lymph ducts to the bloodstream

The major function of the lymphatic system is to assist in preventing the spread of infection and disease by straining out foreign particles and bacteria as the lymph passes through special lymphoid tissue (such as tonsils, adenoids, and lymph nodes) (Marieb & Hoehn, 2007).

The Blood-Vascular System

The human blood-vascular organizational plan is a closed system in which damage to any part will ultimately affect the entire system. The major components of the blood-vascular system are:

1. The heart, a pumping organ.
2. The arteries, tubes that conduct blood from the heart to body cells. The smallest artery branches are called arterioles.
3. The veins, tubes that conduct blood from body tissues back to the heart. Many veins contain one-way valves to prevent blood from flowing backward and thus help return blood to the heart. Valves are most common in veins of the limbs. The smallest vein branches are called venules.
4. The capillaries, minute blood vessels connecting arterioles and venules.

The Heart

The pump of the blood-vascular system is the heart, a hollow organ with highly muscular walls, which is situated within the thorax (chest) between the lungs in the space that separates the right and left pleural cavities. In complex organisms such as humans, the heart has four chambers: two *atria* (upper chambers) and two *ventricles* (lower chambers). A thick partition, the *septum*, separates the left side of the heart from the right. The largest artery of the body, the *aorta*, leads out of the left ventricle, and the *pulmonary artery* emerges from the right ventricle. The largest veins of the body (*superior* and *inferior vena cavae*) enter the right atrium, whereas the *pulmonary veins* enter the left atrium.

The atria and the ventricles are separated by atrioventricular (A-V) valves that control both the location and the amount of blood in each of the four chambers of the heart. The left valve is called the *mitral* or *bicuspid*, and the right valve is called the *tricuspid*. Other valves separate each ventricle from its specific artery (aorta or pulmonary); no valves are found between the atria and their respective veins (venae cavae or pulmonary).

Since the heart is composed of muscle tissue, it needs a rich blood supply in order to maintain proper functioning. *Coronary circulation* involves specific coronary arteries branching from the base of the aorta and distributing blood to the heart muscle. Veins collect the blood to

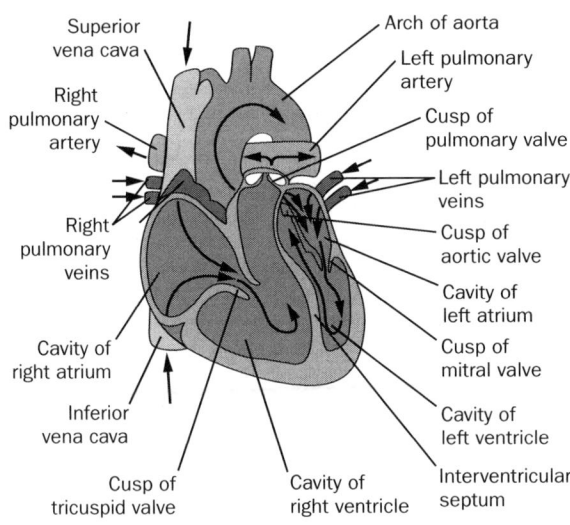

Figure 8.1. Anatomy of the heart and great vessels

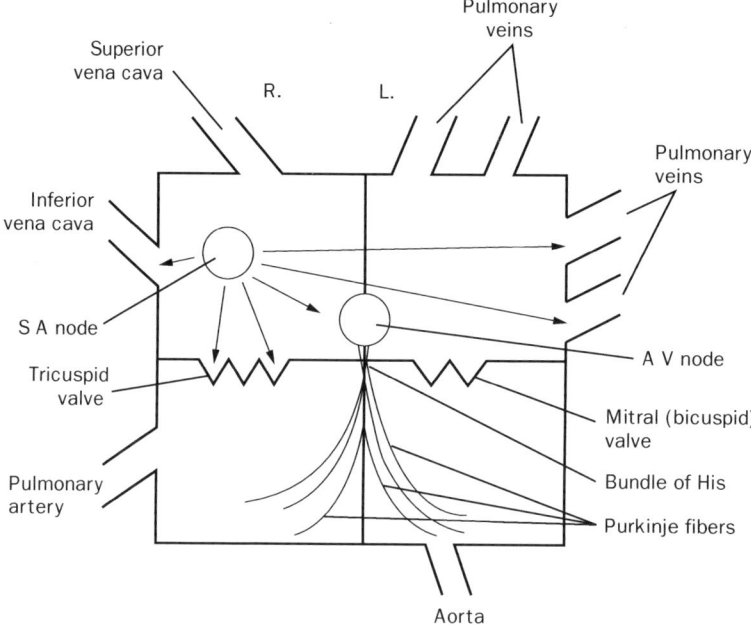

Figure 8.2. Schema of the electric conduction system of the heart

be returned to the right atrium through a large vein called the coronary sinus. If a coronary artery becomes occluded and blocks the supply of oxygen and nutrients to the heart muscle, a heart attack results.

Blood Circulation

In addition to coronary circulation, there are two blood circuits, one called systemic, which supplies all body parts with blood, and the other called pulmonary, which circulates blood through the lungs to purify it. The right side of the heart receives oxygen-poor blood from body tissues, whereas the left side of the heart receives oxygen-rich blood from the lungs.

Systemic Circulation

This part of the cycle begins as oxygen-rich blood from the lungs enters the left atrium via the pulmonary veins. When the atrium fills with blood, it contracts. The mitral valve opens, and blood flows into the left ventricle. Because the valve is a one-way device, blood normally flows only from the left atrium to the left ventricle. When the left ventricle fills with blood, the mitral valve closes, the ventricle contracts, the aortic valve opens, and blood is forced into the aorta, after which the aortic valve closes so blood cannot re-enter the ventricle. Blood circulates throughout the body by way of the aorta and other arteries, connects with veins at the level of the capillaries, and returns, depleted of oxygen and carrying carbon dioxide to the heart via various sized veins ending in the largest veins, the inferior and superior vena cavae, which empty into the right atrium. When the right atrium fills, the tricuspid valve opens, and the deoxygenated blood passes into the right ventricle.

Pulmonary Circulation

This part of the cycle begins after blood fills the right ventricle. The tricuspid valve closes, the ventricle contracts, and the pulmonary valve opens, forcing blood into the pulmonary artery to be carried to the lungs

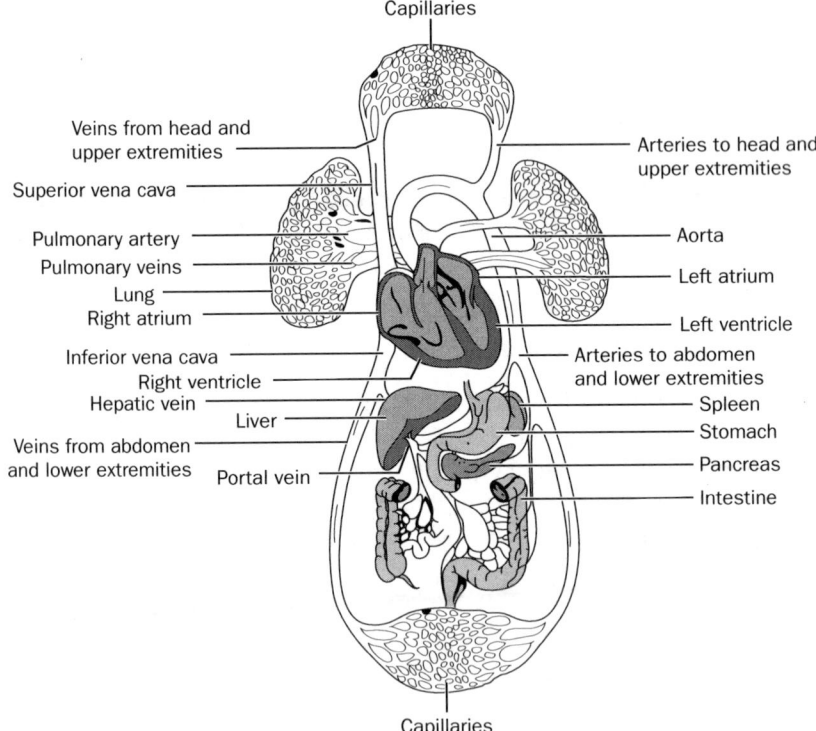

Figure 8.3. Diagram of the pulmonary and systemic circulations

The Cardiovascular System

to be oxygenated. The pulmonary valve closes so that blood cannot re-enter the ventricle. Oxygenated blood returns to the left atrium via the pulmonary veins, and the cycle begins again.

Various estimates suggest the body contains about 70,000 miles of blood vessels, most of which are capillaries. The heart beats at a rate of about 72 times a minute, or about 100,000 times a day. More than 4,000 gallons of blood are pumped through the heart each day.

The normal heart sounds, S1 ("lub") and S2 ("dub") are produced by the closure of the heart valves. The first heart sound (S1) is produced by the closing of both the mitral (bicuspid) and the tricuspid valves. The second heart sound (S2) is produced by the closure of the aortic and pulmonary valves. These sounds help health professionals assess the functional status of the heart.

Maintenance of Circulation

Circulation is maintained through the continuous rhythmic action of the heart. Although the nervous system affects heart rate, heart muscle is unlike other muscle because it is self-excitatory and has its own built-in pacemaker mechanism to maintain rhythmic and coordinated activity. Specifically, the heart beat is initiated by a segment of tissue in the right atrium designated as the sinoatrial (S-A) node. Excitation begun at the S-A node spreads to similar nodal tissue, the atrioventricular (A-V) node at the junction of the right atrium and right ventricle, and then through a bundle of fibers, (the bundle of His) to the ventricle walls, causing the heart to beat. Normally the atria and ventricles beat in a coordinated rhythm at approximately 72 times a minute. If injury or disease interferes with impulse transmission between the S-A and the A-V nodes, the atria and ventricles beat at different rates and heart block results. Sometimes if heart rhythm is disrupted random contractions (fibrillation) occur.

Blood Pressure

The contraction of the left ventricle forces blood into the aorta with a definite force or pressure. The pressure resulting from ventricular contraction is called systolic and represents the upper number of a blood pressure reading. During the subsequent brief relaxation of the ventricle, pressure decreases, representing the diastolic pressure (or resting phase), the lower number of a blood pressure reading.

According to most authorities, average blood pressure for a healthy young or middle-aged person at rest should be less than 120/80, although blood pressure fluctuates according to the individual's physiological and psychological status at the moment, and a variation of readings occurs throughout the day. High blood pressure is defined as a systolic reading of 140 mm Hg or higher over a diastolic reading of 90 mm Hg or higher or if the person uses anti-hypertensive drugs (Davis, 2008). The National Institutes of Health 7th Report of the Joint National Committee on Prevention, Detection, Evaluation, and Treatment of High Blood Pressure (2003) reports that the target blood pressure goal is a systolic reading less than 140 mm Hg over a diastolic reading of less than 90 mm Hg for those without other complicated illnesses and less than 130 mm Hg over less than 80 mm Hg for those with chronic kidney disease or diabetes. Several blood pressure readings need to be taken at different times before hypertension or hypotension (too high or too low blood pressure) can be diagnosed. Some of the factors influencing blood pressure are: (a) age (blood pressure tends to increase with age); (b) pumping action of the heart (this varies with age and health); (c) blood volume (the amount of blood pumped); (d) elasticity of arterial walls (which determines how easy or difficult it is for blood to flow); (e) thickness or thinness of the blood (this affects the rate of blood flow); and (f) peripheral resistance (especially in the limbs).

AGE-RELATED CARDIOVASCULAR CHANGES

While some cells, such as skin or blood cells, are self-replenishing, cardiac (heart) cells are not replaced once damaged or destroyed. In spite of this, it is especially difficult to determine which changes in the circulatory system are "normal" aging changes and which are pathological. More research on healthy older adults is needed to clarify this issue. Therefore, changes commonly reported in the literature are included with the acknowledgment that the distinction between aging and disease is not completely clear at this time.

Age-Related Structural Changes

Substantial evidence now indicates that the overall heart size in healthy older adults does not change significantly with age. Contrary to some popular opinion, an enlarged heart is not normal in older age and may instead suggest pathology. Age-related changes commonly occurring include:

1. Increase in fatty tissues in the outermost layer of the heart muscle.
2. Minimal increase in the thickness of the left ventricular wall (Lakatta, 2000).
3. Increase in collagen and elastin tissues in the heart and arteries, which causes the vessels to become more rigid and thick.
4. Decreased efficiency in the contractile strength of the heart muscle and decreased maximum heart rate, stroke volume, cardiac output, ejection fraction (the percentage of blood leaving the heart during a contraction), and oxygen uptake (Oskvig, 1999).
5. Accumulation of lipofuscin, a pigment giving a brown appearance to heart myocardium (middle layer of heart muscle).
6. Thickening and sclerosis (hardening) of the valve flaps of the heart, especially the tricuspid and mitral (bicuspid), but also in the aortic and pulmonic valves. This causes them all to be less efficient and possibly results in heart murmurs.
7. Pacemaker cells (cells that generate impulses and determine the rate of heart activity in the S-A node) decrease in significant numbers with a concomitant decrease in the S-A node rate. A 75 year old has only 10% of the S-A node cells that a 20 year old has (Taffet & Lakatta, 2003). There is some loss of muscle cells in the A-V node and the bundle of His and an increase in fatty fibrous tissue and amyloid (starch-like protein) infiltration, which is associated with degeneration. Elastic collagen type tissue increases in all parts of the conduction system (Lakatta, 1999).
8. Veins dilate and stretch. Valves in the veins function less efficiently, slowing down return of blood through the veins to the heart.
9. Coronary arteries may become dilated, twisted, and calcified. Circulation decreases about 35% in most adults after age 60 (Jett, 2008).

While not substantiated as an age-related change, both arteriosclerosis (lessened elasticity of artery walls) and atherosclerosis (fatty deposits on inner walls of arteries) are associated with age. Additional factors such as lack of exercise, smoking, obesity, and other diseases contribute to these vascular changes (Ferebee, 2006; House-Fancher & Lynch, 2007).

Age-Related Functional Changes in the Cardiovascular System

The following functional age-related changes in the cardiovascular system have been identified:

1. Longer recovery. Older heart muscle requires a longer time to recover after each heartbeat; in other words, the heart requires a slightly longer rest period between beats. This fact is not significant in most activity, but it may limit behavior in situations where the heart is stressed and required to beat faster than normal. Maximum attainable heart rate declines, but those who exercise do not show as much decline (Marieb & Hoehn, 2007). Generally, though, older people may be more prone to heart failure than younger adults who have a greater reserve capacity in heart functioning.
2. Slight arrhythmias. At rest, heart rate in older people is essentially the same as in younger people; however, some evidence suggests arrhythmias such as skipped or extra beats become more common with age. Arrhythmias sometimes produce anxiety in older adults who fail to understand it is not necessarily indicative of heart disease.
3. Decline in cardiac output. Cardiac output (the amount of blood pumped from the heart in one minute) declines somewhat with age, causing less oxygen to be delivered to body tissues and organs (Oskvig, 1999). Reduced cardiac output occurs both at rest and with exercise, but the decline usually has little significance for normal, everyday behavior. Nevertheless, this fact may help to explain why most older adults tire more quickly than the young, and why endurance, especially when doing strenuous work, tends to decline with age.
4. Increase in atrial fibrillation (irregular, rapid heart beat) and incidence of heart block (a blockage of the impulse conducted from the atria to the ventricle). These are related to age-related changes in the conduction system (which controls the rate and coordination of the heart beat).
5. Changes in arteries and veins. The arteries, and to a lesser extent the veins, become more rigid, less elastic and flexible. Elasticity of arteries is a major factor in regulating blood pressure. For instance, in excitement the heart beats faster and more blood is

pumped through the body at an increased rate. The elastic arterial walls normally expand to accommodate the greater force of blood pushed through, and thus arterial resistance is decreased, but if the arterial walls are rigid and cannot expand, the heart must pump harder to move more blood through the system quickly. Blood pressure increases as arterial resistance is increased. Such increases in blood pressure are a common corollary of the aging process. Changes in the veins predispose individuals to a slower return of venous blood to the heart, venous stasis (stagnation of venous blood), varicose veins, and thrombophlebitis (clotting in a vein due to phlebitis).

6. Blood components. Only slight changes are evident in the blood components with age. The volume of blood decreases as it relates to a lower plasma volume. Hemoglobin and hematocrit levels are only minimally diminished, and the red and white blood cells and the prothrombin (coagulation) time remain unchanged (Moore, 2006; House-Fancher & Lynch, 2007).

In summary, in non-stressful conditions the normal aging heart functions quite adequately unless there is severe damage to the heart from disease. Under stress, however, the effects of age become increasingly more obvious and gradually lead to limitations in activity. Current research recommends regular systematic exercise to promote continued adequate cardiac functioning in the later years. Walking is one of the best and safest ways for elders to exercise and needs no expensive equipment or special locations.

AGE-RELATED DISORDERS OF THE CARDIOVASCULAR SYSTEM

Arteriosclerosis and Atherosclerosis

Arteriosclerosis (hardening of the arteries) is the most common disease of arteries and involves a lessened elasticity and a thickening of the walls of the arteries, especially the small arteries and arterioles. This causes high blood pressure. *Atherosclerosis,* the most prevalent type of arteriosclerosis, involves small white patches that thicken (atheromas) and protrude into the blood vessel. Fatty, fibrous lesions and complicated plaques of scar tissue, calcium salts, and blood clot formation in the vessel cause hypertension, myocardial infarcts (heart attacks), strokes, aneurysms, and angina attacks (Marieb & Hoehn, 2007). Arteriosclerosis and atherosclerosis usually occur together, and it is rare to find one without the other. Their progress is not continuous but involves a building up and a breaking down of plaques. An increased level of low density lipoproteins (LDLs) influences the building up of the fatty streaks on the vessel walls, causing atherosclerosis, while high density lipoproteins (HDL) transport excess lipids from the peripheral tissues to the liver (Ralston, 2004). Atherosclerosis is often found in the aorta (which emerges from the heart and supplies blood to the entire body), the coronary vessels (which supply blood to the heart muscle), and the arteries that supply blood to the brain, abdomen, and legs.

Risk factors include age, gender, ethnicity, and a family history of the disease. Reversible risk factors include cigarette smoking, obesity, diabetes, elevated lipids, hypertension, homocysteine level, psychological state, and inactivity. Prevention should begin early in life, but it is never too late to initiate healthy behaviors.

Diagnosis is made through cholesterol and C-reactive protein levels and electron beam computed tomography (EBCT) that identify the presence of plaques. Treatment includes regular exercise, a low-fat, low-cholesterol diet, cholesterol reducing medications, baby aspirin (81 mg), balloon angioplasty, stents, and bypass surgery.

Both arteriosclerosis and atherosclerosis lead to ischemic heart disease (lack of adequate blood supply to the heart) as well as cerebral ischemia. They also cause increased blood pressure, produce extra stress on the heart muscle, and set the stage for other diseases of the cardiovascular system. The heart must work harder, but with less overall effectiveness resulting in insufficient oxygen delivered to body cells and decreased efficiency of body organs in performing their necessary functions.

Hypertension

Hypertension (HTN) is defined as a systolic blood pressure (SBP) greater than 140 mm Hg or a diastolic blood pressure (DBP) greater than 90 mm Hg on two separate occasions, or if the individual uses antihypertensive drugs. One in three adult Americans has hypertension although many do not know it until they experience a heart attack, stroke, heart failure, or it is discovered during a physical examination. Other complications of hypertension are peripheral vascular disease, chronic kidney disease, and retinal damage; thus early diagnosis and treatment are imperative.

The classification system identifies normal blood pressure as less than 120 mm Hg systolic and less than 80 mm Hg diastolic; pre-hypertension as 120 to 139 mm Hg systolic and 80 to 89 mm Hg diastolic; stage 1 HTN as 140 to 159 mm Hg systolic or 90 to 99 mm Hg diastolic; and Stage 2 HTN as at or above 160 mm Hg systolic or at or above 100 mm Hg diastolic (National Institutes of Health; Seventh Report of the Joint National Committee on Prevention, Detection, Evaluation, and Treatment of High Blood Pressure (2003). Early treatment of pre-hypertension is highly recommended since it can readily progress to Stage 1 and Stage 2 causing serious health complications (Hernandez, 2008). African-Americans have the highest incidence of HTN in the world. About two thirds of individuals age 65 and over experience HTN (Yen, 2004). More older women than men are affected, but males have a higher mortality rate (American Heart Association. Heart Disease and Stroke Statistics–2007 Update, 2007). As one ages, blood pressure increases but levels off in the 60s (Meyyazhagan & Messinger-Rapport, 2004).

Subtypes of HTN include:

(a) Isolated systolic hypertension (ISN), which occurs when the average SBP is 140 mm Hg or more and the average DBP is less than 90 mm Hg. It is more common among older adults and often due to decreased elasticity of the large arteries caused by atherosclerosis.

(b) Pseudohypertension, or false hypertension, which is caused by arteries that are sclerotic and do not compress when the blood pressure cuff is inflated fully (Bradley, 2007).

The etiology (cause) of hypertension is differentiated into:

(a) Primary (essential) hypertension, in which there is no obvious or apparent explanation for the sustained elevation in blood pressure. Approximately 90% of those diagnosed as hypertensive have essential hypertension.

(b) Secondary hypertension is high blood pressure caused by such entities as endocrine, neurologic, renal, and liver disorders as well as certain medications (Ferebee, 2006; Bradley 2007).

Persistent, abnormally high blood pressure, prevalent in many middle-aged and older adults, can be associated with other factors or systems involved in regulating blood pressure. These include: (a) the circulatory or cardiovascular system, because of its tendency toward sclerosis (hardening of the arteries); (b) the endocrine system, when it acts to retain sodium chloride in the body; (c) the excretory system, when renin (an enzyme involved in raising blood pressure) is released into the blood or when the kidneys do not excrete sodium chloride and water is drawn back from the urinary tubules into the blood; and (d) the nervous system, because it responds to excessive and prolonged emotional tension by increasing peripheral resistance to blood flow, often reflected as high blood pressure. Unfortunately, many individuals have hypertension but do not experience symptoms ("silent") until body functions become impaired. Even if they experience headaches, dizziness, or fatigue, these may or may not be associated with hypertension. Blood pressure should be checked regularly at each health care visit and at opportunities that are available at churches, senior centers, clinics, and other locations.

Risk Factors for the Development of Cardiovascular Disease

Non-Modifiable

Age. Blood pressure tends to increase gradually with age until in the 60s, when it tends to level off.

Gender. Men are more likely to be hypertensive in early and middle age, and women are more likely to develop hypertension after age 55.

Heredity. A family history of hypertension and heart disease increases the risk of other family members also developing hypertension.

Ethnicity. African-Americans have the highest incidence of hypertension and suffer from more cardiovascular and major organ complications than Caucasians do.

Diabetes. Diabetics are especially prone to hypertension and cardiovascular disease. When these co-exist the risk for complications is greater.

Modifiable

Obesity. Overweight individuals have a greater tendency to develop hypertension than those of average weight.

Alcohol. Excessive ingestion of alcohol increases the incidence of hypertension. Older persons with hypertension should limit their intake of alcohol to one ounce per day.

Smoking. Numerous research studies associate cardiovascular disease with smoking, and those with hypertension are at greater risk for cardiovascular disease.

Elevated lipids and cholesterol. A diet high in lipids and cholesterol increases the incidence of atherosclerosis, which narrows blood vessels and causes both hypertension and cardiovascular disease.

High sodium intake. Sodium intake promotes fluid retention and increases the likelihood of developing hypertension.

Stress. Prolonged high stress may increase blood pressure. The length of time the stress exists, the intensity of the stress, and the individual's response to stress are all modifiable factors.

Sedentary lifestyle. Regular, systematic exercise can reduce blood pressure and weight as well as the risk of developing cardiovascular disease (Bradley, 2007).

Prevention and Treatment of Hypertension

Early diagnosis and treatment are imperative to prevent extensive damage to major organs. Initially, non-pharmacologic measures are usually prescribed, but this depends on the blood pressure reading. Non-pharmacologic measures include weight reduction if obese, 30 minutes of daily systematic, aerobic exercise, moderate alcohol consumption, reduced sodium and caffeine intake, and no smoking. The Dietary Approaches to Stop Hypertension diet (DASH) limits sweets and meats, is rich in calcium and potassium while reducing total and saturated fats, and includes stress reduction and pharmacologic treatment (Hernandez, 2008).

If lifestyle changes are not effective, medications are prescribed. Initially a thiazide diuretic is usually the drug of choice; however, individuals taking these non-potassium-sparing drugs should be encouraged to take potassium supplements or eat potassium-rich foods such as bananas, oranges, dried prunes, or raisins. Beta blockers, angiotensin-converting enzyme (ACE) inhibitors, angiotensin receptor blockers (ARB), and calcium channel blockers (CCB) may be used alone or in combination to reduce blood pressure levels. A new class of antihypertensive drugs, the first in more than a decade includes Aliskiren (tekturna), the only drug presently in this class. Teaching older adults about the particular drug, its action, side effects, how and when to take it, what foods and drinks are not compatible, and the need to check blood pressure levels frequently is necessary. Many of these drugs may not be stopped suddenly, so contact with a primary care provider is very important if one has questions or unexpected drug reactions.

Postural Hypotension

Postural hypotension (orthostatic hypotension) occurs when systolic and diastolic blood pressure drops at least 20 to 10 mm Hg, respectively, within one to four minutes of standing after being in a recumbent position for a minimum of five minutes (Miller, 2009). Thirty to forty percent of elders over age 75 experience postural hypotension. It may be caused by age-related changes such as reduced sensitivity of the baroreceptors (receptors that sense blood pressure) and a decreased responsiveness of the sympathetic autonomic nervous system. Other prime causes include medications such as diuretics, antihypertensives, vasodilators, anti-depressants, alpha and beta blockers, and calcium channel blockers. Certain disease states such as hypertension, atherosclerosis, Parkinson's disease, arrythmias, anemia, dehydration, and fluid and electrolyte imbalance might also precipitate the symptoms (House-Fancher & Lynch, 2007). Symptoms include dizziness, lightheadedness, fainting, impaired vision, inability to walk properly, fatigue, and confusion, all of which may predispose elders to fall or experience other types of accidents.

Preventive Measures

Care must be taken to prevent blood pressure from falling too low and impairing coronary circulation. Medication regimens need to be continually monitored and evaluated. In addition, elders should be taught to rise slowly from a lying position and to sit for a short time before standing. Putting on elastic stockings prior to getting out of bed and reducing physical activity for an hour following a meal are also helpful. Other preventive measures include sleeping with the head of the bed elevated about 10 inches and avoiding hot baths (Walczak, 1991).

Acute Coronary Syndrome

Even though large amounts of blood continually pass through the heart, this blood does not provide the heart muscle with nutrients and oxygen. Instead, this function is carried out by a group of arteries called coronary arteries that branch off the aorta and envelop the heart. Coronary heart disease results when the blood supply through these arteries is reduced or blocked in any of the following ways:

1. Too high blood pressure in the coronary arteries may result in hemorrhage if a coronary blood vessel should rupture.
2. An aneurysm (a weakened area in the coronary arterial wall) may protrude and rupture causing a hemorrhage.
3. If blood clots form, they may restrict or block blood flow through the coronary arteries, depriving the heart muscle of blood.
4. Fatty deposits (atherosclerosis) in the inner walls of coronary arteries may interfere with blood flow to the heart muscle; this is the most frequent cause of heart disease in older persons.

Angina Pectoris

The term angina pectoris is Latin for "chest pain." It occurs when the heart muscle is not receiving an adequate blood supply for effective functioning due to occlusion (closure) or vasospasm (spasm of a blood vessel) of the coronary arteries. Attacks usually last three minutes or less, and are characterized by radiating pain primarily down the left side of the jaw, neck, between the shoulder blades, and down the arms. Pain, however, may also be on the right side and individuals may complain of feelings of tightness or pressure in the chest over the sternum or feelings of suffocation. These classic symptoms of angina may not be experienced by older adults, but weakness, fatigue, and difficulty breathing may be more likely (Wenger, 1997).

Chronic stable angina (exertional angina) is described as episodic (3–5 minutes) chest pain that occurs over a long time period. The symptoms, onset, intensity, and duration are similar but increase when causative factors such as cold weather, physical exertion, or a heavy meal are present (Martinez & Bucher, 2007). Because of decreased subcutaneous fat, older adults can develop symptoms of angina more rapidly than younger individuals, and should therefore wear an extra layer of clothing in cold weather.

Unstable angina is characterized by pain while at rest and with the slightest provocation. It occurs with increasing frequency and represents an emergency requiring immediate attention (Martinez & Bucher, 2007).

Diagnosis involves a careful history, observing whether the pain is relieved by nitroglycerin, an electrocardiogram, stress testing, and ambulatory heart monitoring. If medications are not effective, cardiac catheterization, angioplasty (a procedure by which a catheter is inserted into a coronary vessel and plaque is compressed against the vessel wall by the inflation of a balloon), placing a stent in the coronary artery to open up an occlusion in the vessel, or coronary bypass surgery may be indicated.

The initial treatment consists of 325 mg of aspirin with nitroglycerin. This is considered the cornerstone of anginal therapy because it inhibits spasms of the coronary vessels and improves collateral circulation to the heart muscle. Nitroglycerin is placed under the tongue and relief should occur in about three minutes. If not, the dosage is repeated up to three times. Medical attention is advised if the medication is not effective in relieving the discomfort. Long-acting nitrates are also prescribed to reduce or prevent episodes of angina.

Beta-adrenergic blockers, calcium channel blockers, and Ace inhibiters may also be prescribed. Three hundred and twenty-five mg or less of aspirin each day may be recommended because it thins the blood and can help prevent a myocardial infarction. Stress reduction and avoiding caffeine, heavy meals, and physical exertion is also advised.

Instructing older adults regarding precipitating factors, signs and symptoms of angina, and how and when to take medication or seek medical care are important. If sublingual nitroglycerin is prescribed it should be carried by the person at all times, stored in a capped dark glass bottle, and a new supply obtained every three months.

Myocardial Infarction (MI)

A myocardial infarction results when there is reduced or no blood flow to the heart muscle from the coronary arteries, which deprives the heart muscle of oxygen and causes the heart rhythm to become erratic or cease altogether. It may cause contained or extensive damage. Older adults are more likely to develop complications such as heart failure, dysrhythmia, pulmonary edema, and rupture of the heart (House-Fancher & Lynch, 2007). Those with an MI require close observation in an intensive care unit to prevent further complications.

Typical symptoms of an MI include severe, vice-like, continuous, constrictive, chest pain that frequently radiates to the jaw, neck, arm, and back. The pain often occurs in the early morning, is unrelieved by nitrates, position change, or rest, and lasts about 20 minutes or more. Other signs and symptoms include profuse perspiration, moist, clammy skin, pallor, nausea, and vomiting. Anxiety, restlessness, drop in blood pressure, arrhythmias, shock, and heart failure may also be present (Martinez & Bucher, 2007). Twenty-five to sixty-eight percent of MIs are not identified as an MI; this "silent MI" occurs most frequently in older adults and women who may not display the usual clinical symptoms of a heart attack. Instead of the classic symptoms, these populations may have gastric disturbances, dizziness, nausea and vomiting, fatigue, behavioral or mental changes, or a dysrhythmia (Arnow, 2006; Miller, 2009). The course of the illness is more complex and the mortality rate is higher among elders, so early definitive diagnosis and treatment are imperative (House-Fancher & Lynch, 2007).

Early treatment is vital but is sometimes delayed due to the atypical presentation of symptoms in elders. An electrocardiogram, various scans, serum cardiac markers and other blood tests, an angiogram, or stress test may be used to diagnose an MI. The treatment may involve fibrolytic therapy, such as t-PA, administered within a rigid time frame; however, these drugs have multiple contraindications. Seeking medical attention immediately is crucial because these drugs should only be administered within three hours of the symptoms' first appearance. Other treatments include IV nitroglycerin, morphine sulfate, ACE inhibitors, B-adrenergic blockers, anticoagulants, antidysrhythmias, and cholesterol lowering agents. Coronary angioplasty, intracoronary stents, and coronary bypass surgery are other treatment options (Martinez & Bucher, 2007).

Rehabilitation

Cardiac rehabilitation, along with dedication to a healthy lifestyle, is paramount in preventing coronary artery disease. Cardiac rehabilitation programs are now widely available throughout the country. These programs introduce individuals to monitored exercise and educate them about the benefits of stress reduction, smoking cessation, modified alcohol ingestion, and weight control. Dietary teaching includes reducing sodium and fat consumption and increasing servings of high-fiber foods like fruits, vegetables, and whole grains. (Sherman, 2008). Psychosocial issues such as risk modification, psychological support, socialization, and resuming sexual activity are also considered.

Congestive Heart Failure (CHF)

Congestive heart failure occurs when the heart is no longer able to pump adequate blood and oxygen to body tissues during exercise or even at rest. There may be left-sided (diastolic) heart failure due to the failure of the left ventricle to adequately pump the blood it is receiving from the lungs, which results in a build-up of fluid in the lungs. Right-sided (systolic) heart failure occurs when the right side of the heart cannot empty itself adequately of the blood coming from the venous circulation, which produces a back-up of fluid (edema) in the extremities or in the abdominal cavity (ascites). The signs and symptoms include coughing, shortness of breath, wheezing, edema, loss of appetite, nausea, and tachycardia. Atypical signs include fatigue, disorientation, and weakness (Mauk, 2006). Diagnosis involves a history, a physical examination assessing pulmonary and systemic congestion and measuring the output of the heart, a chest X-ray, an echocardiogram, an electrocardiogram, blood chemistries, exercise, stress testing, nuclear imaging studies, and cardiac catheterization (Martinez & Bucher, 2007; Jett, 2008).

Two-thirds of those with CHF are over age 65. Congestive heart failure usually develops gradually and progresses over time with a high morbidity and mortality rate. It frequently is undetected in the early stages because symptoms of fatigue and shortness of breath may be expected and equated with growing older (Jett, 2008).

Risk Factors for CHF

Cardiac factors. Coronary artery disease, myocardial infarction, hypertension, and valvular heart disease all reduce the efficiency of the pumping action of the heart.

Non-cardiac factors. Pathologies increasing the risk for CHF are chronic obstructive pulmonary disease, pulmonary emboli, kidney disease, liver disease, and anemia.

Iatrogenic factors (caused as a result of treatment). Medications used by elders, such as beta blockers, digoxin, steroids, hormones, and anti-inflammatory drugs, often increase the risk of CHF.

Other factors such as malnutrition severe enough to produce fluid and electrolyte imbalances, obesity, and prolonged high stress situations may also cause CHF.

Treatment of CHF

Treatment includes medications, lifestyle and dietary management, and rest. The goals of treatment are: (a) to reduce the body's demand for high cardiac output (through a balanced exercise/rest program and weight reduction); (b) to increase the cardiac output if possible (usually through the use of medication); and (c) to reduce body congestion (water and sodium retention) by sodium restriction and medications such as diuretics. Digoxin (digitalis) is used to increase the force of the heart's contractions and slow down the heart rate. It is important to teach individuals how to take an accurate pulse and not to take digoxin if the pulse rate is below 60 unless otherwise instructed by a primary care practitioner. Digitalis toxicity is common among older adults, so blood levels need to be monitored regularly. Other drugs prescribed for CHF include diuretics, morphine sulfate, vasodilators, B-adrenergic blockers, positive inotropes, angiotensin-converting enzymes, and angiotensin II receptor blockers.

If prescribed diuretics deplete potassium, foods rich in potassium such as bananas should be encouraged. Sodium restriction helps to decrease the work load on the heart. For CHF to be adequately managed, older adults and family need to understand as much as possible about the disease, its treatment, medications, and a healthy lifestyle. Ongoing education and monitoring, in addition to psychological support, is crucial in preventing exacerbations of the disease. The prognosis in older adults is guarded since CHF is an end-stage heart disease reflecting the accumulative effects of other serious pathologies.

Heart Valve Disease

The incidence of heart valve disease is increasing as larger numbers of people are living longer and have degenerative heart diseases. Heart valve disease is thought to be due to valvular or muscle dysfunction, endocarditis (inflammation of the lining of the heart), and/or rheumatic diseases. Mitral valve disease causes mitral regurgitation and is usually related to rheumatic heart disease that occurred in childhood. Aortic stenosis, often seen in older adults, is caused by sclerosis of the aortic cusps.

Cardiac Arrhythmias and Conduction Disorders

With aging, cardiac arrhythmias (irregular heartbeats) become more common, although they may not always be clinically significant (Horowitz & Lynch, 1991). Arrhythmias and conduction disorders (disorders affecting the heart's ability to regulate a synchronized heartbeat) are more serious in older adults because vital body functions are already less efficient, and reduced blood supply to tissues is less well tolerated. Disturbances found more often in the older age group include premature atrial and ventricular contractions, atrial fibrillation (extremely rapid incomplete contractions), and abnormal rhythms of the atrial pacemaker mechanism. Impaired functioning of the SA node may cause "sick sinus syndrome" resulting in dysrhythmias, sinus bradycardia (slow heart beat), heart block, and/or palpitations (rapid throbbing pulsations), weakness, dizziness, or fainting. These disorders are frequently first identified during a routine health examination.

Treatment involves antiarrhythmic drugs such as digoxin, beta blockers, sodium, potassium or calcium channel blockers, B-adrenergic blockers, and other medications. Sometimes the use of a manual or automatic external defibrillator or a synchronized cardioversion is warranted to interrupt the dysfunctional rhythm and restore normal heart rhythm. A permanent pacemaker or an implantable cardioverter-defibrillator may also be implanted to maintain or restore normal heart rhythm.

Transient Ischemic Attack (TIA, Mini-Stroke)

A TIA is an early warning of impairment in the blood supply to the brain and, potentially, of an imminent major stroke. One third of those who have a TIA will eventually have a stroke, which most likely occurs within two to seven days after a TIA; however, Giles and Rothwell (2007) report individuals treated immediately after a TIA by a specialist had a lower stroke risk than those who were not treated. TIAs are caused by a sudden interruption in the circulation of blood and oxygen to the brain usually lasting less than 24 hours, with no permanent brain injury. At risk for TIAs are those age 60 and over with hypertension, obesity, diabetes, cerebrovascular insufficiency, and cardiovascular disease. Also at risk are smokers, alcoholics, and those with sleep apnea (Louden, 2007). New Guidelines of the American Stroke Association (2006) recommend treating a TIA in the same way as an ischemic stroke. Initially there should be a complete diagnostic workup and the same preventive treatments used for a stroke should be prescribed. Various medical options should be considered including the use of blood thinners and interventional therapies such as endarterectomy (surgical removal of a blood clot from the carotid artery), angioplasty (when a balloon attached to a catheter is blown up to compress the plaque against the vessel wall), or the placement of a stent in the carotid artery. Such interventions carry some risk of a stroke; thus it is important to select a surgeon who has a low rate of complications and who has performed large numbers of these procedures. Individuals on blood thinners should be carefully monitored for signs of bleeding in the urine, feces, or under the skin. The individual should also be counseled to adopt healthy behaviors such as a low-cholesterol, low-fat diet, no smoking, minimal alcohol intake, and a consistent exercise regimen.

Symptoms last from a few minutes to 24 hours, with recovery often occurring in 3 hours. TIAs frequently go unnoticed because symptoms are minimal and of short duration. Typical signs of a TIA are: (a) sudden, temporary weakness or numbness of the face, arm, or leg; (b) difficulty understanding speech; (c) brief vision loss in one or both eyes; (d) double vision; (e) unexplained headaches or a change in the type of headache; (f) temporary dizziness or unsteadiness; and (g) change in personality or mental abilities (Louden, 2007).

If TIAs lead to small strokes, tissue damage will accumulate and eventually produce changes in behavior. Sometimes behavioral changes following accumulated mini-strokes are so slight that only close family members realize the subtle changes taking place in personality or mood. Any unusual or persisting change in normal behavior patterns, or other unusual symptoms, should be evaluated immediately by a professional because early diagnosis and treatment are important.

Cerebrovascular Accident (CVA, Stroke)

A cerebrovascular accident (CVA, stroke) results when the blood supply to any part of the brain is reduced or completely shut off. The majority of elders experience an *ischemic stroke,* which includes either a thrombotic or embolic stroke. A thrombotic stroke occurs when a cerebral artery is narrowed by plaque (fatty deposits) in the artery, which causes a clot to form (cerebral thrombosis) that either reduces or closes off the blood flow to an area of the brain. An embolic stroke is caused by air, fat tissue, blood clot, or other foreign matter circulating in the blood that blocks blood flow in a cerebral vessel. A *hemorrhagic stroke* occurs when a weak spot in a blood vessel of the brain bursts causing bleeding into the brain tissue. The most common location of a stroke is the middle cerebral artery and at the bifurcation of the common carotid artery (House-Fancher & Lynch, 2007).

Significant risk factors associated with a stroke include hypertension, heart disease, previous TIAs, smoking, diabetes, atherosclerosis, high cholesterol, and a family history of strokes. Those of African ancestry have a higher incidence of strokes, and more men than women have strokes. Individuals with one or more of these risk factors should be especially attentive to their health and lifestyle, because the best treatment for stroke is prevention.

Strokes affect behavior in many different ways depending upon the location and the amount of brain tissue damaged. Injury to the right half of the brain may result in impaired movement and sensation on the left side of the body, spatial-perceptual difficulties, and memory problems. Conversely, strokes on the left half of the brain affect movement and sensation on the right side of the body. Language or speech aphasia, impaired vision, reduced comprehension, or emotional problems may also result.

Following a thorough history and physical examination, careful screening must begin immediately using angiography, CT, PET, MRI, or other scans, and laboratory tests. If the individual has an ischemic stroke and meets the specific criteria, tPA (tissue plasminogen activator) or other drugs may be given intravenously (IV) to help re-establish blood flow through the occluded artery. This therapy must be initiated within three hours of the time the individual shows the first clinical signs of a stroke. Thus calling an emergency number such as 911 and getting the individual to a designated stroke center or an acute care hospital is necessary. Initially the person's status is stabilized in ICU. Depending on the type, location, and extent of tissue damage, post-stroke management can include anticoagulants or anti-platelet therapy and prolonged physical and psychological rehabilitation to help improve functioning and to prevent the many complications of a stroke. A team approach is initiated involving medical and nursing care and physical, occupational, speech, psychological, and social therapy, ideally at a rehabilitation center. Most neurological recovery takes place within the first three to six months following a stroke. Family functioning is greatly affected following a stroke in a family member. Since the healing process is often prolonged, family need to assume added responsibilities of caregiving, managing a household, transportation, cooking, and managing finances. The family experiences many of the same psychological responses as the patient; thus they too need continual social and psychological support. Patient/family teaching is paramount to assist them in understanding the importance of a healthy lifestyle regarding diet, exercise, medication adherence, and stress free living.

VASCULAR DISORDERS

Peripheral vascular disease is primarily a result of generalized atherosclerosis, causing a narrowing of the arteries in extremities as well as the neck, head, abdomen, and legs. Both aneurysmal and occlusive vascular disease result from atherosclerosis.

Aneurysm

Aneurysms tend to occur after age 60, with males more likely candidates than females. Those with hypertension and atherosclerosis are more prone to aneurysms. Aneurysm is the term for a "pouch" formation in a weakened arterial wall. The pouch fills with blood and may burst, especially if the arterial wall is weak and blood pressure is high; the larger the aneurysm the more likely it is to rupture. When aortic and cerebral aneurysms rupture, shock and death often result. Other areas commonly affected include the femoral and popliteal arteries in the leg. While significant pain does not always accompany an aneurysm, some individuals experience chest, back, and abdominal pain, or leg weakness. Some individuals also experience cramping when walking that is relieved by rest. Treatment involves supportive treatment and dissection of the aneurysm that replaces the area with a synthetic graft material.

Arterial Occlusion

The major causes of arterial occlusion are thrombosis, embolism, and trauma. An occlusion develops inside an artery near an area having plaque formation. Most often they occur in the coronary vessels, causing a coronary infarction, or perhaps in the legs. When the legs are involved they become cold, pale, and bluish colored; severe pain is present along with intermittent cramping, especially after walking. Diagnosis utilizes vascular studies, scans, ultrasound, a thorough history, and a physical examination.

Treatment involves increasing the flow of blood to the area through exercise, anticoagulant therapy, or surgery. Elders should be advised not to cross their legs or wear tight clothing, and shoes should be made of leather, well fitted, and comfortable. Feet should be kept clean and dry with foot care provided by a podiatrist. Any trauma, blister, or break in the skin needs to be immediately reported to a primary care practitioner.

Varicose Veins

Varicose veins are caused by the inefficiency of one-way valve peripheral veins that return blood from the peripheral to the central circulation. Blood then pools, especially in the lower extremities, vein walls become weak, and swollen, "knotted" veins result from the slowed circulation. Varicose veins are more prevalent in females and the obese, with a predisposition to varicosities occurring in families. Treatment involves keeping the affected limb elevated, avoiding trauma to the leg, wearing support hose, and the use of sclerotherapy, laser, high-intensity pulsed-light therapy, endovenous occulsion, or saphenofemoral ligation. Varicose veins in the lower part of the rectum and anus are called hemorrhoids.

Phlebitis and Deep Vein Thrombosis

Phlebitis is an inflammation of a vein, often in the leg, producing conditions favorable for the formation of blood clots (thrombi) that can break loose and occlude a major vessel in the lungs (pulmonary embolism), heart, or brain and may be life threatening. Particularly at risk are postoperative knee or hip surgery patients who are elderly or obese and those who smoke, are dehydrated, or have major heart or circulatory problems. Signs and symptoms include a leg that is bluish-red in color, warm to touch, tender, swollen, and painful, especially when the toe is pointed toward the heart (Homan's sign). Appropriate leg exercises, anti-embolic stockings, intermittent compression devices (ICDs), and anticoagulant therapy are among the appropriate treatment choices.

SUMMARY

Heart disease remains the most common cause of death in individuals over age 65, but it is often preventable, especially if health promotion behaviors are initiated early in life. Nevertheless, positive results can be attained even if they are begun later in life. Maintaining an active exercise regimen, controlling weight, and managing stress are all necessary for optimal cardiac health.

Cardiovascular disease frequently leads to fear and anxiety, increasing self-preoccupation, and impatience with those who are healthy and active. It is important that efforts be directed toward assuming a normal lifestyle following each episode of cardiac dysfunctioning. Many individuals with cardiovascular disease live normal, well-balanced lives under medical supervision. Participation in a cardiac rehabilitation program is especially recommended to promote a longer, healthier life.

REFERENCES

American Heart Association. *Heart Disease and Stroke Statistics-2007 Update.* Dallas, TX: American Heart Association.

Arnow, W.S. (2006). Heart failure guidelines focus on prevention, new therapies. *Geriatrics, 61*(1), 14.

Bradley, E.G. (2007). Nursing management: Hypertension. In S. L. Lewis, M. M. Heitkemper, S.R. Dirksen, P.G. O'Brien, and L. Bucher (Eds.), *Medical-surgical nursing* (7th ed., pp. 761–783). St. Louis: Mosby Elsevier.

Davis, L. L. (2008). Blood pressure in America: The magnitude of the problem. In L. L. Davis, R. J. Trupp, & E. J. Valezquez (Eds.), *Getting to goal in hypertensive treatment: Practical strategies* (pp. 4–7). Montvale, NJ:Haymarket Medical Education.

Ferebee, L. (2006). Cardiovascular function. In S. E. Meiner, & A.G. Lueckenotte (Eds.), *Gerontologic nursing* (3rd ed., pp. 468–503). St. Louis: Mosby Elsevier.

Giles, M. F., & Rothwell, P. M. (2007). Risk of stroke early after transient ischemic attack: A system review and meta-analysis. *Lancet Neurology, 6*(12), 1063–1072.

Hernandez, J. (2008). Prehypertension: Why should we worry? *Advance for Nurse Practitioners, 16* (1), 65–73.

Horowitz, L.N., & Lynch, R.J. (1991). Managing geriatric arrhythmias: General considerations. *Geriatrics, 46*(3), 31–38.

House-Fancher, M. A., & Lynch, R. J. (2007). Cardiovascular system. In A. D. Linton, & H.W. Lach (Eds.), *Matteson & McConnell's gerontological nursing* (3rd ed., pp. 313–352). St. Louis: Saunders.

Jett, K. (2008). Chronic disease in later life. In P. Ebersole, P. Hess, T. A. Touhy, K. Jett, & A. S. Luggen (Eds.), *Toward healthy aging* (7th ed., pp.222–268). St. Louis: Mosby Elsevier.

Lakatta, E. G. (1999). Circulatory function in younger and older humans in health. In W. R. Hazzard, J. P. Blass, W. H. Ettinger, J. B. Halter, & J.G. Ouslander (Eds.), *Principles of geriatric medicine and gerontology* (4th ed., pp. 645–660). New York: McGraw-Hill.

Lakatta, E. G. (2000). Cardiovascular aging in health. *Clinics in geriatric medicine, 16,* 419–444.

Louden, K. (2007). Transient ischemic attack: A medical emergency. *Nursing Spectrum, 17*(24), 8.

Mareib, E. N., & Hoehn, K. (2007). *Human anatomy and physiology* (7th ed.). San Francisco: Pearson Benjamin Cummings.

Martinez, L. G., & Bucher, L. (2007). Nursing management: Coronary artery disease and acute coronary syndrome. In S. L. Lewis, M. M. Heitkemper, S. R. Dirksen, P. G. O'Brien, & L. Bucher (Eds.), *Medical-surgical nursing* (7th ed., pp. 784–820). St. Louis: Mosby Elsevier.

Mauk, K. (2006). Management of common illnesses, diseases, and health conditions. In K. Mauk (Ed.), *Gerontological nursing* (pp. 391–474). Sudbury, MA: Jones & Bartlett.

Meyyazhagan, S., & Messinger-Rapport, B. (2004). Hypertension. In C. S. Landerfeld (Ed.), *Current geriatric diagnoses and treatment* (pp. 183–190). New York: McGraw-Hill.

Miller, C. (2009). *Nursing for wellness in older adults* (5th ed.). Philadelphia: Wolters Kluwer/Lippincott Williams & Wilkins.

Moore, S. A. (2006). Laboratory and diagnostic tests. In S.E. Meiner, & A.G. Lueckenotte (Eds.), *Gerontologic nursing* (3rd ed., pp. 427–446). St. Louis: Mosby Elsevier.

National Institutes of Health: Seventh Report of the Joint National Committee on Prevention, Evaluation, and Treatment of High Blood Pressure (2003). Bethesda,MD: National Institutes of Health.

National Heart, Lung, and Blood Institute (2006). New Guidelines, American Stroke Association. *Stroke, 37,* 577–617.

Oskvig, R.M. (1999). Special problems of the elderly. *Chest, 115* (suppl. 2), 158–164.

Ralston, A. (2004). Cardiovascular system. In S. L. Lewis, M. M. Heitkemper, S. R. Dirksen, P.G. O'Brien, J. F. Giddens, & L. Bucher (Eds.), *Medical-surgical nursing* (6th ed., pp. 756–776). St. Louis: Mosby Elsevier.

Rich, M. (2004). Cardiac disease. In C. S. Landerfeld (Ed.), *Current geriatric diagnoses and treatment* (pp. 156–182). New York: McGraw-Hill.

Sherman, C. (2008). Reducing the risk of heart disease in women. *The Clinical Advisor, 11*(1), 49–53.

Taffet, G. E., & Lakatta, E. G. (2003). Aging of the cardiovascular system. In W. R. Hazzard, J. P. Blass, J. B. Halter, J. G. Ouslander, & M. Tinetti (Eds.), *Principles of geriatric medicine and gerontology* (5th ed., pp. 403–421). New York: McGraw-Hill.

Walczak, M. (1991). The prevalence of orthostatic hypotension in high risk ambulatory elders. *Journal of Gerontological Nursing, 17*(11), 26–29.

Wenger, N. K. (1997). Cardiovascular disease. In C. K. Cassel, H. J. Cohen, E. B. Larson, D. E. Meier, N. M. Resnick, L. Z. Rubenstein, & L. B. Sorensen (Eds.), *Geriatric medicine* (3rd ed., pp. 357–374). New York: Springer-Verlag.

Yen, P. (2004). Nutritional treatment of coronary artery disease. *Geriatric Nursing, 25*(4), 246–247.

17 Health Promotion and Exercise

Health is defined by the World Health Organization (1946) as "a state of complete physical, mental, and social well-being not merely the absence of disease or infirmity" (p.100). Health and wellness for older adults can be best described as a potential balance between a person's internal and external environment plus an individual's physical, social, emotional, and cultural functioning (Touhy, 2008).

Older adults often view themselves as healthy when they are able to carry out the activities of daily living, and they live full productive lives despite the presence of disability and disease. In this light an appropriate definition of health for elders is not necessarily total freedom from disease, but rather the ability to live and function in society and to exercise self-reliance and autonomy to the maximum extent possible (Filner & Williams 2000).

Hansen-Kyle (2005) describes health in the latter years as "a process of slowing down, physically and cognitively, while resiliently adapting and compensating in order to optimally function and participate in all areas of one's life–physical, cognitive, social, and spiritual" (p. 52). Rather than continuing the more traditional health care modalities of managing disease and illness, the focus must be on diminishing risks for illness, maintaining maximal functioning, and lessening illness-associated disabilities (Touhy, 2008).

Older age is often considered to be a time of illness, disability, and pain, yet based on current evidence it is reasonable to suggest that many of the health problems commonly associated with older age need not exist, or at least may be delayed to old-old age. Kligman (1992) cites Fries' "compression of morbidity theory," which proposes that life-threatening chronic problems can be delayed to the very end of the life span by judicious use of preventive health measures. The population of elders then would be larger and healthier than previously, but there would also be a larger number coping with age-related and age-determined disability, frailty, and comorbidity (Nakasato & Carnes, 2006). Among the leading causes of illness and death in people over age 65 are strokes, cancer, coronary heart disease, lung disease, falls and fractures, depression, dementia, influenza, and pneumonia. Many of these conditions could be prevented or their progress slowed, resulting in a significantly improved quality of life.

HEALTH PROMOTION

Health promotion focuses on assisting individuals to achieve maximum health status and is closely linked to successful aging (Resnick, 2006). Rowe & Kahn (1998) define successful aging as the ability to maintain three important states: low risk for disease or disabilities; high level of physical and mental functioning; and engaging actively in life. Resnick (2006) identifies significant areas of health promotion for older adults as: control of smoking; mind-body health; maximal nutritional status; weight control; social health; medical self-care; spiritual health care; and environmental health. Addressing health in a holistic manner should involve incorporating all these aspects into the older person's life. Maintaining a positive attitude and living life to the fullest while realistically facing concomitant age-related changes and diseases can result in a happy, fulfilled, transcendent life throughout the latter years.

DISEASE PREVENTION

Chronic and even communicable diseases in older age pose a tremendous financial burden on society and constitute a large percentage of the national health budget. As increasing numbers of people live to older age, this percentage will escalate unless health promotion and disease prevention measures and programs are adopted by individuals of all ages.

Healthy People 2010 (2000) is a comprehensive plan for the nation regarding health promotion and disease prevention. Its purpose is to achieve two goals: first, to increase the quality and years of healthy life; and second, to eliminate health disparities. These goals are supported by 28 focus areas and 467 objectives; targets are to be achieved by 2010. The focus areas are related to 10 major health indicators: physical activity; overweight and obesity; tobacco use; substance abuse; responsible sexual behavior; mental health; injury and violence; and environmental quality. Healthy People 2010 is available from the U.S. Government Printing Office.

Hickey & Stilwell (1991) discuss the differences between health promotion for the young and the old. For youth, the focus is primarily on exercising regularly, eating a good diet, and not smoking, goals which are also appropriate for elders. For elders, the focus is more on early treatment and modification of lifestyle to slow the progression of chronic diseases, minimizing disability, and maintaining functional independence for as long as possible.

Ideally, those who arrive at old age in a healthy state will be able to maintain their health for a long time. Preventive health strategies are important, though, and beneficial for individuals in all stages of life. Fried (1990) describes the various health issues specifically affecting older adults as the presence of new chronic or acute diseases; diseases already present that will result in death; and the dependence, disability, functional losses, hospitalizations, and eventual death which are the outcomes of chronic illnesses. According to Lach (2007) these issues are best approached by using the following preventive measures:

1. Primary prevention. These measures involve identifying and targeting risk factors in individuals and preventing disease before it starts, for example, eating a diet with lower levels of fat and salt to reduce the incidence of cardiovascular disease and getting recommended immunizations.
2. Secondary prevention. The goal of secondary prevention is to prevent disease while it is still asymptomatic or unreported, and identify unrecognized health problems in the early stages by screening and assessment. Examples include identifying high cholesterol levels or blood pressure during a routine visit to the primary care practitioner.

Physical Change & Aging

3. Tertiary prevention. This measure involves minimizing the overall effects of disease by accurate diagnosis, appropriate treatment, and rehabilitation that aims to prevent the progression of symptoms.

Health promotion and disease prevention measures are valuable no matter when in life they are initiated.

Primary and Secondary Prevention Guidelines

The following are more specific primary and secondary prevention guidelines for attaining optimal health in older age:

1. Dental check-ups are recommended annually or biannually.
2. Immunizations for influenza should be obtained yearly; pneumococcal pneumonia vaccine once, with a one time revaccination if the prior vaccination occurred 5 or more years previously and the person was under age 65 at the time of the primary vaccination; tetanus diphtheria (TD) one dose every 10 years: and the shingles vaccine once in a lifetime. Other vaccines are recommended for elders who are at risk for developing a specific disease or who are exposed to a specific disease. These include hepatitis A, hepatitis B, varicella, and meningococcal vaccines (Lach, 2007).
3. Recommended screenings include an annual preventive health examination in which blood pressure, height, and weight are measured; mammogram and breast clinical examination annually with a monthly self-breast exam; and a Papanicolaou (Pap) smear yearly until three normal ones and then once every 3 years; a periodic bone density scan for women; digital rectal examination; and an annual prostate-specific antigen assay for men. In addition, one should have colon and rectal cancer screening beginning at age 50, fasting cholesterol screening every 5 years, eye examinations every 1 to 2 years, a hearing examination every 3 years, and skin examination yearly. Other types of recommended health assessments include diabetic and thyroid testing, cognitive impairment screening, depression screening, and HIV testing as indicated.
4. Periodic assessments are advised regarding the health habits and behaviors of elders including tobacco use, drug or alcohol

abuse, sexual behavior, food intake, exercise regimen, sleep patterns, mental health status, and quality of their living environment, particularly regarding injury and violence (Mauk, 2006; Resnick, 2006).

Tertiary Prevention Guidelines

Secondary and tertiary prevention often overlap. Tertiary preventive measures are directed toward maintaining functional autonomy and enhancing quality of life when disease is already present. The following are recommended:

1. Evaluation of the individual's physical and functional impairments. This might include assessing drug use and side effects, incontinence, falls, foot problems, depression, immobilization, disorientation, visual or hearing impairments, and how dependent the person is on others.
2. Assessment of factors in the person's environment such as room temperature; accessibility of bathroom, kitchen, and bedroom; the presence of safety hazards (such as scatter rugs); ability to contact others in emergencies; ability to secure food and maintain an adequate diet; the availability of adequate clothing; and knowledge of and ability to contact support services.
3. Continual monitoring of rehabilitative therapies such as physical, occupational, or speech therapy to restore and maintain functional capabilities for as long as possible.
4. Monitoring health status and personal hygiene by health care providers.
5. Assessment of family and social services available in the community to assist the elder in compensating for losses.

Fried (1990) suggests that tertiary prevention is the most important focus of care for older adults because it deals with preventing dependency and disability, maintaining functioning, and improving quality of life in the latter years. She believes, however, that all three types of prevention (primary, secondary, and tertiary) can have a significant impact on the lives of older adults and advocates an approach based on the use of risk profiles and individual health assessments to determine the best possible outcomes.

STRATEGIES FOR CHANGE

Healthy People 2000 (1992) states that the responsibility for adopting health-protective behaviors must be shared by:

1. The individual. The individual is the starting point and the major target of a health promotion campaign. Disease can best be prevented and health best promoted when individuals take responsibility for their own health behavior. Such health behaviors include changes in alcohol and drug use, diet, exercise, sexual habits, engaging in injury prevention behaviors, and using health screening and immunizations.
2. The family. The family is seen as the major context in which health promotion behaviors occur. Here attitudes and behaviors concerning hygiene, smoking, alcohol, drug use, physical activities, and diet are initially learned and reinforced by parents. Parents also have the responsibility for initiating essential preventive care such as immunizations, health screening, and teaching children about health risks and behaviors.
3. The community. Within the community local health officials, voluntary and business organizations, community leaders, schools, and churches can all play a part in keeping the nation healthy. They can assure the maintenance of public sanitation and a pure water supply, sponsor education and health promotion programs, promote safe environments, encourage healthy foods, and offer special support for disadvantaged groups.
4. Health professionals. Health professionals are the major source of information concerning health. In collaboration with individuals, families, and community groups, they are responsible for screening, immunizations, health teaching, and counseling.
5. The media. Media partnerships with health professionals and voluntary organizations offer powerful health promotion messages via the printed word, television, radio, computer, and audiovisuals.
6. The government. Policy decisions from governmental bodies assist public and health care professionals to achieve national health goals. Federal, state, and local governments support health promotion programs and assure that surveillance systems regarding the incidence of disease, delivery of services, and exposure to risks are operational and efficient.

BARRIERS TO HEALTH PROMOTION

Some common barriers to older adults' interest and participation in health promotion activities include:

1. Cost of preventive health services may be prohibitive for those already on a fixed income (Meiner & Lueckenotte, 2006).
2. Difficulty in obtaining adequate treatment for existing illnesses that results in a sense of futility about seeking additional services for health promotion and disease prevention.
3. Ethnic and cultural influences regarding health-seeking behavior vary greatly and are complex. Diversity has not always been considered or even recognized by many health care policy makers or providers.
4. Both the availability and the cost of transportation constitute a very real barrier for some older adults (Meiner & Lueckenotte, 2006).

For most older adults, promoting and maintaining health means making major changes in lifestyle and habits formed over many years. Behavior modification (which includes motivation and incentives), counseling, and consistent support from others are often necessary for such changes to occur. Sennott-Miller & Kligman (1992) discuss specific strategies to prevent relapses into former unhealthy behaviors. These include locating a successful role model, identifying the health risks of the former behavior, imagining the risks of a relapse, regularly practicing relaxation techniques, deciding what to do in case of a relapse, and developing an attitude of distancing oneself from urges and cravings leading to the unhealthy behavior. Vigilance in maintaining the new behavior is imperative for success, and health care professionals can be potent motivators in facilitating behavior change.

EXERCISE

Regular, systematic, appropriate exercise is one of the best anti-aging agents known. Research documents its positive influence on the older population. Physical fitness maintained by a consistent exercise regimen can substantially reduce the behavioral impact of many age-related changes that limit mobility, reduce independence, and affect the enjoyment of life in older age. Yen (2005) describes a term created by health professionals called "sedentary death syndrome" that refers to the many diseases and life-threatening problems brought on by an inactive lifestyle. Inactivity is known to be a major risk factor for the development of obesity, diabetes, cardiovascular disease, respiratory disease, and musculoskeletal disease, as well as a host of others. It is now established that many common physical changes long regarded as an inevitable part of growing older are in reality mostly due to inactivity and a sedentary life style (disuse, or hypokinetic disease). The adage "use it or lose it" becomes even more true as attention is increasingly focused on the study of normal aging rather than on disease and pathology.

AGE-RELATED CHANGES MODIFIED BY EXERCISE

Aerobic Capacity and Cardiovascular–Pulmonary Functioning

Maximal oxygen consumption or VO_2 max is the most frequently used measure of exercise capacity. VO_2 max is an indicator of the ability of the cardiovascular system to deliver blood and oxygen to the muscles and the ability of the muscles to use oxygen in performing work. VO_2 max declines with age; however, exercise research indicates a 10% to 30% VO_2 max improvement with exercise training (Emery, Burkes, & Blumenthal, 1991). Similarly, other studies indicate an increase in pulmonary function with systemic exercise.

Muscle Strength

Both muscle mass and strength decline with age (sarcopenia), and the decline is generally greater in weight-bearing muscles. These changes can have a significant impact on the ability to carry out daily activities and increase the possibility of falls and other accidents. Research shows impressive results of muscle strengthening and muscle functioning in older adults following an appropriate program of strength training, and the literature on exercise in older age emphasizes the importance of strength training for older adults including the oldest-old (Schwartz & Buckner, 1999; Fahlman, Tapp, McNevin, Morgan, & Bradley, 2007).

Flexibility and Balance

Joint flexibility tends to decline with age, especially in the shoulder, elbow, wrist, hip, knee, ankle, and spine. Flexibility is needed to perform activities of daily living and also for gait and locomotion. Studies report improved flexibility in older adults who participate in exercise programs that include a flexibility component (Kart, Metress, & Metress, 1992). Postural control declines with age, as does vibratory sense in the feet. Furthermore, there is a decreased stride, gait changes, and lessened ability to raise foot height, all of which influence balance. Medications also may impact balance and postural control (Baum, Capezuti, & Driscoll, 2002). Tsang & Hui-Chan (2004) report joint proprioception (awareness of the body in space) and balance improved in elders who took part in Tai Chi and golf.

Bone Mass

Osteopenia, or decrease in bone mass, is common in older adults, especially women. When osteopenia is severe enough to cause fractures the condition is known as osteoporosis. Stressing bones with weight-bearing exercises increases bone mass and muscle strengthening exercises reduce the risk for osteoporosis (Sebastian, 2007). Vigorous flexion exercises are not recommended for older persons because they may contribute to compression fractures of the vertebrae, but increasing bone mass, muscle strengthening, balance, and gait stability reduce the risk of future falls and fractures.

Metabolic Functioning (Glucose and Lipoproteins)

Some variability in metabolic functioning in older age has a genetic component; other aspects of age-related metabolic change are influenced by obesity, diet, smoking, medications, physical activity, fluid and electrolyte balance, and central nervous system functioning. A number of these factors are based on lifestyle and therefore can be modified by choice. Strength training positively influences glucose metabolism and resistance training escalates glucose uptake as well as sensitivity to insulin in the skeletal muscles (Sebastian, 2007).

Changes in glucose and lipoprotein metabolism predispose older adults to diabetes and high levels of fats in the blood. These disorders increase the likelihood of coronary artery disease, the leading cause of death in this age group. Regular systematic exercise has been shown to improve glucose tolerance, lipoprotein levels, and weight loss for those who also eat a healthy diet (Fleg & Goldberg, 1990).

Blood Pressure

Elders who maintain physical fitness through exercise have lower blood pressure and heart rate, improved cardiac output, and more efficient skeletal muscles, all of which reduce the workload of the heart. Goldberg & Hagberg (1990) conclude that older adults with hypertension can safely participate in exercise programs if heart rate and blood pressure are carefully monitored.

Psychological Benefits

Systematic studies regarding the psychological effects of exercise on elders are sparse and inconsistent. Nevertheless, numerous research findings report a more positive mood, improvement in cognitive functioning (such as memory), a sense of improved self-esteem and body image, more meaningful social relationships, and a general feeling of well-being resulting from a regular exercise regimen.

EXERCISE PROGRAMS

Exercise programs usually include a variety of different types of exercise. Several of the most recommended types of exercise are identified and discussed here.

Types of Exercise

Isometric

In isometric exercise, very specific muscles are contracted for a short period of time (5 to 8 seconds) without joint movement. For example, clasp your hands and then try to pull them apart. Considerable effort can be expended, but there is no movement of a joint. Isometric exercises are appropriate for building the strength of specific muscles and are used to rehabilitate muscles after an injury, but they do not provide cardiovascular conditioning.

Isotonic

Isotonic exercise produces muscle contraction and movement at adjacent joints, but the activity is not maintained consistently enough for significant cardiovascular and respiratory conditioning. Bowling and golf are examples of isotonic exercise.

Aerobic

Aerobic exercise requires the body to use oxygen to produce the energy needed to carry out the activity. It involves rhythmic or repetitive activity using several large muscle groups (as in walking) for 20 to 30 minutes of sustained exercise. Both the pulmonary system and the cardiovascular system are conditioned with aerobic exercise. Ideally, aerobic exercise programs should be tailored to the individual's abilities. Activities involved in the program should be varied to prevent boredom and to encourage cross training, which uses various muscle groups rather than the same ones over and over again.

Strength Training (Resistance)

These exercises involves muscles contracting against a type of resistance greater than normally experienced such as using resistance bands or hand/ankle weights. Muscle groups are exercised resulting in increased muscle strength and muscle building. These should ideally be performed at least 2 times a week (Miller, 2009; Touhy, 2008).

Endurance

Endurance exercises are individual movements of large muscle groups in 10 minute segments. Examples of endurance exercises are swimming, dancing, walking briskly, and playing tennis. Initially these exercises should be started for a short period of time and gradually increased as tolerated (Struck & Ross, 2006; Touhy, 2008).

Flexibility/Stretching

These exercises put the joints through their full range of motion, keeping the body flexible and limber. Yoga is a type of exercise that stretches and flexes the muscles. Flexibility and stretching exercises are recommended 2 to 4 times a week (Sebastian, 2007; Miller, 2009).

Balance

Balance exercises are important for maintaining standing and walking. They also help prevent falls and accidents and should be done 3 times a week (Sebastian, 2007; Miller, 2009).

The American Heart Association (AHA) (Williams et al., 2007) and the American College of Sports Medicine (ACSM) (2006) updated the 1995 exercise recommendations for adults. In doing so they outlined the benefits of physical activity, which include a reduced risk for hypertension, cardiovascular disease, thromboembolic stroke, obesity, colon cancer, breast cancer, type 2 diabetes, depression, and anxiety. They recommend adults ages 18 to 65 undertake moderate intensity aerobic (endurance) exercise for 30 minutes 5 days a week or 20 minutes of intense aerobic physical exercise 3 days a week. Moderate aerobic exercise results in a noted increase in heart rate and breathing, yet does not prohibit conversation. AHA and ACSM also outline exercise guidelines for elders age 65 and above and for those 50 to 64 with clinically significant chronic health problems and/or functional disabilities.

GENERAL RECOMMENDATIONS FOR EXERCISE PROGRAMS FOR OLDER ADULTS

1. Since cardiovascular, pulmonary, and musculoskeletal disease are so common in older adults, a physical examination is recommended before embarking on an exercise program. In addition to the physical exam, a medical history, pertinent laboratory testing, and a stress test (if necessary) should be performed. Existing medical conditions should be monitored for stability prior to exercising (Struck & Ross, 2006).
2. It is helpful for the older adult to learn how to monitor heart rate. The maximum heart rate is found by subtracting the person's age from 220. The target heart rate to be reached while exercising is usually considered to be 60% to 75% of the maximum heart rate; however, it is now recognized that any exercise program using the target heart rate to monitor intensity of exercise is not appropriate for elders. Instead, they can use their perceived level of exertion (for example, when they feel tired) as a guide for regulating the intensity of exercise. Larson and Bruce (1997) advocate teaching elders guidelines for self-pacing during exercise. Using the "talk

test," individuals know they are exercising at a comfortable rate when they can carry on a conversation while exercising. Being too breathless to talk while exercising is an indication that the exercise is too strenuous. An exercise program should be started slowly and the exercise time and challenge gradually increased. Being aware of how you feel during exercise is very important. Signs of too strenuous exercise include wheezing, coughing, difficulty breathing, chest discomfort, excessive sweating, feeling faint or dizzy, exhaustion, and local joint or muscle pain. These and other symptoms are an indication to slow down or stop the exercise.

3. For fitness conditioning and safety, an exercise program should include three components: a warm-up period, an aerobic component, and a cool-down period. The warm-up and cool-down periods consist of gentle stretching exercises to warm muscles up before strenuous activity and to allow them to cool down slowly following strenuous activity. Gentle stretching for approximately 5 minutes is important for elders to prevent injury and also to improve flexibility.

Walking is considered to be one of the best and safest aerobic activities for older adults. Other activities to consider are swimming, cross-country skiing, bicycling, water aerobics, and aerobic dancing. Research indicates exercise does not have to be intense or exceptionally vigorous to provide physical fitness. A moderately paced walk for approximately 20 to 30 minutes each day can promote cardiovascular conditioning and be effective for general physical fitness. Mall walking has become quite popular with the older age group since it provides a climate-controlled, safe environment in which to exercise and also promotes social interaction.

Activities involving straining or breath-holding are dangerous as they may increase the possibility of causing cardiovascular problems. Exercises should always be gentle with no bouncing, twisting, or heavy straining. Injury prevention is paramount, because muscle soreness and fatigue usually lead to permanent withdrawal from an exercise program.

SUMMARY

In summary, an effective exercise program for older adults increases conditioning (especially endurance), minimizes risk, improves muscle strength, and promotes enjoyment without excessive fatigue or discomfort (Larson

& Bruce, 1997). The MacArthur studies of successful aging found physical fitness to be the single most important factor in remaining healthy in old age (Rowe & Kahn, 1998).

REFERENCES

American College of Sports Medicine. (2006). *ACSMS guidelines for exercise testing and prescription* (7th ed.). Philadelphia: Lippincott Williams & Wilkins.

Baum, T., Capezuti, E., & Driscoll, G. (2002). Falls. In V. T. Cotter, & N. E. Stumpf (Eds.), *Advanced practice nursing with older adults: Clinical guidelines*. New York: McGraw-Hill.

Emery, C. F., Burkes, E. J., & Blumenthal, J. A. (1991). Psychological and physiological effects of exercise among older adults. In K. W. Schaie, & M. P. Lawton (Eds.), *Annual review of gerontology and geriatrics* (pp. 218–238). New York: Springer.

Fahlman, M. M., Tapp, R., McNevin, N., Morgan, A. L., & Bradley, D. J. (2007). Structured exercise in older adults with limited functional ability. *Journal of Gerontological Nursing, 33,* 32–39.

Fleg. J. L., & Goldberg, A. P. (1990). Exercise in older people: Cardiovascular and metabolic adaptations. In W. R. Hazzard, R. Andres, E. L. Bierman, & J. P. Blass (Eds.), *Principles of geriatric medicine and gerontology* (2nd ed., pp. 85–100). New York: McGraw-Hill.

Filner, B., & Williams, R. (2000). Health promotion for the elderly: Reducing functional dependency. In *Healthy people 2010*. United States Government Printing Office: Washington, D.C.

Fried, L. P. (1990). Health promotion and disease prevention. In W. R. Hazzard, R. Andres, E. L. Bierman, & J. P. Blass (Eds.), *Principles of geriatric medicine and gerontology* (2nd ed., pp.192–200). New York: McGraw-Hill.

Goldberg, A. P., & Hagberg, J. M. (1990). Physical exercise in the elderly. In E. L. Schneider, & J. W. Rowe (Eds.), *Handbook of the biology of aging* (3rd ed., pp. 407–428). San Diego, CA: Academic Press.

Hansen-Kyle, L. (2005). A concept analysis of healthy aging. *Nursing Forum, 40,* 45–57.

Healthy People 2000. (1992). U.S. Department of Health and Human Services. Public Health Service. Boston: Jones & Bartlett.

Healthy People 2010. (2000) U.S. Government Printing office web site at http://bookstore.gpo.gov/.

Hickey, T., & Stilwell, D.L. (1991). Health promotion for older people: All is not well. *Gerontologist, 31,* 822–829.

Kart, C. S., Metress, E. K., & Metress, S. P. (1992). *Human aging and chronic disease*. Boston: Jones and Bartlett.

Kligman, E. W. (1992). Preventive geriatrics: Basic principles for primary care physicians. *Geriatrics, 47,* 39–49.

Lach, H. W. (2007). Health promotion and health education for older adults. In. A. D. Linton, & H. W. Lach (Eds.), *Matteson & McConnell's gerontological nursing* (3rd ed., pp. 785–809). St. Louis: Saunders Elsevier.

Larson, E. B., & Bruce, R. A. (1997). Exercise. In C. K Cassel, H. J. Cohn, E. B. Larson, D. E., Meier, N. M., Resnick, L. Z. Rubenstein, & L. B. Sorensen (Eds.), *Geriatric medicine* (3rd ed., pp. 815–821). New York: Springer Verlag.

Mauk, K. (2006). *Gerontological nursing.* Sudbury, MA: Jones & Bartlett.

Meiner, S. E., & Lueckenotte, A. G. (2006). *Gerontologic nursing* (3rd ed.). St. Louis: Mosby Elsevier.

Miller, C. (2009). *Nursing for wellness in older adults* (5th ed.). Philadelphia: Wolters Kluwer/Lippincott Williams & Wilkins.

Nakasato, Y. R., & Carnes, B. A. (2006). Health promotion in older adults: Promoting successful aging in primary care settings. *Geriatrics, 61,* 27–31.

Resnick, B. (2006). Health promotion and illness disability prevention. In S. E. Meiner, & A. G. Lueckenotte (Eds.), *Gerontologic nursing* (3rd ed., pp. 162–175). St. Louis: Mosby Elsevier.

Rowe, J. W., & Kahn, R. L. (1998). Successful aging. *Geriatrics, 37,* 433–440.

Schwartz, R. S., & Buchner, D. M. (1999). Exercise in the elderly: Physiologic and functional effects. In W. R. Hazzard, J. P. Blass, W. H. Ettinger, J. B. Halter, & J. G. Ouslander (Eds.), *Principles of geriatric medicine and gerontology* (4th ed., pp. 147–158). New York: McGraw-Hill.

Sebastian, L. A. (2007). Exercise recommendations. *Advance for Nursing, 8,* 27–29.

Sennott-Miller, L., & Kligman, E. W. (1992). Healthier lifestyles: How to motivate older patients to change. *Geriatrics, 47,* 52–59.

Struck, B. D., & Ross, K. M. (2006). Health promotion in older adults: Prescribing exercise for the frail and homebound. *Geriatrics, 61,* 22–27.

Touhy, T. A. (2008). Health and wellness. In P. Ebersole, P. Hess, T. A. Touhy, K. Jett, & A. S. Luggen (Eds.), *Toward healthy aging* (7th ed., pp. 43–64). St. Louis: Mosby Elsevier.

Tsang, W. W., & Hui-Chan, C. N. (2004). Effects of exercise on joint sense and balance in elderly men: Tai Chi versus golf. *Medical Science Sports Exercise, 36,* 658–667.

Williams, M. A., Haskell, W. L., Ades, P. A., Amsterdam, E. A., Bittner, V., Franklin, B. A., Gulanick, M., Laing, S. T., & Stewart, K. J. (2007). Resistance exercise in individuals with and without cardiovascular disease: 2007 update: A scientific statement from the American Heart Association Council on Clinical Cardiology, and Council on Nutrition, Physical Activity, and Metabolism. *Circulation, 116,* 572–584.

World Health Organization (1946). *Preamble to the Constitution of the World Health Organziation as adopted by the International Health Conference, New York, 19–22 June, 1946.* Official Records of the World Health Organization, no. 2, p. 100. New York: World Health Organization.

Yen, P. K. (2005). Physical activity—the "New" nutrition guideline. *Geriatrics, 26,* 341–342.

19 Nutrition

Health, vigor, and quality of life from infancy to old age depend upon adequate nutritional intake. Eating patterns of older adults are an outcome of lifelong experiences with foods. The human body needs certain basic nutrients such as carbohydrates, fats, proteins, vitamins, minerals, and water to build and repair tissues, to supply energy, and to regulate vital body processes. The National Center for Health Statistics (1997) states that poor dietary habits are linked with four of the ten leading causes of death in the United States: coronary heart disease, stroke, some types of cancer, and noninsulin-dependent diabetes mellitus.

Healthy older adults generally require fewer calories than younger persons and the same or higher levels of nutrients. A calorie is the quantity of heat energy in a food. Older adult males require about 2,900 to 3,000 calories and older women 1,600 to 2,300 calories of carbohydrates, fats, and protein daily (Baker, 2007). Energy requirements change with age due to reduced physical activity; decrease in metabolic rate; altered body weight and composition; and prevalence of multiple disabilities and diseases. Dwyer, White, Ham, Lipschitz, and Wellman (1991) suggest that older people are indeed at greater risk for a poor nutritional state because of dependency or disability, social isolation, acute or chronic diseases, poverty, inappropriate or excessive food intake, and chronic medication use. Nutritional needs are also influenced by age-related changes in various body systems such as diminished enzyme production and mucosal changes in the digestive system; loss of nephrons and altered kidney function; blood vessel changes and decreased cardiac output; alterations in lung function; and glucose intolerance and insulin response decline due to altered carbohydrate metabolism. Less total body water and protein, loss of lean body mass, and more fragile temperature regulation are characteristic of the older body. These, in addition to other age-related changes, influence digestion, absorption, utilization, and excretion of food in the older person.

As a society Americans consume more calories than needed as well as an excess of saturated fats, cholesterol, salt, and sugars. Concomitantly, recommended amounts of vegetables and fruits are not eaten, all of which result in fiber, calcium, potassium, magnesium, and vitamins A, C, and E deficiencies (Tufts University Health and Nutrition Newsletter, 2008). Healthy People 2010 (2000) recommends increasing daily fruit and vegetable intake to two servings of fruits for 75% of the U.S. population and at least three servings of vegetables. In spite of these recommendations, national reports indicate that only about 30% to 40% of Americans meet these goals.

About 45 chemical compounds and single elements from foods are required for human cell functioning. They include carbohydrates, fats, proteins, vitamins, and minerals. There are also 13 vitamins essential for healthy human functioning. Vitamins A, D, E, and K are fat-soluble vitamins; the water-soluble vitamins include vitamin C and eight B vitamins: biotin, thiamine, folate, B_6, B_{12}, riboflavin, niacin, and pantothenate. Linoleic, and possibly linolenic acid, must be obtained from food. Seventeen minerals and trace elements complete the required nutrients. These include iron, magnesium, calcium, chlorine, potassium, phosphorus, sodium, chromium, sulfur, copper, cobalt, fluorine, manganese, iodine, selenium, molybdenum, and zinc. Neglecting to ingest even one of these may lead to illness or even death (Baker, 2007).

Dietary standards are essential to determine which foods to eat and in what amounts to maintain a healthy lifestyle. The Recommended Dietary Allowance (RDA) was initially developed in 1941 to help protect individuals from deficiency diseases and inadequate diets. When observing the outcome of dietary excesses it was deduced that the focus should not only be on avoiding excesses, but also on achieving maximal health, thus the RDAs have been replaced by the Dietary Reference Intakes (DRIs) (Dudek, 2006). Included under the umbrella of the DRIs are the RDAs, Adequate Intake (AI), Tolerable Upper Intake Level (UL), and Estimated Average Requirement (EAR) indices. The DRIs recognize the special nutritional needs of older adults and include recommendations for the 51 to 70 age group and those ages 71 and over. A second kind of nutritional guide, *The Dietary Guidelines for Americans* published by the U.S. Department of Agriculture (2005), focuses on health as it relates to nutrients, food, and lifestyle practices that prevent chronic disease and help to promote health. A federal document, it is updated every five years and used as the basis for federal nutrition policy and government food and nutrition programs such as school meals, Head Start, and older adult nutrition programs.

PSYCHOSOCIAL AND CULTURAL ASPECTS OF NUTRITION

Food plays a major role in the lives of humans. From the beginning of time food not only provided sustenance, but was also part of religious and cultural rites. Eating is a social event usually shared and enjoyed with others; however, the social aspect becomes increasingly limited for older persons who are handicapped, live alone, or who are institutionalized. There may be difficulties in purchasing, storing, and preparing food, or little incentive to shop or prepare food only for oneself. A sense of well-being and sharing stimulates interest in shopping, preparing, and eating well-balanced meals.

Food has symbolic meaning for individuals and may represent reward or punishment, security, sociability, age, and sex symbolism. A unique and important part of every culture is the particular food that is prepared and enjoyed by family and friends; people share memories, seek comfort and belonging, and thrive on foods that are culturally relevant. Food and drink are served at a variety of gatherings such as meetings and receptions, and throughout life satisfying foods are associated with security. Children are often rewarded with food or punished by not being given a treat; these relationships carry over into adulthood when eating becomes a coping mechanism for pain, stress, or loss. Foods are associated with age; for instance, low salt, low fat, or low cholesterol foods are often linked with older persons, whereas fast foods such as hamburgers and hot dogs are associated with the young. Food also symbolizes affection, as when a box of candy or fruit basket is given to a friend or we take someone to dinner. Candy, cookies, cakes, and special foods are an integral part of celebrating holidays, birthdays, weddings, and anniversaries.

Psychological states such as feelings of loneliness often influence one's interest in shopping or cooking. Individuals who are depressed and those experiencing loss and grief frequently have poor eating patterns, whereas those who are neurotic, psychotic, or demented typically modify the kinds and amounts of food eaten.

Limited funds and habits such as alcoholism, drug overdosing, or even smoking negatively impact food intake. Some older persons live in restricted space with limited cooking or refrigeration; others may have little or no access to transportation or are not physically able to shop or carry groceries. These and other variables all influence older adults' eating patterns to a greater or lesser degree.

Cultural practices are gradually learned by individuals in childhood through both conscious and unconscious learning. Food preferences and eating habits are among the most deeply rooted aspects of one's culture. Certain foods have deep symbolic meaning within each culture. Older family members are usually the transmitters of these preferences, which have been passed from generation to generation as special food served at family, community, and religious gatherings. Such foods bind people together; they are served at rites of passage, soothe those who are grieving, and are an integral part of celebrations (Guthrie & Picciano, 1995).

Cultural food preferences may also impact methods of handling, storing, and cooking food, as well as the types of food eaten, attitudes toward food, and how food relates to health. Cultures often identify specific staple foods, times for meals, as well as special feasts for various holidays. Certain foods are even identified in the treatment of disease. Meeting specific cultural food needs and individual preferences are complex challenges that are best accomplished through the services of a registered dietitian. Another resource is the food guide pyramid, called MyPyramid, which is available in many languages on the internet and can be accessed by http://www.mypyramid.gov. Food preferences of elders need to be reviewed to better understand how their dietary intake relates to the maintenance of good health. Changing cultural eating patterns may be very difficult and sometimes impossible. If a dietary change is necessary, including familiar foods if possible may increase compliance to a therapeutic diet.

PHYSIOLOGICAL ASPECTS OF NUTRITION

Aging is accompanied by physiological changes; however, when recommending nutritional approaches and requirements it is necessary to differentiate between a healthy older adult and one who has an acute or chronic disease (Orr, 2000). Food is one of the primary sources of satisfaction and contentment in the later years, even though sensory losses associated with aging often influence the ability to gain as much pleasure and satisfaction as formerly.

The number of taste buds declines with age, taste perception declines, and decrements have been reported in all four taste qualities: salty, bitter, sweet, and sour (Ship, 1999). Consequently many elders use additional seasoning on foods to obtain a satisfying taste. The sense of smell is closely allied to the sense of taste. As smell acuity decreases with age, it may be necessary to increase olfactory stimulation. Additionally, medications, periodontal disease, mouth infections, ill-fitting dentures, and decreased salivation may alter both taste and smell.

Consequently, methods of enhancing the appearance, taste, and smell of food are needed when cooking for older persons. The liberal use of foods of different colors, allowing cooking odors to permeate the eating area, and preparing foods with more definite taste by using taste enhancers like herbs may improve elders' enjoyment of food. Be aware, also, that spoiled foods are more likely to be ingested by those whose taste and smell acuity has decreased.

Other physiological age-related changes possibly affecting nutritional status are decreased lean body mass, increased fatty tissue, and lower metabolic rate; thus, older adults require fewer calories to maintain their optimal body weight (Siegler & Hark, 1996). Recent RDAs recommend a 10% reduction in the amount of caloric intake for individuals over age 51 (Baker, 2007). There is some atrophy of tissues in the mouth, decreased salivation, and reduced sensation of thirst, which may also contribute to less effective processing and enjoyment of food (Granville & Musson, 1999). Chewing and swallowing are less efficient, and if the older person also has poorly fitting dentures or missing teeth, the initial processing of food in the mouth will be affected (Ship, 1999). Decreased enzyme secretion in the mouth, stomach, and intestines tends to reduce the nutritional value of food.

Health problems related to range of motion, coordination, or ambulation influence shopping for food, cooking, and eating. Arthritis, a disease prevalent among the elderly, makes handling food in the grocery store, pushing a cart, and transporting food difficult. Removing food from bags, opening boxes and cans, and storing food can all become arduous tasks for those with musculoskeletal limitations. Disabilities related to lung disease, cancer, heart disease, and fractures can also affect food intake. Many chronic diseases require special diets and changing lifelong eating habits is a challenge some elders find difficult or impossible. The palatability of food and food preparation methods often determine whether food is appealing to the individual and will be eaten.

Certain drug therapies affect the appetite by altering taste perceptions or by causing an unpleasant aftertaste or dry mouth. Other medications stimulate or decrease appetite. Some cause nausea, diarrhea, or constipation, which can interfere with the absorption of nutrients. Psychotropic drugs reduce mental acuity, causing drowsiness and ultimately lessened food intake. Lethargy or weakness caused by drugs may impede the ability to shop for or cook foods. All of the above contribute to a tendency for older adults to adopt a "tea and toast" regimen or to consume diets high in refined sugars and fats.

WATER AND BODY FLUIDS

Water is essential in maintaining life; in fact, six to eight glasses are needed daily to maintain stable body temperature, efficient cell metabolism, and to give form and structure to the body (Chernoff, 1991). Homeostatic mechanisms regulate fluid supply, and the amounts taken in and excreted should be equal. Fluids are excreted through the lungs, skin, kidneys, and intestines and also lost through diarrhea, vomiting, fever, and hemorrhage. Dehydration caused by limited fluid intake is one of the most common fluid and electrolyte imbalances observed in older adults; it impairs homeostasis, disrupts functions in many major body organs such as those in the circulatory and urinary systems, causes mental confusion, and elevates body temperature. Sufficient fluid intake is equally as important as food for older adults (Luggen, Bernstein, & Touhy, 2008).

Many elders have a decreased ability to detect thirst and may not even realize they need to drink fluids; others may voluntarily limit their fluid intake to prevent frequent urination. Physical limitations may prevent individuals from obtaining needed fluids, and those with altered mental processes may not recognize when they are thirsty, or lack the motivation to drink fluids. Demented individuals, those with ambulation problems, and the old-old are especially vulnerable to fluid imbalances (Larson, 2003). Warm temperatures can also increase older adults' vulnerability to dehydration. Signs of dehydration include constipation; weakness; thromboembolism; dizziness; agitation or confusion; dark, concentrated urine; and dry mouth. These factors necessitate increasing fluid intake to 1,500 to 2,500 cc daily unless medically contraindicated. It is extremely important that caregivers monitor fluid intake, especially for disabled older adults, and make a variety of fluids available to prevent fluid imbalance. Use of air conditioners, fans, and shades all help to diminish fluid loss. Rubbing the skin with creams, olive oil, or vegetable shortening, especially after bathing, aids in hydrating the skin and providing comfort.

PROTEIN

Protein is essential to preserve lean body mass, to maintain organ system performance, and for adequate functioning of the immune system (Chernoff, 1990). Protein intake should be 0.8 grams per kilogram of body weight (Biggs, 2007). This amounts to 20% to 30% of total caloric intake, with preference given to complete protein foods. The RDA for older men is 56 gms daily and for older women 46 gms daily. Amino acids are the structural units of proteins, and both essential (those supplied by food) and nonessential (those produced by the body) amino acids are necessary to maintain health. Nitrogen and both types of amino acids are provided by protein of animal origin, including meat, fish, poultry, eggs, milk, and cheese. Grains and vegetables, though, are deficient in one or more of the essential amino acids. Protein is necessary for growth and maintenance of body tissue, as well as for other physiological and metabolic activities, and must be continually replenished in the body by an adequate intake. Unfortunately, the high cost of meat and other animal products often prohibits those on restricted incomes from purchasing protein-containing food. Substituting chicken, fish, soy products, or nuts for red meat may be healthier choices. Elderly persons are at risk for protein-calorie malnutrition because many eat fewer calories and less protein; a low protein diet is likely to contain fewer minerals and vitamins.

Rosenberg (1991) states that one third of those over age 70 lose their ability to secrete sufficient amounts of stomach acid, which influences the absorption of folic acid, calcium, and iron. These persons are more likely to become anemic because reduced hydrochloric acid in the stomach and loss of the intrinsic factor (a protein in the gastric juice) lead to poor iron and vitamin B_{12} absorption. Foods rich in iron and vitamin $B_{12,}$ such as liver, fortified cereal, and red meats, should be included in most diets to avoid the iron deficiency anemia caused by the reduced meat intake that is quite common in this age group (Yen, 2000). Individuals with high cholesterol are encouraged to eat lean meat, egg whites, low fat desserts, and breads, and to drink fat-free milk (Lutz & Przytulski, 2006).

Older adults with infections, trauma, burns, fever, and malignancies, as well as those under stress or undergoing surgery, require greater protein and calorie intake because these conditions can produce a negative nitrogen imbalance resulting in lowered body resistance and slower wound healing (Dudek, 2006). Skin breakdown and the formation of pressure ulcers are especially related to low protein ingestion. Overall, the protein intake of older adults should reflect individual needs at a particular time. Dietitians can greatly assist in assessing and recommending the best food to ensure adequate protein levels, and sometimes liquid protein supplements are prescribed to maintain adequate protein ingestion.

CARBOHYDRATES AND FIBER

Carbohydrates are the preferred source of energy for the majority of body functions. Older adults should obtain about 50% to 60% of their total calorie intake from carbohydrates, which are necessary for various physiological activities such as contraction of muscles, transmission of nerve impulses, and brain and lung functioning (Lutz & Przytulski, 2006). Complex carbohydrates found in whole-grain cereals and breads, fruits, and vegetables are rich in vitamins, fiber, and minerals. Refined carbohydrates such as crackers, cookies, candies, and pastries are said to contain "empty calories" because they only contribute calories to a diet and may cause malnutrition if eaten at the expense of other nutrient and fiber-rich foods.

Fiber, an indigestible complex carbohydrate, has limited nutritive value in itself, but cereal fiber (fiber in grains) absorbs many times its weight in water and helps to move food through the digestive system more rapidly, aiding in the elimination of wastes. Soluble or gel-forming fiber found in peas, beans, and some fruits, though, actually slows down transit time and may contribute to constipation. There is increasing evidence that cereal fiber is helpful in preventing constipation, cancer of the colon, hiatal hernia, appendicitis, hemorrhoids, and diverticular disease, and in lowering serum lipoproteins (fatty proteins in the blood). Prudent increases in fiber are recommended as a substitute for laxatives and as a means of improving intestinal musculature; however, individuals must drink sufficient quantities of water or the fiber may actually cause constipation. Eating too much fiber is not recommended because it may impede the absorption and digestion of other nutrients. Recommended daily dietary fiber intake is 20 to 35 gms, which ought to include ample fresh fruits and vegetables, high fiber cereals and whole grains, and legumes (Chernoff, 2006; Lutz and Przytulski, 2006).

Older adults have a reduced tolerance for glucose and are more likely to experience fluctuations of high or low blood sugar. Elevated blood sugars usually decline more slowly in older people than in the young. These changes are thought to be due to the "secondary aging phenomena" of physical deconditioning caused by decreased activity, obesity, improper diet, reduced muscle mass, and the use of various medications, all of which possibly influence reduced glucose tolerance and insulin action (Goldberg, Andres, & Bierman, 1990). Decreasing intake of refined sugars and substituting complex carbohydrates are suggested to avoid such sudden fluctuations and high blood sugar levels. Increasing dietary fiber can lower blood sugar levels and reduce or even eliminate the need for insulin or oral anti-diabetic medications in some diabetics. Moderating the intake of carbohydrates is especially important for older diabetics. Those who are overweight should reduce calorie intake, monitor blood sugar, and carefully regulate carbohydrate, fat, and protein intake.

FATS

Fats are a member of the class of compounds commonly call lipids. A concentrated form of energy, fats yield twice as many calories as equal amounts of carbohydrates and proteins. In addition to energy, fats form an integral part of the cell membrane; they help the body absorb vitamins A, D, E, and K and promote healthy body functioning. Fat also serves other purposes in the body; it cushions and protects the body and insulates it from extremes of heat and cold. Fats are also a major source of flavor in food and contribute to feelings of fullness and satiation. In addition, fats contribute to oils in the skin and scalp that facilitate a healthy look.

Older adults may have a reduced ability to utilize fats, which is reflected in high cholesterol levels. Serum cholesterol levels peak between 50 and 59 years of age for men and 60 and 69 years in women. Serum triglycerides, however, continue to rise, possibly due to a lessened ability to remove dietary fat from the blood. Unsaturated fats from vegetable sources are likely to lower cholesterol levels, whereas saturated animal fats tend to raise cholesterol levels. Twenty to thirty percent of calories ideally should come from fats, but trans-fats are to be avoided and preference given to polyunsaturated and mono-saturated fats from non-animal sources such as olives, peanut butter, and nuts. Cholesterol ingestion of less than 300 mg daily is advised (Dietary Guidelines for Americans USDA, 2005; Biggs, 2007).

Long implicated as a potential cause of obesity, research documents the association of fat ingestion with high cholesterol levels and coronary artery and cardiovascular disease. Likewise, a high-fat diet has been linked to cancer of the colon and breast. Individuals with high blood pressure, diabetes, obesity, or those who smoke should adhere to a low-cholesterol diet, as should those with elevated cholesterol levels, or who have a family history of atherosclerosis.

VITAMINS AND MINERALS (MICRONUTRIENTS)

Vitamins are necessary in small amounts for the physiological functioning of the body because of their coenzyme (enzyme activating) activity in the metabolic process as they promote biochemical reactions in the cells. Eliopoulos (1997) states that about one half of older adults in this country take vitamin and mineral supplements daily. Vitamins and minerals together are micronutrients the body needs to prevent specific diseases. Most of these deficiency-caused diseases can be cured when appropriate amounts of micronutrients are restored. Both vitamins and minerals must come from food or supplements because the body usually cannot manufacture them.

Vitamins and minerals likely to be deficient in the diets of older persons include vitamins C, B_6, B_{12}, folic acid, calcium, and zinc. There is some evidence that with age C, D, B_6, B_{12}, folic acid, and zinc may be less well absorbed and utilized in the body (Rowe & Kahn, 1998; University of California, Berkeley, Wellness Letter, 1999). Older adults in acute or long-term care institutions are especially vulnerable to vitamin and mineral deficiencies because of acute or chronic illnesses, eating insufficient amounts of food, or taking various prescribed medications.

Vitamin deficiency in older adults results from a lack of meat, fish, fresh fruits, vegetables, milk, and eggs. Adequate vitamin intake can only be assured if the required foods from each food group are eaten daily. A daily multivitamin is recommended for elders, especially those who do not eat a balanced diet. Multivitamins enhance the immune system and decrease the likelihood of developing various infections.

Vitamins are either fat-soluble or water-soluble. The water-soluble vitamins, B and C, are readily eliminated from the body through urine and perspiration, whereas fat-soluble vitamins A, D, E, and K are eliminated only when used up by the body. Because they remain in the body much longer before depletion occurs, vitamin toxicity is more likely with fat-soluble vitamins.

WATER SOLUBLE VITAMINS

Vitamins B and C, the water soluble vitamins, are primarily located in the watery portions of food and distributed to the body's cells, tissues, and organs. They are readily absorbed into the blood stream and excreted if their levels in the blood become too high.

Vitamin B

Vitamin B, important in preventing deficiency diseases, also serves vital control-agent roles in building tissue and in energy metabolism reactions as coenzyme partners with critical cell enzymes. There are eight B vitamins: thiamin, riboflavin, niacin, vitamin B_6, folic acid, vitamin B_{12}, pantothenic acid, and biotin. These vitamins do not provide energy per se, but they help burn carbohydrates, fats, and proteins. Deficiencies in B vitamins are reflected in skin changes such as flaking, dermatitis, or roughness. Mucous membranes may atrophy and become painful. Anemia, convulsions, constipation, diarrhea, anorexia, heart abnormalities, irritability, seizures, depression, and confusion progressing to psychosis have all been attributed to a lack of vitamin B.

Age-Related Changes Related to Vitamin B

Thiamine, riboflavin, and vitamin B_6 deficiencies have been noted among older adults, even those taking supplements. Decreased hydrochloric acid secretion in the older adult's stomach may deactivate thiamine, causing a thiamine deficiency. Reduced levels of riboflavin usually accompany decreases in the other B vitamins and are also linked to protein metabolism. The need for riboflavin is based upon protein need. Lower niacin levels are more prevalent among those who are chronic alcoholics, on low incomes, or are institutionalized. Symptoms of niacin depletion include diarrhea, dementia, and dermatitis.

Vitamin B_6 is found in many foods, yet many older adults are deficient in this vitamin, which can lessen their ability to ward off disease, increase homocysteine levels, and increase the risk for stroke or heart disease (Rowe & Kahn, 1998). The RDA for vitamin B_6 is 1.7 mg daily for older men and 1.5 mg per day for older women.

Folic acid is not as readily accessible in foods as other B vitamins, and is more readily excreted from the body. Individuals taking anticonvulsant medications and those who are alcoholics may have reduced levels of folic acid. Atrophic gastritis in older adults results in reduced folic acid and vitamin B_{12} absorption (Rowe & Kahn, 1998). Mental confusion, anemia, fatigue, apathy, and increased homocysteine levels predisposing one to stroke or heart disease can result from folic acid deficiency.

Reduced vitamin B_{12} seems to be observed more in those over age 60. This may be due to minimal intake of red and organ meats and green, leafy vegetables; lessened intrinsic factor, a protein secreted by the stomach that makes absorption of vitamin B_{12} possible; ingesting certain medications; and the presence of intestinal diseases. Symptoms of vitamin B_{12} deficiency include a lemon-yellow skin tint; smooth, beefy, red tongue; anemia; depression; confusion; psychosis; and reduced pain and temperature sensations. Individuals are usually given monthly injections of vitamin B_{12} as replacement therapy, to be continued for life.

Food sources of vitamin B_{12} and folic acid are leafy green vegetables, yeast, some fruits, legumes, liver, red meats, soy, and fortified breads. The RDA recommendation for vitamin B_{12} is 2.4 mcg daily for both older men and older women. Both folic acid and vitamin B_{12} supplements are recommended for most older adults (Oakley, Adams, & Dickinson, 1996).

Vitamin C

Vitamin C (ascorbic acid), an antioxidant, plays an important role in building and maintaining tissues, overall body metabolism, strengthening resistance to infections, and helping the absorption of iron. It must be replenished daily, and the body's stores of vitamin C can become depleted from smoking, stress, fever, hemorrhage, infection, burns, wound healing, and inadequate intake (Dudek, 2006). Suter (2006) reports there are no age-related changes in the metabolism of vitamin C, but an adequate intake is necessary as vitamin C deficiency may play a role in the development of certain diseases, such as cancer of the esophagus, stomach, and colon, all of which are quite common in older adults. The RDA recommendation for vitamin C is 90 mg daily for older men and 75 mg per day for older women.

Major sources of vitamin C are citrus fruits, tomatoes, potatoes, cabbage, cantaloupe, and peppers. With aging, increased vitamin C is needed for adequate body functioning because of its importance in tissue healing, resisting infections, collagen repair, and aiding in response to stress.

FAT SOLUBLE VITAMINS

Fat soluble vitamins include vitamins A, D, E, and K. Most often they occur together in oils and fats in foods and are absorbed by the body from the gastrointestinal tract. They are not readily excreted and can build up to toxic levels. Deficiencies in fat soluble vitamins are linked to diets low in fats, diseases interfering with transport, absorption, and storage of these vitamins, and over-ingestion of laxatives such as mineral oil.

Vitamin A

Vitamin A is necessary for healthy epithelial tissues in the skin, eyes, gastrointestinal, genitourinary, and respiratory systems. It is also needed for visual light and dark adaptation, reproduction and growth, bone growth, and energy regulation (Lutz & Przytulski, 2006). Major food sources include liver; beef; dark, green, leafy vegetables; yellow or orange vegetables; milk; cheese; and eggs. Symptoms of deficiency include night blindness, sensitivity to glare, corneal ulceration, and rough, dry skin.

Absorption of vitamin A does not seem to be appreciably impaired in older adults, and for most, levels of vitamin A appear to be adequate (Suter, 2006). Some research, however, does indicate that an increased absorption of vitamin A in older adults could produce toxicity if excessive amounts are taken as a supplement (Lipschitz, 1997). On the other hand, alcoholics, or those with respiratory, circulatory, or nervous system disease may need vitamin A supplementation (Suter, 1991). Vitamins A, E, and C are antioxidants and serve to neutralize free radicals in the body. Recommended RDA amount of vitamin A is 900 mcg for older men and 700 mcg for older women.

Vitamin D

Vitamin D is essential for calcium and phosphorus absorption and for bone mineralization. The principal sources of vitamin D are sunshine, fortified milk, yeast, deep-sea fish, and fish liver oils. Because only minimal amounts of vitamin D are found in most foods, fortified sources such as milk and margarine, as well as eggs, liver, and fish are advised. Six hundred IU are recommended daily or up to 1,000 IU if individuals are not exposed to sun (Yen, 2003). Elders may not be exposed to sun, especially if they live in northern climates or if they are institutionalized. Exposure to sunlight must be twice as long for an older person as for the young to produce equivalent amounts of vitamin D in the skin. Those confined indoors need at least 15 minutes of sun exposure twice a week to help ensure adequate vitamin D levels, but wearing sun screen with an spf of 8 or more inhibits the production of vitamin D by blocking ultraviolet rays (Lutz & Przytulski, 2006). Individuals with inadequate intakes of vitamin D or with chronic digestive diseases, as well as alcoholics and those exposed to little or no sun, may be at high risk for developing osteomalacia or osteoporosis.

Vitamin E

Vitamin E maintains cell membrane structure and integrity by safeguarding fatty acids and other lipids from the damage of oxidation and by protecting red blood cell membranes. There is also speculation that it protects white blood cells and participates in the immune defenses of the body (Cataldo, DeBruyne, & Whitney, 1992). Vitamin E is an important antioxidant. Current data suggest that the absorption of vitamin E in older adults is not impaired (Suter, 2006). Major sources of vitamin E are wheat germ and soy bean oil, vegetable oils, nuts, whole grains, legumes, milk, eggs, fish, leafy vegetables, and fortified cereals.

The major symptoms of vitamin E deficiency include anemia, reduced blood clotting time, neuromuscular degeneration, weakness, leg cramps, difficulty walking, and fibrocystic disease. A vitamin E overdose may result in fatigue, muscle weakness, reduced thyroid hormone concentrations, general gastrointestinal discomfort, and an enhanced effect of anti-blood clotting medication. The RDA recommendation for vitamin E is 15 mg daily for both older men and women.

Vitamin K

The major function of vitamin K is to help speed up the synthesis of several blood-clotting factors, such as prothrombin, in the liver; it also plays a role in bone metabolism (Lutz & Przytulski, 2006). Food sources of vitamin D include green, leafy vegetables, milk, cheese, eggs, and liver. Diseases interfering with fat and bile absorption impede vitamin K absorption, resulting in a greater tendency to bleed. Anticoagulant drugs also inhibit vitamin K action. The AI for vitamin K is 120 mcg daily for older men and 90 mcg for older women.

MINERALS

There are 16 essential minerals in the body. They consist of 7 major minerals needed daily in amounts of 100 mg or more each, and 9 trace minerals, also necessary daily in amounts of less than 100 mg each (Lutz & Przytulski, 2006). Minerals are responsible for a variety of vital metabolic body processes such as building bone mass, nerve and muscle functions, and regulating body fluids. Examples include maintaining acid-base balance and controlling the movement of water in body compartments. Calcium, chloride, magnesium, phosphorus, potassium, sulfur, and sodium are macronutrients present in large quantities in the body.

Adequate absorption of minerals is essential if the body is to utilize them properly. Absorption is often impaired in older adults because of diarrhea; excess or deficiency of one nutrient, which diminishes another's absorption time; and certain minerals, such as iron and calcium, in combination with chemical compounds contained in some foods, which become insoluble compounds and are excreted from the body. The minerals that have the greatest influence on body functions in elders are calcium and iron, but sodium, chloride, and potassium are important in maintaining electrolyte balance. Medications such as diuretics (non-potassium-sparing, or those that deplete potassium) are often implicated in causing electrolyte imbalance.

Calcium

Calcium balance is necessary throughout life because calcium is a significant mineral in maintaining bone structure and vital metabolically for certain enzyme activities. The most abundant mineral in the body is calcium. Ninety-nine percent of all calcium, in the form of calcium salts, is found in bones and teeth where it also serves as the body's calcium bank in case blood calcium levels drop. Once deposited in bone, calcium does not remain there forever because bones are continually in a state of flux with ongoing building up (bone deposition) and tearing down (bone resorption) processes. Both hormones and vitamin D promote deposition of calcium in bone. About 30% of the calcium taken in daily is retained in the body; the remainder is excreted in feces.

Calcium absorption decreases with age, especially in postmenopausal women. Absorption is decreased by insufficient vitamin D intake, excessive fiber intake, large amounts of phosphorus and magnesium, and a sedentary lifestyle. Osteoporosis is more common among women than men because body mass is usually less in women, and men generally eat twice as much calcium-containing foods as women. Both smoking and long-term excessive alcohol intake increase the risk of osteoporosis. Several lifestyle modifications can prevent or retard calcium loss: increasing dietary calcium; taking calcium supplements (calcium citrate is the most readily absorbed in the GI tract); regular exercise; estrogen replacement therapy or other medications; maintaining health status; and taking adequate amounts of vitamin D, protein, phosphorus, lactose, magnesium, and fluoride. Milk and milk products are the best sources of calcium. Adequate intake (AI) of 1,200 mg per day is recommended with 1,500 mg for post menopausal women.

Phosphorus, Potassium, Sodium, Chloride, Magnesium, Sulfur

Phosphorus is found in all body cells and is needed for all growth processes. The second most abundant mineral in the body, it is important for energy transfer in cell metabolism and in the development of bones and teeth. Eighty-five percent of phosphorus is found in bones and teeth. Fats (lipids) also contain phosphorus (phospholipids) and aid in carrying lipids in the blood and in the transport of nutrients in and out of cells. Milk is the best source of phosphorus; other sources include eggs, meat, fish, and carbonated beverages. The RDA recommends 700 mg daily for both women and men.

Potassium, sodium, and chloride are involved in primary body functions such as fluid, electrolyte, and acid-base balance, as well as muscle irritability. These are all vitally important in maintaining health in older age. Loss of potassium through the use of non-potassium-sparing diuretic drugs, surgery, injury, or diarrhea may have serious consequences such as weakness, heart irregularities, or muscle impairment. Potassium sources are fruits, milk, vegetables, and meat. The recommended AI is 4,700 mg daily.

Sodium levels are often too high among Americans, but certain sodium-restricted diets, diuretic medications, vomiting, diarrhea, or excessive perspiration may result in sodium depletion. Neither extreme is desirable for good health. The estimated minimum requirement for sodium is approximately 1/4 tsp daily. The recommended AI is 1,200 mg per day.

Chloride is found in body fluids and makes up a portion of gastric secretions. The RDA is 750 mg.

Magnesium is essential in the bones, where it combines with calcium and phosphorus, and also in body tissues and fluids as an agent to control metabolic activity. Available in many green vegetables and whole grains, deficiencies are rare except in certain intestinal disturbances and in alcoholism. Older adults may develop magnesium deficiencies due to disease and poor diet (Linderman, 2006). The RDA recommendation is 320 mg daily for older women and 420 mg for older men.

Sulfur is present in the protein of all body cells. It maintains the structure of nails, skin, and hair. If diets are adequate in protein, sulfur levels will usually be sufficient.

Iron, Copper, Iodine, and Zinc (Trace Elements)

Iron is important in the formation of hemoglobin in the red blood cells. Hemoglobin is critical to body functioning because it distributes 98.5% of the blood's oxygen. Iron levels may be low in the older population due to inadequate intakes of iron-containing food such as meats, altered absorption of iron, or blood loss. Nutritional anemia results from lack of iron, ascorbic acid, protein, folic acid, vitamin B_{12}, diminished acidity of the stomach, or combinations of these factors. Iron deficiency may also result from using aspirin, NSAIDs (non-steroidal anti-inflammatory drugs), or anticoagulants, all of which cause gastrointestinal (GI) bleeding. Stomach ulcers, hemorrhoids, pressure sores, infection, surgery, or cancer also deplete iron levels in the body.

Symptoms of low levels of iron are weakness, fatigue, anemia, pallor, atrophy of the tongue, and spoon-shaped nails. Poor nutrition seems to account for some of the unexplained anemia often observed in older adults; however, much is attributable to blood loss (Lipschitz, 1991). Increased meat intake, enriched grains, and green vegetables are recommended and iron supplements may be necessary. The RDA recommendation is 8 mg daily.

Copper is an important element in body functioning because it operates synergistically with iron in the iron absorption process. Copper deficiency in older age, however, is rare. Food sources include seafood, organ meats, whole grains, and nuts. The RDA for copper is 900 mcg daily.

Iodine is most highly concentrated in the thyroid gland, with varying amounts in other body tissues. Iodine is important in regulating vital metabolic activities. Individuals deficient in iodine often develop a goiter. Food sources of iodine include iodized table salt, seafood, milk and milk products, and bread. The RDA for iodine is 150 mcg daily.

Zinc, present in all body tissues, is important in growth and tissue repair, in metabolic activities such as collagen formation, and as a complement to critical enzymes. Grodner, Anderson, & DeYoung (2000) report that over 200 enzymes in the body are dependent on zinc. It enhances the ability to taste and smell, assists in immune system efficiency, and is significant in healing, carbohydrate metabolism, and the growth process. The Age-Related Eye Disease Study (2001) found that a high intake of zinc, vitamin C, vitamin E, and beta carotene lowers the risk of developing age-related macular degeneration (AMD) and also slows the rate of vision loss for those who have AMD. Deficits in zinc are found in elders with inadequate diets. Stress, diabetes, alcohol consumption, surgery, and burns increase zinc excretion and may produce abrupt zinc losses. Food sources include meats, shellfish, milk, eggs, and whole-grain foods. RDA for zinc is 11 mg for older men and 8 mg for older women.

Other trace elements such as fluorine, selenium, nickel, and chromium are necessary in very small amounts to maintain normal body functioning. Selenium is an antioxidant that, together with vitamin E, collaborates in the prevention of cell and lipid membrane damage by free radicals. It also plays a role in thyroid functioning. Some evidence suggests that those with low levels of selenium seem to be at greater risk for cancer. The RDA for selenium is 55 mcg daily.

MALNUTRITION

Malnutrition is defined as deficiencies in dietary intake (undernutrition), or over-consumption of food that increases the risk of developing disease. Nutrient imbalances interfere with normal functioning in cells, tissues, and organs, setting the stage for illness. Diagnosis of malnutrition is especially important in older adults because losing weight and being underweight increase both morbidity and mortality in this age group (Lipschitz, 1997).

Malnutrition is often overlooked in older adults who seek medical care, leading to incorrect diagnoses or to assuming that ailments such as headaches, skin rashes, insomnia, fatigue, confusion, debilitation, and general malaise are part of the aging process when in actuality these symptoms reflect malnourishment. Morley (1991) believes malnutrition is often not given high priority by physicians because they may lack the knowledge to diagnose malnutrition and recognize those at risk; they seem unaware that protein-energy malnutrition may be the first symptom of a treatable disease; or they generally are not aware of the best methods to manage individuals who have protein-energy malnutrition. Protein-energy malnutrition (PEM) is a metabolic response to stress in which there are increased requirements for protein and calories (Lipschitz, 1997).

About 50 % of those over age 65 have dietary intakes of less than the daily recommended levels. Some factors thought to contribute to malnutrition include poverty or near poverty; obesity; polypharmacy; lack of ability to shop for or prepare food because of physical or mental impairments; social isolation caused by loneliness, depression, or apathy; alcohol abuse; ignorance about adequate dietary requirements; poor teeth or ill-fitting dentures; digestive system disease; and bereavement (Luggen, Bernstein & Touhy, 2008).

UNDERNUTRITION

Older adults are especially prone to undernutrition (less than body requirements) for a variety of reasons including living alone, eating empty calories rather than nutritious food, poor fluid intake, medications, depression, malignancy, and bereavement. Although many factors such as medications, mood, lack of socialization, and diminished sense of taste and smell alter appetite, psychological aspects also inhibit appetite. Appetite plays a significant role in causing malnutrition. Lessened motivation to eat due to decreased neurotransmitter activity or changes in certain gastrointestinal hormones may also decrease appetite (Ebersole, Hess, Touhy, & Jett, 2005). Orexigenic medications are now available to stimulate appetite to prevent malnutrition. Caregivers are not always alert to preventing malnutrition by monitoring food intake, feeding elders, and developing effective strategies to ensure adequate nutrition. Institutional malnutrition is also a common occurrence. Seventeen to sixty-five percent of older adults in hospitals and long-term care settings experience undernutrition (Luggen, Bernstein, & Touhy, 2008). Individuals in acute care settings may be on NPO (nothing by mouth), receiving intravenous fluids, or have medical or surgical conditions that interfere with nutritional intake.

Undernutrition can result in agitation, depression, dementia, anemia, inadequate wound healing, weakness, fatigue, increased incidence of pressure sores, impaired elimination, and immunological functions. High mortality rates are associated with inadequate nutritional levels.

Silver (1993) believes the key to treating malnourished individuals is to intervene as early as possible by increasing protein intake during periods of stress; promoting exercise to enhance appetite; encouraging fluid intake to normal levels; increasing the diet to a minimum of 2,000 calories per day; avoiding constipation by adequate fluid intake and drinking prune juice instead of taking cathartics; reviewing the drug regimen including OTC (over the counter) drugs, vitamins, minerals, and alcohol; screening for depression; promoting a more independent and active lifestyle; and routinely examining the person's mouth for lesions or dental needs. Specific dietary management techniques to promote eating, such as environmental modifications to enhance the pleasantness of eating, focusing on methods to stimulate the appetite, and ongoing monitoring of nutritional status, are useful and effective. Underweight older adults may be given a high-fat diet including milk, cream, red meats, and ice cream (unless other health issues prohibit these choices). In addition, they may eat frequent, small meals along with high calorie and protein supplements. Regular nutritional screening is highly recommended along with biochemical assessments, especially for those who are most vulnerable. It is important to keep in mind that undernutrition may be confused with the normal aging process, thus continued vigilance is essential (Furman, 2006).

OVERNUTRITION

Many people, including older adults, are considerably overweight in the United States. It is estimated that overweight Americans age 65 and over will escalate from 10.3 million to 14.3 million by 2010, which is an average of 400,000 new individuals each year who are obese (Arterburn, Crane, & Sullivan, 2004). This represents a real epidemic of obesity with all its concomitant health issues. Patterns of overeating developed in childhood often continue into old age; more often, though, eating habits leading to obesity are related to sedentary lifestyle. Other reasons for overeating include anxiety, a sedentary occupation, a difficult life situation, mental illness, glandular imbalance, and grief or loss.

The dangers from overeating are many. Healthy People 2010 (2000) relates overnutrition to high blood pressure, coronary heart disease, stroke, type 2 diabetes, some cancers, gallbladder disease, osteoarthritis, and sleep apnea. Nevertheless, some believe it may not be harmful for older adults to be slightly overweight.

While crash or extreme diets are not recommended, reduction in calorie intake, not eating empty calories, and including all the food groups in the diet are appropriate weight loss plans. Older adults who need to lose weight should have specific and realistic dietary guidance. Weight loss programs of every kind are available, but it is prudent to seek a primary care practitioner's advice before embarking on any specific program. A physical examination is advised as is consultation with a dietitian and pharmacist before starting a formal diet program (Flood & Newman, 2007). Diets that call for less than 800 calories a day should be avoided; the recommended weight loss is from one half to one pound per week, but fluctuating weight gain and loss patterns are not desirable. Exercise is important for weight reduction as it not only burns calories but also enhances feelings of well-being.

FAILURE TO THRIVE

"Failure to thrive" has long been associated with infants who do not gain weight. In frail older people, it is a syndrome defined as a gradual decline in physical and/or mental functioning along with weight loss, decreased appetite, and withdrawal from social interactions in the absence of an explanation for these symptoms (Palmer, 1990; Rourke, 2006).

FTT is a syndrome often used as an admission diagnosis to hospitals and nursing homes. Verdery (1997) found that more than 50% of adults over 65 hospitalized with a history of weight loss continued to lose weight after discharge and 75% of them died within one year. The most common causes of FTT in elders are depression, delirium, dementia, drug reactions, chronic inflammation, and disease. Economic factors often contribute to the problem (Sarkisian & Lachs, 1996; Marcus & Berry, 1998). Normal aging changes such as impaired sensory systems or lower homeostatic reserves also contribute to FTT. Individuals display multiple problems including physical, social, mental, and environmental difficulties along with severely diminished coping abilities and functional capacities. FTT is not considered to be a normal age-related change nor is it necessarily exhibited in all older individuals who have a chronic disease.

Newbern (1992) and Rourke (2006) recommend an in-depth evaluation including assessments of nutritional and mental status, relational attachments, and the use of a genogram to assess the behavioral, cultural, and social development of the older person's family. Other useful evaluations include a medical history; a physical assessment (especially of the special senses-vision, hearing, taste, and smell); pulmonary, musculoskeletal, cardiovascular and neurological examinations; interviews with family members or caregivers; and selected laboratory studies. Osato, Stone, Phillips, & Winne (1993) argue that when treating the underlying cause of an individual's FTT is not possible, concern should be directed to his or her symptoms and the prevention of complications. Furthermore, prevention of complications, providing comfort, decreasing symptoms, and restoring and/or preserving functioning as much as possible is paramount. Attention should focus on dietary needs, education, functional status, special equipment necessary, and development of a coordinated plan for discharge and aftercare. Priority should be given to older high-risk individuals in an effort to prevent FTT.

FOOD LABELS

Food labeling provides a major source of information for consumers when choosing a healthy diet. The Nutrition Labeling and Nutrition Act allowed the Food and Drug Administration (FDA) to develop and enforce specific labeling. Uniform and mandatory nutrition labeling is now required for most prepared food, raw vegetables, fruits, and meat. Food packages must list the total calories from fat (both saturated and transfats) plus the amounts of cholesterol, total carbohydrates, fiber, sugar, and protein. Major nutrients must be listed in grams or milligrams, and also as a percentage of the total recommended intake of an individual consuming 2,000 calories a day. The FDA also regulates health claims (relationships between food and a specific disease or illness). Furthermore, they regulate structure and function claims (those claims that the nutrients or ingredients are intended to influence structure and function in human beings) such as "helps to lower cholesterol." Descriptions such as free, high, low, light, and lean that are used on food must meet the specific legal definition of the words (Lutz & Przytulski, 2006). Elders should be instructed how to read labels and to choose and shop for healthy foods based on content.

OLDER ADULTS AND INSTITUTIONAL DIETS

About 5% of adults over 65 are in nursing homes, and many have health problems that necessitate special diets. Most states require consulting dietitians and trained food service managers to plan and prepare diets served to institutional populations. There are policies that control the frequency with which the same foods are served, and in most cases weekly menus must be posted. Because food is extremely important to most elders, facilities should offer opportunities for varied food selection. The quantity and quality of food served in these settings is highly variable; some facilities serve nutritious and tasty meals whereas meals at other institutions need decided improvement.

All nursing home residents are assessed upon entrance into the nursing home setting using the Minimum Data Set (MDS). The MDS includes a nutritional assessment portion in which percentage of meals eaten, disabilities, age, and weight status are assessed and appropriate interventions initiated (Furman, 2006). Other useful information includes current diagnoses, sex, height, appetite, dietary history, pattern of weight gain or loss, food preferred or disliked, types and amounts of food eaten at every meal, pattern of snacking, ethnic and religious food preferences, food intolerances, special therapeutic diets, current medications, diagnostic laboratory test results, and emotional states. It is also important to determine the person's ability to feed him or herself and to chew and swallow. Using these data, preferences and problems can be identified and a dietary plan including goals is developed to ensure a pleasant and adequate diet for the resident. Periodic dietary evaluations are essential because both physical and mental status change over time.

Various health problems of many institutionalized elderly necessitate assistance with feeding. Suggestions for caregivers assisting the elderly with eating include:

1. Allow sufficient time for eating; do not hurry the person.
2. Attempt to offer a diet as close as possible to the person's accustomed diet.
3. Encourage the person to eat a substantial and healthy breakfast because the appetite is usually best at this time of day.
4. Inquire whether the family or significant others, when available, might like to feed the person, then instruct them on proper feeding techniques.

For severe undernutrition, using feeding tubes in conjunction with high caloric and protein diets or hyperalimentation may help stabilize the person's nutritional state. Some elders may require modified diets because of chronic or acute diseases. For instance, diabetics require a reduced carbohydrate diet, and those with cardiovascular problems often need a low-fat, low-cholesterol, or low-sodium diet. Individuals with cancer may require vitamin and nutritional supplements to assure adequate dietary nutrition. Certain drugs, such as diuretics and antidepressants, also make dietary modifications necessary. Regimens of strict therapeutic diets such as low-cholesterol or low-salt may contribute to a decreased food intake and are not advised for frail elders (Morley, 2003).

BASIC FOOD GROUPS

Adequate nutrition is based on the five food groups and adequate amounts of fluids. The primary food groups include:

1. Meat, poultry, fish, and alternatives such as eggs, dried peas, and beans. Protein, iron, fat, thiamine, and other nutrients are available from these foods. Daily requirements: 5 1/2 ounces.
2. Milk, butter, and other milk products including ice cream, cheeses, and yogurt made from skim, whole, dried, or evaporated milk,

according to dietary requirements. These foods supply calcium, protein, riboflavin, and fat. Daily requirements: 3 cups.
3. Vegetables such as carrots, cabbage, brussel sprouts, cucumbers, green or yellow beans, potatoes, corn, leafy greens (collards, spinach, mustard, lettuce), tomatoes, winter or summer squash, and mushrooms. These foods supply vitamin A, folic acid, and other nutrients. Daily requirements: 2 1/2 cups.
4. Fruits such as oranges, grapefruit, cantaloupes, peaches, strawberries, watermelon, pears, apples, and bananas. Vitamin A and vitamin C, potassium, and other nutrients are available from these foods. Daily requirements: 2 cups.
5. Breads and cereals such as whole grain or enriched breads, rolls, tortillas, cereals, rice, pastas, bagels, muffins, cornbread, pancakes, and biscuits. Thiamin, riboflavin, niacin, iron, and other nutrients are obtained from these foods. Daily requirement: 6 ounces.

Although fluids are not part of these groups, water, juices, and other liquids are necessary to maintain life processes. Daily requirements: 8 servings. Fluids may be more acceptable when taken in the form of tea, coffee, soups, fruit juices, milk, or gelatin.

THE FOOD GUIDE PYRAMID

In 2005 the United States Department of Agriculture developed MyPyramid (Figure 19-1), which includes recommendations for a healthy diet along with appropriate activity (http://www.mypyramid.gov). Foods are grouped into categories: grains; vegetables; fruits; oils; milk; and meat and beans. The width of the bands indicates general amounts of a particular type of food that should be eaten. It is recommended that individuals limit the use of sugars, fat, and salt. The figure climbing the stairs is a reminder to balance physical activity with caloric intake.

The Modified MyPyramid for Older Adults

In 2007 Tufts University updated the Food Guide Pyramid for 70+ Adults, now called the Modified MyPyramid for Older Adults, (Figure 19-2), which is consistent with and to be used in conjunction with MyPyramid. It is intended for individuals age 70 or above who lead independent, active lifestyles. In the diagonal sections, whole

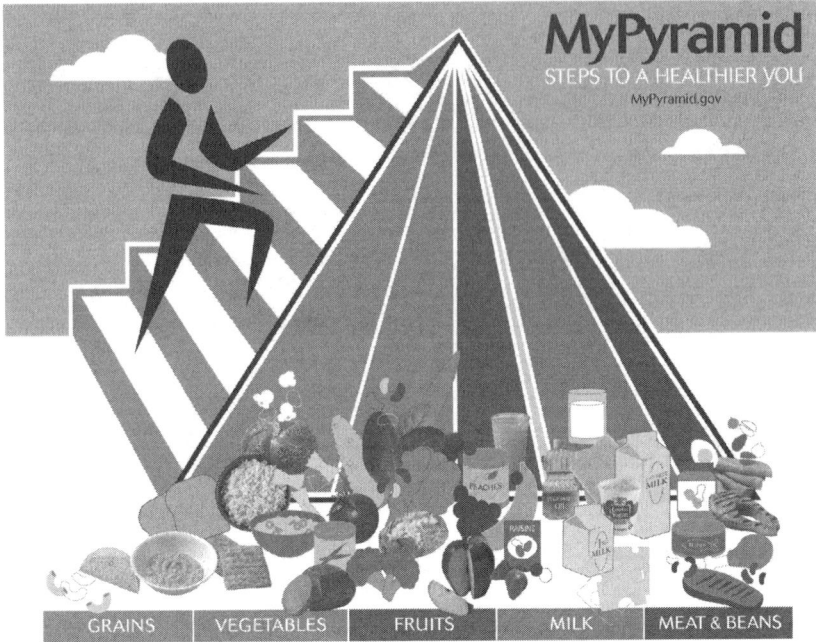

Figure 19.1. MyPyramid: Steps to a Healthier You. U.S. Department of Agriculture, 2005. http://mypyramid.gov.

grains; bright-colored vegetables; deep-colored fruits; low or no-fat dairy products; lean meats, eggs, nuts, or dry beans; and vegetable oils and soft spreads low in saturated and trans fats are depicted. More accessible forms of food that meet the special needs of elders, such as frozen fruits and vegetables, are pictured. A horizontal line near the bottom of the pyramid shows a row of glasses indicating the importance of adequate fluid intake for this age group. Physical exercise is highly recommended in various forms and is depicted at the bottom of the pyramid. Last, the flag on top of the pyramid is a reminder that some older individuals may need more calcium and vitamins D and B_{12} because they are not consuming sufficient amounts, especially when their caloric needs are reduced (Lichtenstein, Rasmussen, Yu, Epstein, & Russell, 2008). (Also available at http://nutrition.tufts.edu/.)

National nutrition programs for elders encourage use of the Food Guide Pyramid. In addition, some national groups, as well as manufacturers, use the food pyramid in advertising and on food labels.

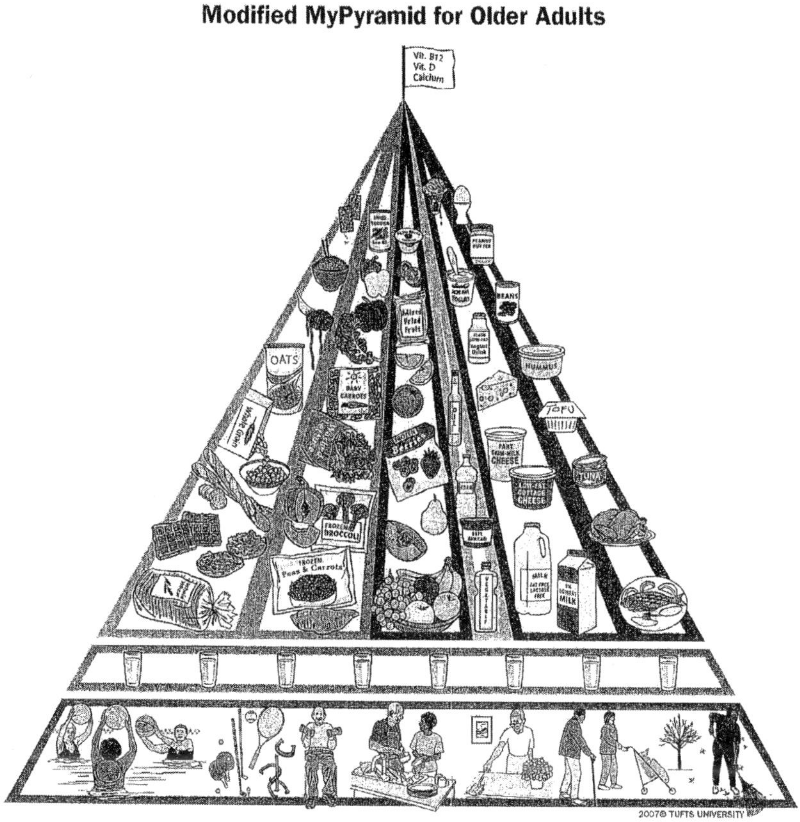

Modified MyPyramid for Older Adults

Figure 19.2. Modified MyPyramid for Older Adults. Reprinted with permission from Lichenstein et al., 2008.

NUTRITIONAL RECOMMENDATIONS FOR OLDER ADULTS

- Consume fewer calories, because older adults tend to have a reduced metabolism and lower levels of activity.
- Consume a variety of food daily.
- Reduce fat intake to 20% to 30% of total calories consumed; substitute unsaturated fats for saturated ones and limit cholesterol intake to 300 mg a day or less.
- Daily protein consumption should total 0.8 gms per kilograms of body weight for a healthy older person and 20% to 30% of the total caloric intake.
- Carbohydrate consumption should make up about 50% to 60% of the total caloric intake, with the major part coming from complex

sugar sources such as fresh fruits, vegetables, cereals, and breads. Few calories should come from simple sugars such as sugar, candy, preserves, and syrup.
- Consume six or more servings of grain products, especially whole grains.
- Vitamin intake should be adequate, especially vitamins A, B complex, C, D, E, and K.
- Ensure adequate mineral intake, including 1,200 to 1,500 mg of calcium daily plus sufficient amounts of phosphorus, potassium, zinc, iron, and other minerals.
- Consume three servings of milk daily.
- Prevent constipation by ingesting adequate amounts of fiber-rich food and water. Food such as fresh fruits and vegetables provide important roughage in the diet. Three or more servings of fruits and two or more of vegetables daily are necessary.
- Plan regular daily physical activity to prevent constipation and assist in the digestive process. Thirty to sixty minutes a day is advised by the 2005 Dietary Guidelines.
- Eat in moderation to maintain ideal weight and prevent or decrease obesity.
- Avoid junk foods.
- If alcoholic beverages are consumed, they should be used only in moderation.
- Consume smaller, more frequent meals help to prevent snacking. Frequent, small meals serve as a source of greater satisfaction for some individuals.
- Moderate or decrease salt intake.
- Be aware of harmful food and drug interactions.
- Store foods at the proper temperature and wash hands frequently when handling food (Yen, 2005).
- Follow instructions for specialized therapeutic diets.
- Diet planning should take into account individual preferences for ethnic and other foods, specific nutritional needs, and idiosyncratic intolerances of various foods.

EDUCATION

Educating older adults and their caregivers is one of the most important factors in promoting adequate nutrition. Teaching should focus on the meaning of food for people, its various functions in the body, food groups, food pyramid, major vitamins and minerals, food selection and preparation, drug-food interactions, methods of healthy cooking, food storage, specific therapeutic diets, diet preparation that takes into consideration ethnic and individual food preferences, and selected methods for assuring adequate food intake for individuals with disabilities. Most congregate nutrition sites offer some type of nutrition education to their participants. The purposes of a nutritional education program are as follows:

1. To assist the individual in selecting the required food for good health from the best sources, and for the least money.
2. To explain methods of identifying and obtaining various nutritional services such as home health aides or homemaker services.
3. To increase the older person's awareness of nutrition programs, such as Meals on Wheels or congregate dining in the community, and inform them about the availability of food stamps.
4. To provide information about special diets or menus needed for good health.

Using creative approaches to nutrition education in an environment promoting enjoyment, socialization, and support should help ensure improved dietary intake as well as increased compliance with various necessary dietary modifications.

SUPPLEMENTAL NUTRITION

If the older adult cannot, or refuses to, eat the necessary food to sustain adequate nutritional intake, supplementation with vitamins and minerals may be necessary. Although supplementation can treat an individual with less than needed nutritional intake, it cannot provide all the needed nutrients found in food (Yen, 2005). Supplemental feedings are available for those who cannot or will not ingest a balanced diet. Four types of supplements are available and used as oral feedings: modular supplements containing only one nutrient such as a carbohydrate or protein; intact or "polymeric" formulas, such as Ensure, Meritene and Sustacal, to be used when the elder needs all nutritional requirements within a specific amount; easier to digest elemental or "predigested formulas," such as Vivonex or Flexacal; and disease-specific formulas,

Hepatic-Aid or Pulmocare, designed for individuals with specific metabolic problems such as a kidney or lung disorder. When individuals are unable to eat in the usual manner or in sufficient amounts, enteral (tube feedings) may be administered via a tube inserted through the nose into the stomach or through a surgically inserted tube into the stomach. Intermittent or continuous formulated liquid foods help meet the necessary nutrition for each person. In the case of an individual with more serious and immediate nutritional requirements an IV infusion (hyperalimentation) of needed nutrients may be administered (Lutz & Przytulski, 2006).

COMMUNITY-BASED NUTRITION PROGRAMS FOR OLDER ADULTS

A variety of programs aimed at promoting improved and accessible nutrition at minimum cost are available. In 1972, the Older Americans Act (OAA) of l965 was amended, establishing the National Nutrition Program for Older Americans. A national network of programs for home-delivered and congregate dining was made available to the states and U.S. territories through Title 111c of the OAA. It requires food be provided five days a week with at least one meal per day that meets a third of the recommended dietary allowances (RDA). Also available is the Nutrition Assistance Program for Seniors (NAPS) extension program. The Senior Farmer Market Nutrition Program offers coupons to purchase fresh locally grown fruits and vegetables to those age 60 and above. The Supplemental Food Commodity Program is available in some states and distributes commodity foods such as cereals, cheese, flour, fruits, and vegetables (Yen, 2004). Meals on Wheels America is a national program supported by private funds to provide food on days when food is not served through governmental programs. Various other services may be offered to serve the frail elderly such as weekend meals, multiple daily meals, or liquid supplemental snacks. Even diets to meet specific health needs may be offered along with special ethnic or Jewish foods (Krinke, 2005).

The 1964 Food Stamp Act offers the USDA food stamp program to individuals in low-income households by issuing an electronic benefit card to purchase food. Certain third-party payers such as Medicare, Medicaid, Veterans Affairs, and insurance carriers offer and reimburse the cost of nutritional support and teaching. Nutritional counseling is offered in acute and long-term care settings, home health, and hospice care, as well as in ambulatory care settings (Blumberg & Suter, 1991).

Volunteers play important roles in delivering food to the homebound or those eating at congregate dining sites. In both settings they offer socialization and someone to show concern and caring. A registered dietitian develops the dietary plan, including specific therapeutic diets. Sites such as churches, schools, social halls, and other settings are used for congregate dining and also offer opportunities to participate in various recreational, educational, and counseling programs. Similar programs are offered at adult day care centers. In addition, homemaker services are available through governmental and private sources to assist older persons with shopping, food preparation, and even light housekeeping. Homemakers are specially trained in meal preparation and diet modification, and a dietitian or nutritionist is usually available for consultation. Other specific programs are offered by county extension services throughout the country.

SUMMARY

The importance of an adequate diet throughout life cannot be overestimated. We are indeed what we eat. The prevention of chronic and life-threatening illnesses, rapid recovery from surgery or disease, and optimal physical and psychosocial functioning depend on the ingestion of necessary amounts of carbohydrates, proteins, fats, vitamins, minerals, and fluids. Many older adults do not have a nutritionally sound diet because they are unable to shop for, pay for, or prepare and eat proper food. All who work with older persons have a responsibility to assess dietary intake, teach about nutrition, and refer individuals to the various nutritional programs and to qualified professionals in the local community.

REFERENCES

Age-Related Eye Disease Study Research Group (2001). A randomized placebo-controlled clinical trial of high dose supplementation with vitamins C and E, beta carotene, and zinc for age-related macular degeneration and vision loss. *AREDS Report No. 8. Archives of Ophthalmology, 119,* 1417–1436.

Arterburn, D., Crane, P., & Sullivan, S. (2004). The coming epidemic of obesity in elderly Americans. *Journal of the American Geriatrics Society, 52,* 1907–1912.

Baker, H. (2007). Nutrition in the elderly: An overview. *Geriatrics, 62*(7), 28–31.

Biggs, A. J. (2007). Nutritional considerations. In A. D. Linton, & H. W. Lach (Eds.), *Matteson & McConnell's gerontological nursing* (3rd ed., pp. 161–197). St. Louis: Saunders.

Blumberg, J. G., & Suter, P. (1991). Pharmacology, nutrition, and the elderly: Interactions and implications. In R. Chernoff (Ed.), *Geriatric nutrition: The health professional's handbook* (pp. 337–362). Gaithersburg, MD: Aspen Publications.

Cataldo, C. B., DeBruyne, L. K., & Whitney, E. N. (1992). *Nutrition and diet therapy: Principles and practice* (3rd ed.). St. Paul, MN: West Publishing.

Chernoff, R. (1990). Nutrition, health promotion, and aging. *Topics in Geriatric Rehabilitation, 6*(1), 19–26.

Chernoff, R. (Ed.). (1991). *Geriatric Nutrition: The health professional's handbook*. Gaithersburg, MD: Aspen Publications.

Chernoff, R. (2006). Carbohydrate, fat, and fluid requirements in older adults. In R. Chernoff (Ed.), *Geriatric nutrition: The health professional's handbook* (2nd ed., pp. 23–30). Sudbury, MA: Jones & Bartlett.

Dudek, S. (2006). *Nutrition essentials for nursing practice* (5th ed.). Philadelphia: Lippincott.

Dwyer, J., White, J., Ham, R., Lipschitz, D., & Wellman, N. S. (1991). Screening older Americans' nutritional health: Future possibilities. *Nutrition Today, 26*(5), 21–25.

Ebersole, P., Hess, P., Touhy, T. A., & Jett, K. (2005). *Gerontological nursing and healthy aging* (2nd ed.). St. Louis: Mosby.

Eliopoulos, C. (1997). *Gerontological nursing* (4th ed.). Philadelphia: Lippincott.

Flood, M., & Newman, A. M. (2007). Obesity in older adults. *Journal of Gerontological Nursing, 33*,(12), 19–34.

Furman, E. F. (2006). Undernutrition in older adults across the continuum of care. *Journal of Gerontological Nursing, 32* (1), 22–27.

Goldberg, A. P., Andres, R., & Bierman, E. L. (1990). Diabetes mellitus in the elderly. In W. R. Hazzard, R. Andres, E. L. Bierman, & J. P. Blass (Eds.), *Principles of geriatric medicine and gerontology* (2nd ed., pp. 739–758). New York: McGraw-Hill.

Granville, L. J., & Musson, N. (1999). Eating abnormalities: Disorders of self-feeding and swallowing. In W. R. Hazzard, J. P. Blass, W. H. Ettinger, J. C. Halter, & J. G. Ouslander (Eds.), *Principles of geriatric medicine and gerontology* (4th ed., pp. 1455–1490). New York: McGraw-Hill.

Grodner, M., Anderson, S. L., & DeYoung, S. (2000). *Foundations and clinical applications of nutrition: A nursing approach* (2nd ed.). St. Louis: Mosby.

Guthrie, H. A., & Picciano, A. (1995). *Human nutrition*. St. Louis: Mosby.

Healthy people 2010: Understanding and improving health (2000). Boston: Jones & Bartlett.

Krinke, U. B. (2005). Nutrition and the elderly. In J. E. Brown, J. S. Isaacs, U. B. Krinke, M. A., Murtaugh, C. Sharbaugh, J. Strang, & N. H. Woolridge (Eds.), *Nutrition through the life cycle* (2nd ed., pp. 420–449). Belmont, CA: Thomson Wadsworth.

Larson, K. (2003). Fluid balance in the elderly: Assessment and intervention-important role in community health and home care nursing. *Geriatric Nursing, 24*(5), 306–309).

Lichenstein, A. H., Rasmussen, H., Yu, W. W., Epstein, R., & Russell, R. M. (2008). Modified MyPyramid for older adults. *Journal of Nutrition, 138*(1), 5–11.

Linderman, R. D. (2006). Mineral requirements. In R. Chernoff (Ed.), *Geriatric nutrition: The health professional's handbook* (2nd ed., pp. 77–93). Sudbury, MA: Jones & Bartlett.

Lipschitz, D. A. (1991). Impact of nutrition on the age-related declines in hematopoiesis. In R. Chernoff (Ed.), *Geriatric nutrition: The health professional's handbook* (pp. 271–287). Gaithersburg, MD: Aspen Publications.

Lipschitz, D. A. (1997). Nutrition. In C. K. Cassel, H. J. Cohen, E. B. Larson, D. E. Meier, N. M. Resnick, L. Z. Rubenstein, & L. B. Sorensen (Eds.), *Geriatric medicine* (3rd ed., pp. 801–813). New York: Springer.

Luggen, A. S., Bernstein, M. J., & Touhy, T. A. (2008). Nutritional needs. In P. Ebersole, P. Hess, T. A. Touhy, K. Jett, & A. S. Luggen (Eds.), *Toward healthy aging* (7th ed., pp. 194–221). St. Louis: Mosby Elsevier.

Lutz, C., & Przytulski, K. (2006). *Nutrition and diet therapy: Evidence-based applications* (4th ed.). Philadelphia: F.A. Davis.

Marcus, E. L., & Berry, E. M. (1998). Refusal to eat in the older adult. *Nutrition Review,* 56, 163–171.

Morley, J. E. (1991). Why do physicians fail to recognize and treat malnutrition in older persons?. *Journal of the American Geriatrics Society,* 39(11), 1139–1140.

Morley, J. E. (2003). Anorexia and weight loss in older persons. *Journals of Gerontology Series A: Biological Sciences and Medical Sciences,* 58(2), 131–137.

National Center for Health Statistics (NCHS). (1997). Report of mortality statistics (1995). *Monthly Vital Statistics Report,* 45(11), Suppl. 2.

Newbern, V. B. (1992). Failure to thrive: A growing concern in the elderly. *Journal of Gerontological Nursing,* 18(8), 21–25.

Oakley, G. P., Adams, M. J., & Dickinson, C. M. (1996). More folic acid for everyone now. *Journal of Nutrition,* 126, 751–755.

Orr, M. (2000). Nutrition. In A. G. Lueckenotte (Ed.), *Gerontologic nursing* (2nd ed., (pp. 181–198). St. Louis: Mosby.

Osato, E. E., Stone, J., Phillips, S. L., & Winne, D. M. (1993). Clinical manifestations: Failure to thrive in the elderly. *Journal of Gerontological Nursing,* 19(8), 28–34.

Palmer, R.M. (1990). Failure to thrive in the elderly: Diagnosis and management. *Geriatrics,* 45(9), 47–55.

Rosenberg, I. (1991). Nutrition and aging. In G. E. Gaull, F. N. Kostsonis, & M. A. Mackey (Eds.), *Nutrition in the 90's: Current controversies and analysis* (pp. 41–49). New York: Marcel Dekker.

Rourke, K. M. (2006). Nutrition. In S. E. Meiner, & A. G. Lueckenotte (Eds.), *Gerontologic nursing* (3rd. ed., pp. 210–228). St. Louis: Mosby.

Rowe, J. W., & Kahn, R. L. (1998). *Successful aging.* New York: Pantheon Books.

Sarkisian, C. A., & Lachs, M. S. (1996). "Failure to thrive" in older adults. *Annals of Internal Medicine,* 124, 1072–1077.

Ship, J. A. (1999). The oral cavity. In W. R. Hazzard, J. P. Blass, W. H. Ettinger, J. B. Halter, & J. G Ouslander (Eds.), *Principles of geriatric medicine and gerontology* (4th ed., pp. 591–602). New York: McGraw-Hill.

Siegler, E., & Hark, I. (1996). Older adults. In G. Morrison, & L. Hark (Eds.), *Medical nutrition and disease* (pp. 142–155). Cambridge, Mass: Blackwell Science.

Silver, A. J. (1993). The malnourished patient: When and how to intervene. *Geriatrics,* 48(7), 70–73.

Suter, P. M. (1991). Vitamin requirements. In R. Chernoff (Ed.), *Geriatric nutrition: The health professional's handbook* (pp. 25–51). Gaithersburg, MD: Aspen Publishers.

Suter, P. M. (2006). Vitamin metabolism and requirements in the elderly: Selected aspects. In R. Chernoff (Ed.), *Geriatric nutrition: The health professional's handbook* (2nd ed., pp. 31–76). Sudbury, MA: Jones & Bartlett.

Tufts University Health and Nutrition Newsletter. (2008). 26(5), 1–4.

University of California, Berkeley (1999). Should you take a multivitamin? And which one? *Wellness Letter, 15.*

U.S. Department of Agriculture. (2005). *Dietary Guidelines for Americans.* Retrieved from http://www.health.gov/dietary guidelines

Verdery, R. B. (1997). Failure to thrive in old age: Follow-up on a workshop. *Journal of Gerontology, 52,* M333–M336.

Yen, P. K. (2000). Nutritional anemia. *Geriatric Nursing, 21*(2), 111–112.

Yen, P. K. (2003). Vitamins and disease prevention. *Geriatric Nursing, 24*(5), 316–317.

Yen, P. K. (2004). Community food assistance improves older adults' nutrition. *Geriatric Nursing, 25*(3), 182–183.

Yen, P. K. (2005). Food and supplement safety. *Geriatric Nursing, 26*(5), 277–280.

20. Medications and the Elderly

Multiple health problems are often concomitant with aging; those over 65 are likely to have one to three chronic diseases involving major body systems. The use of prescribed medications is often necessary to manage the various disease entities; many elders take six to ten medications simultaneously (Rolita & Freedman, 2008). Thus polypharmacy, "the use of one or more medications concurrently," especially multiples of the same drug, is commonplace in this age group. In addition, many take readily available over-the-counter (OTC) drugs for a variety of ailments such as headache, colds, arthritis, constipation, or indigestion. Another significant issue is the use of herbal products or nutritional supplements. Healthy People 2010 (2000) stipulates decreasing polypharmacy as a national priority.

Older adults, who constitute about 13% of the population, take at least one third of all prescription drugs and about 40% of all nonprescription drugs used by the general population (Maiese, 2002). It is not unusual for some elders to ingest 10 to 20 pills each day. As the number of drugs taken increases, so does the likelihood of drug-drug reactions. Furthermore, the incidence of medication errors escalates as inappropriate dosages are taken at the wrong times for the wrong ailment, often causing hospitalizations (Mauk, 2006). A national study of elders (average age 75) on Medicare reveals that 40% did not take medications as prescribed over the prior 12 months. Reasons cited were prohibitive cost and belief they did not need them or that they were taking more than necessary (Wilson, Schoen, Neuman, Strollo, Roger, Chang, & Safran, 2007). At times contraindicated medications, such as those that are outdated, duplicated from different physicians, or shared with a neighbor, are ingested. These behaviors often result in a litany of adverse reactions and interactions such as gastric irritation and bleeding, electrolyte imbalance, heart irregularities, orthostatic hypotension, nausea, altered mental states, constipation, movement disorders, falls, and urinary retention (Kane, Ouslander, & Abrass, 1999; Pepper, 1999). The likelihood of adverse drug reactions are further enhanced by alterations in pharmacodynamics, pharmacokinetics, lower body fat and body mass, reduced liver size, and lessened blood flow, as well as multiple and increasingly severe health problems (Rolita & Freedman, 2008).

Drug side effects are responsible for at least 30,000 deaths and 1.5 million admissions to hospitals each year, and elders are much more likely to experience toxic effects from drugs than are younger people. It is interesting to note that the standard normal adult dosage cited in drug literature is developed for 150-pound males, 22 to 26 years old. This standard adult dosage, however, can easily be an overdose for an older person with various age-related changes in body composition. Certain age-related changes decrease the ability of the body to utilize medications as effectively as in the younger years. In addition, drug studies on which standard dosages are based often include few or no older adult subjects, and if older persons are included they tend to be healthy individuals of the young-old group. The outcome of such studies can hardly be applied to the old-old who have multiple health problems and who take multiple medications (Shorr, 2007).

Sherman (2007) considers lack of adherence to medication schedules a national epidemic among older adults. Noncompliance is influenced by a variety of factors such as complex medication schedules, lack of doctor-patient discussion, memory impairment, inability to hear or see well, loss of hand and finger dexterity, and not being given adequate information about the drug. Other issues leading to noncompliance include uncomfortable drug side effects such as dry mouth or frequency of urination, lack of literacy skills, or the inability to organize the drug regimen and clearly understand how drugs are to be taken. It is essential to consider these and other reasons for noncompliance when teaching and assessing the ways elders take their prescribed medications.

CULTURAL RESPONSES TO DRUGS

Our country includes increasing numbers of individuals from diverse cultural backgrounds. Each culture brings with it beliefs and practices that influence the health of its members. Treatment of illness through the use of medications and other practices is deeply rooted in each tradition and passed on from one generation to the next. A variety of regimens used by cultural groups to treat disease are use of herbal and home remedies exclusively; use of Western medicine and medical practices exclusively; combining prayer and certain rituals along with vegetable drugs; use of Western medicine as an adjunct to usual folk practices; and following certain environmental and dietary guidelines. Because the older generation often have closer ties to past generations and cultural practices, it is important to determine the various treatments individuals use. Some of these may influence the effectiveness of prescribed medications and have the potential to cause adverse reactions.

OLDER ADULTS' RESPONSES TO DRUGS

Older adults' unique responses to drugs and their incidence of drug misuse place them at high risk for impaired physical and psychological states, accidents, and even institutionalization. Furthermore, highly variable individual responses to medications appear to increase with aging.

Pharmacokinetics is the study of the time it takes for drugs to be liberated, absorbed, distributed, metabolized, and excreted (LADME) from the body and the correlation between where they are distributed in the body and the duration of the intensity of therapeutic effects (Vestal, 1990). Normal aging influences each drug's pharmacokinetics somewhat differently. Individual responses to drugs vary widely, and sensitivity to drugs may either increase or decrease with age. Factors such as age, disease, the presence of other medications or food in the body, smoking, alcohol ingestion, body weight and composition, genetics, and environment all influence the processing of drugs in the body (Vestal, 1990; Kane, Ouslander, & Abrass, 1999; Shorr, 2007). The effectiveness of a drug depends upon its concentration at the site of action. Thus the rate at which liberation, absorption, distribution, metabolism, and excretion occurs influences the speed at which the drug works, how long it remains in the body, and the blood concentration of the drug.

Liberation

Liberation occurs when the coating of a pill or capsule of a medication dissolves in the mouth, thus liberating the active drug ingredient.

Absorption

Absorption occurs when the medication is ingested and absorbed in the mouth, stomach, or intestinal tract. Drugs must be absorbed in solution into body systems to be effective. Most drugs are absorbed through the gastrointestinal tract into the general blood circulation. Considerable controversy exists regarding the influence of age-related changes on the rate that drugs are absorbed into the body. Possible age-related impediments to drug absorption, though, do exist. A higher pH in the stomach can reduce the absorption and solubility of drugs such as tetracycline and iron preparations, or may inactivate penicillin. Furthermore, a delay in stomach emptying, diminished gastrointestinal blood flow, and changes in the number, structure, and functioning ability of the absorbing cells' surfaces may also influence absorption of drugs. Decreased intestinal motility slows the passage of nutrients and unabsorbed drugs through the intestines, increasing the chance that drugs will become inactive or will not be completely absorbed.

Some medications are best absorbed on an empty stomach, whereas others need the presence of food to reduce gastric irritation. In some situations, a drug and food may interact when taken together; for example, orange juice increases and tea decreases iron absorption, laxatives containing mineral oil reduce the absorption of fat-soluble vitamins in food, and carbonated beverages and fruit juices tend to lessen the action of penicillin. Even though age-related changes in the gastrointestinal tract have minimal influence on drug absorption, the GI tract is a common site for both mild and severe reactions that may lead to hospitalization (Lin & Lin, 1993).

Distribution

The process by which drugs in the bloodstream are sent to various parts of the body is called distribution. Depending upon their chemical characteristics, drugs absorbed from the intestinal tract pass into the portal vein (which carries blood to the liver) and are partly metabolized by the liver prior to entering the blood stream where they are transported to various body sites. The majority of drugs are attached or bound to proteins in the blood, a process that is both reversible and variable. Other drugs are not bound to blood proteins; they are "free" drugs in the blood. Bound drugs serve as a reserve supply of drugs, which are released into the bloodstream as the unbound or "free" drugs are metabolized and excreted.

Blood proteins decline with age, reducing the total number of usable binding sites. Older persons, then, tend to have increased amounts of "free" drug in the body, which can result in elevated drug levels in the blood. Certain drugs such as warfarin (an anticoagulant) and NSAIDs (anti-inflammatory drugs) are highly protein bound. They may displace each other by competing for available protein binding sites. Free drug molecules may then rapidly enter body tissues causing dangerously high drug concentrations (Le Fever-Kee & Hayes, 2000).

Reduced cardiac output and diminished blood flow to various organs decrease the amount of blood reaching body tissues and affect the speed of drug distribution. Drugs are more rapidly transported to organs with a rich blood supply, whereas it may take hours for drugs to reach fatty tissue. The aging process may also cause a greater permeability of the blood/brain barrier, allowing certain drugs to enter the central nervous system and cause unexpected neurological reactions.

Metabolism (Biotransformation)

Most drugs are metabolized in the liver into metabolites (substances produced during metabolism). This process enhances drug excretion through the kidneys. An older person's liver function is reduced due to lessened blood flow in the liver and lessened enzyme activity. Diminished liver function can influence the rate at which drugs are metabolized, creating a potential for drug toxicity. These changes may cause increased blood and tissue concentrations of some drugs, or may prolong the half-life of others (Woodhouse, 1998; Schwartz, 1999). For example, in older adults a specific cardiac medication such as propranolol (Inderal), a bronchodilator such as theophylline (Elixophyllin), certain antidepressants, and narcotics such as meperidine (Demerol) may produce higher blood levels of the drug due to altered liver metabolism. Individuals with liver diseases such as cirrhosis or hepatitis or those with decreased blood flow to the liver are especially sensitive to drugs metabolized by the liver.

Elimination

The kidneys, a major route for excretion of drugs from the body, eliminate metabolites from the liver into the urine as well as drugs not metabolized by the liver. Drugs are also eliminated through feces, exhalation, perspiration, and saliva. With age, there is reduced blood flow to the kidneys, fewer functional nephrons, reduced glomerular filtration rate, and less efficient tubular secretion and reabsorption. Despite these changes, older adults' elimination of waste and fluid is usually adequate for health.

Medications primarily eliminated through the kidneys are thought to have a longer half-life in older persons. Half-life is the time needed for the concentration of the drug in the blood to decrease by 50%. Some medications have short half-lives, others have long half-lives; the longer the half-life of a drug the longer it will remain in the body. For instance chlordiazepoxide's (Librium) half-life is from 5 to 30 hours, and the half-life of digitalis is as long as a week. Drugs with a long half-life should be taken with longer time intervals between doses. If a drug is taken over a shorter time period than 1.5 its half-life time, accumulation will occur. For example, if a drug's half-life is 10 hours, it should not be taken more than every 15 hours to prevent accumulation. Knowledge of the specific half-life of each drug prescribed is very important information to use in preventing toxic reactions. Concomitant kidney diseases further impair drug elimination and increase the likelihood of drug toxicity.

Tissue Sensitivity

Pharmacodynamic interactions are due to the additive, synergistic, or antagonistic effects of drugs (LeFever-Kee & Hayes, 2000). Greater therapeutic effects or likelihood of toxicity can result from age-related changes in pharmacodynamics (Avorn & Gurwitz, 1997). Age-related changes at the site of action determine the individual's responsiveness to the drug. Older adults are more sensitive to certain drugs, whereas sensitivity to other drugs may decrease with age. The actual effects of age-related pharmacodynamics of certain drugs for each person remains relatively unknown (Kane et al., 1999).

OVER-THE-COUNTER (OTC) DRUGS

OTC drugs, those purchased without a prescription, are considered by the Food and Drug Administration (FDA) to be effective and safe therapy if used as indicated on the packaging of the drug. Dosages are usually lower than for prescription drugs and therefore may not be as effective.

Some are single-drug products, whereas others are in combination with other ingredients. Elders treat themselves for mild ailments with OTC drugs 69% to 85% of the time. Six hundred or more of these drugs have the ingredients or prescribed dosages that could only be secured by prescription two decades ago. There are about 100,000 OTC drugs available to the consumer (Amoako, Richardson-Campbell, & Kennedy-Malone, 2003).

Professionals have a responsibility to alert older persons to possible problems associated with OTC drugs, including interactions with other drugs, alcohol, or food. They should be encouraged to become enlightened consumers by using the many reliable sources of information about drugs available in books, health newsletters, and from the internet. Health care providers, particularly pharmacists, are excellent resource persons for up-to-date and accurate information regarding a drug regimen.

Some individuals believe that OTC medications are harmless, or do not even consider them to be drugs, but both OTC and prescription medications are drugs that have the potential for overuse and interaction with other drugs, alcohol, or foods. OTC drugs may also interfere with the accuracy of laboratory tests, alter nutritional states, mask symptoms of a disease, or may even delay a diagnosis. Weight loss, diarrhea, confusion, depression, toxicity, or change in appetite could also result from OTC drug use. Reasons for their use include lack of money to visit a health care professional, lack of a personal physician, a desire to self-medicate, and the presence of an acute or chronic health problem such as a cold, arthritis, indigestion, insomnia, or constipation. OTC drugs most frequently used by older adults include analgesics, laxatives, antacids, cough medications, acetaminophens, milk of magnesia, vitamins, Pepto-Bismol, and non-steroidal topical preparations.

GENERIC DRUGS

Generic drugs are commonly prescribed and used today, but each state has specific regulations as to how they may be dispensed. A generic name is the common chemical name of the active ingredient in a drug product. A drug product includes not only the active ingredient but also several other elements such as coatings, dyes, fillers, and binding agents. The latter cause the equivalency and quality of drug products to vary widely between manufacturers. "Generic equivalent" is defined as two drugs that are chemically the same, but may not be therapeutically the same because of differences in the pharmacokinetics, such as how they are absorbed. Medications are designated as therapeutically equivalent if they have identical active ingredients; are in the same concentration, strength, and dosage form; and follow the same route after they are administered. To be bioequivalent, the extent and route of absorption of a generic drug may not be 20% or less or 25% greater than the drug with the brand name. If a tested drug earns an AB rating, this indicates the drug is therapeutically equivalent to other drugs given the AB rating and it has the same active ingredients. The Federal Drug Administration (FDA) publishes the "Approved Drug Products with Therapeutic Equivalence Evaluation," which rates the therapeutic equivalency of drugs (Ditrapano & Peoples, 2008).

When a drug is discovered it takes about 12 years before it is approved for human use and costs around 800 million dollars (Cuozzo, 2007). Drug patents last for 17 years, but after this period other drug companies may apply to the FDA to manufacture, market, and sell the drug as a generic drug under a different brand name (Ditrapano & Peoples, 2008). The drug manufacturer obtains FDA approval by showing that the drug is safe, effective, and therapeutically comparable to the brand name drug. Nevertheless, some physicians recommend that generic drugs not be used by individuals with diagnoses such as congestive heart failure, diabetes, and depression.

The majority of commonly prescribed drugs are available in generic form at about 30% to 40% less than the cost of brand name drugs. Consumers should ask health professionals about the advisability of using a generic drug and should know when generics are dispensed to them. Currently, many HMOs or insurance companies pay primarily for generic drugs; some states permit substitution of a generic drug when filling a prescription.

ADVERSE DRUG REACTIONS

Adverse drug reactions (ADRs) are a leading cause of morbidity and mortality in the United States. ADRs are unexpected and undesirable pharmacological responses to drugs (Melman, Morrelli, Hoffman, & Nierenberg, 1993; Kane et al., 1999). Many drugs cause not only distressing, but also life threatening reactions. Causes of adverse drug reactions include ingesting the wrong dosage at an incorrect time, stopping a drug too early, not taking the appropriate dose, and prescribing the drug inappropriately (Lefkovitz & Zarowitz, 2007).

Thirty-five percent of older adults who live in non-institutionalized settings experience adverse drug reactions yearly with 29% needing medical attention. If adverse reactions were recognized as a disease in the United States, they would be listed as the fifth leading cause of death (Petrone & Katz, 2005). Frequently reported adverse reactions include dry mouth, blurred vision, delayed voiding, constipation, and tardive dyskinesia (involuntary muscle movements caused by long-term use of antipsychotic drugs). Other commonly reported problems include electrolyte imbalances, a decrease in potassium levels when using some diuretics, gastric bleeding as a result of NSAIDs (nonsteroidal anti-inflammatory drugs), falls, and others. Prescribing appropriate medications is imperative in preventing adverse drug reactions. The Beers List is available to identify medications not appropriate to prescribe for older adults, and it's use can be valuable in prescribing medications less likely to cause adverse drug reactions (Fick, Cooper, Eade, Waller, Maclean, & Beers, 2003). As each group of drugs is considered, adverse reactions will also be discussed.

Consideration should be given to allergic drug reactions because these account for from 6% to 10% of all unusual or unexpected reactions to drugs. Drugs may interact with each other, increasing or decreasing their expected actions. Drugs prescribed for certain diseases, such as liver or kidney diseases, may cause adverse reactions such as confusion, lethargy, agitation, or even seizures.

Drugs and Alcohol

Over the years, alcohol ingestion has become an accepted part of social interaction. Alcohol, however, can be a chronic and progressive addiction causing intoxication, unconsciousness, depression, increasing accidents, and even death. Alcoholism may result in irreparable physical damage and psychosocial pain to the alcoholic as well as to the family. Ten to fifteen percent of males exhibit a rate of unhealthy drinking versus five percent of females (Fleming, 2002). Merrick and colleagues (2008) found that one out of ten older Medicare beneficiaries drank more than the amount of alcohol recommended. Age-related changes enhance the likelihood of older drinkers incurring more physical, psychological, and social problems. Specifically, aging results in decreased lean body mass, and decreased total body water. Since alcohol is dispersed almost entirely in the body's water compartments, there is a higher blood alcohol level per dose of alcohol than for younger individuals. This means that older drinkers are more likely to experience enhanced effects of alcohol and therefore experience more problems associated with alcohol use. Additionally, elders ingest more prescribed and OTC drugs than their younger counterparts. Metabolism is slower and they experience more chronic disease, thus enhancing the potential for greater drug-alcohol interactions (Culberson, 2006).

Older alcoholics are categorized into two groups: two thirds represent "early-onset" drinkers who have survived to what is often an unhappy, unhealthy old age; and one third are those over age 60 who have begun drinking in response to aging or loss. Factors contributing to alcoholism that begins in the older years include recent retirement; older adults' lessened control over their lives and less recognition by others; bereavement after the death of a significant person, usually a spouse; impaired physical or mental health; and relocation to a new environment. Any or all of these factors should alert those working with elders to the possibility of alcoholism and the dangers of mixing alcohol and drugs.

Major groups of drugs, both prescription and OTC medications, that adversely react with alcohol include tranquilizers, anti-diabetic drugs, sleeping pills, antibiotics, anti-infectives, barbiturates, anti-anginal and antihypertensive agents, blood thinners, diuretics, pain medications (both narcotic and non-narcotic), antidepressants, gout medications, muscle relaxants, allergy medications, cough and cold suppressing products, motion sickness drugs, vitamins, antihistamines, central nervous system stimulants, anticonvulsants, and anti-alcoholic preparations. Vigilance on the part of caregivers is necessary because the older alcoholic is not easily detected unless actually seen drinking. Elders and their caregivers should become acquainted with the potentially lethal effects of simultaneously ingesting drugs and alcohol.

Interaction of Drugs with Other Substances

The elderly, because of possible multiple chronic health problems, subclinical malnutrition, excessive use of drugs, poor cooking methods, and alterations in how the body utilizes drugs, represent an at-risk group with respect to drugs, caffeine, food, and tobacco interactions. Such interactions depend upon body size, age, drugs, drug dosages, and current health problems.

The therapeutic action of medication can be adversely affected by nicotine, which alters liver enzyme metabolism, causes vasoconstriction, results in greater amounts of gastric acid secretion in the stomach, and stimulates the central nervous system. To attain the desired therapeutic action of a drug, higher doses may be required; for example, nicotine reduces the effectiveness of diuretics, heparin, and analgesics (Miller, 2009).

Caffeine is present in many drinks, foods, cold preparations, and other medications. Caffeine-medication interactions mostly affect the medication action, not the caffeine's action on the body. Such interactions may reduce the absorption of iron, diminish the effect of antiarrhythmic medications, and increase gastric irritation when taken with corticosteroids or analgesics (Miller, 2009).

The action of medications and nutrients may be affected by medication-nutrient interactions for individuals of all ages. Elders are especially vulnerable due to age-related changes and disease states. A major way that nutrients influence medications is by altering their absorption in the stomach (Miller, 2009). Nutrients can either increase or decrease drug absorption, which could either be serious or beneficial to the individual. Grapefruit can cause serious toxicity with a number of drugs such as simvastatin, amlodipine, or it can increase the action of other drugs such as cyclosporine (Lehne, 2007). Depleted nutritional states are further aggravated by certain medications that alter vitamin and/or mineral absorption. For example, mineral oil when used regularly impairs absorption of vitamin A, D, E, and K. Vitamin B-complex absorption is impaired by digitalis, antiinflammatory drugs, aspirin, and oral hypoglycemic drugs. Vitamin C levels are negatively influenced by both aspirin and alcohol. Many diuretics cause potassium loss, whereas aluminum-containing antacids reduce phosphate and calcium absorption.

Drugs can cause nutritional deficiencies by appetite suppression, changes in nutrient absorption, changes in utilization and metabolism of nutrients, and changes in elimination of nutrients. Certain drugs are known to suppress appetite. These include cancer chemotherapy drugs, alcohol, antacids, antihistamines, narcotics, digitalis, cough medicines, amphetamines, and caffeine. Conversely, some medications, including tranquilizers such as phenothiazines and antidepressants, stimulate the appetite. Recommendations to prevent drug-food interactions include:

1. Drugs and alcohol should never be taken together.
2. Medications should be ingested with sufficient water (preferably a full glass) to allow for complete swallowing.
3. Medications should not be taken with juices, tea, coffee, or soft drinks.
4. The cautions on OTC and prescription drugs regarding food-drug incompatibilities should be read and followed carefully.
5. Persons obtaining a new medication should ask a health care professional or pharmacist about any restrictions regarding food intake and medication use.

Drug-Drug Interactions

Drug-drug interactions are possible whenever the individual takes two or more drugs. When these interactions take place the following may occur: drug A may enhance or lessen the action of drug B, or cause a response not observed with either drug; the larger the number of drugs ingested the greater likelihood of serious drug reactions. When considering the number of prescribed and OTC drugs taken by elders, it is not surprising that there are a large number of identified adverse drug reactions, much less those that are never diagnosed (Lehne, 2007).

Drug Misuse

The following are some of the many factors responsible for misuse of drugs by older adults.

Psychological Factors

1. Cognitive impairments influence the ability to take the correct drugs at appropriate times.
2. Depression or other psychiatric conditions result in less interest and motivation to take medications.
3. Being required to take many medications, especially on complex schedules, may be difficult to understand and manage.
4. Needing to take medications is perceived as a threat to self-esteem and independence.
5. Some may have a fear of becoming addicted to drugs, or fear of taking high-risk drugs.
6. Lack of knowledge about medications and medication management.

Physiological Factors

1. Visual impairment affects the ability to read labels and directions on how to take the drugs.
2. Hearing impairment may hinder understanding instructions regarding how and when to take medications.
3. Health problems such as arthritis and degenerative diseases often cause weakness and pain, making it difficult to open bottles and manipulate medications.
4. Pain, especially chronic pain, may contribute to ingestion of too much medication.
5. Using hypnotic drugs to combat insomnia may result in overmedication.
6. Individuals may be allergic to medications.
7. A weakened, debilitated, fragile state may make it difficult to take the correct medicine at the right time.

Social Factors

1. Reduced financial income may restrict individuals from purchasing needed medications.
2. Religious or cultural belief may influence use, non-use, or disuse of some medications.
3. Using medications may imply to others that the individual has assumed the "sick role."

Other Factors

Research and clinical observations have cited other patterns of drug misuse such as:

1. Failure to have prescriptions filled or refilled.
2. Skipping doses.
3. Ingesting medications at the wrong time.
4. Swapping medications with friends.
5. Stopping medications prematurely.
6. Overdosing.
7. Underdosing.
8. Using outdated medications.
9. Consuming various drugs prescribed by several physicians and purchasing the drugs at different pharmacies.

378 Physical Change & Aging

10. Using alcohol, caffeine, smoking, or certain contraindicated foods with medications.
11. Not understanding the directions on how to take the medication.
12. Using OTC drugs along with prescription drugs.
13. Lack of periodic evaluation and follow-up by the primary care practitioner to assess the need to continue using medication.
14. Having too easy access to prescription drug refills via the telephone.
15. Being unable to open tamper-proof, child-proof drug packaging.
16. Using herbal preparations with prescribed medications.

All of the above possibilities should be considered when monitoring medications used by older adults. Medication misuse has the potential to create mental problems such as confusion or lethargy; physical problems such as unsteadiness and falling; and social impairments such as the inability to engage in everyday activities of daily living (Miller, 2009).

DRUG THERAPY

The treatment of choice for many older persons who have multiple chronic diseases is pharmacological. Drugs, however, can be both helpful and harmful, and should be used with caution. Because all the drugs prescribed for elders cannot be discussed in this chapter, the use of reliable, up-to-date resources on medications is suggested for both professionals and non-professionals interested in geriatric pharmacology. Reference books such as *Davis's Drug Guide for Nurses* (Deglin & Vallerand, 2007), *Physician's Desk Reference (2009)*, and *Drug Facts and Comparisons* (Medline Plus. U.S. National Library of Medicine http://medlineplus.gov) are recommended for reliable accurate information. Newsletters such as *Prescriber's Letter* may also be helpful. The internet, too, can be a valuable resource of drug information through the use of drug company information sites, online pharmacies, and research information. Chat rooms offer the opportunity to communicate with other individuals who are taking a similar drug. Nevertheless, not all online information is reliable because any person can post information regardless of qualifications. Therefore it is important to access medical sources such as http://evolve.elsevier.com/Lehne which is a substantive site for drug information (Lehne, 2007).

COMMONLY PRESCRIBED DRUGS

Cardiovascular Drugs

Digitalis

Digitalis slows and strengthens the heart beat and is the drug of choice in treating congestive heart failure and other heart disorders. The half-life of digitalis may be as long as 36 to 48 hours, thus the likelihood of it causing digitalis toxicity and the necessity of carefully monitoring serum drug levels. Those taking this drug are taught to count their pulse rate regularly and to stop the drug if the pulse is below 60 beats per minute. Nausea, vomiting, and visual disturbances are signs of acute digitalis toxicity. Other symptoms include irregular heart rate, heart block, headache, confusion, agitation, and even psychosis.

Digitalis may depress the appetite and impair nutritional states. Some drugs and foods reduce the absorption of digitalis when taken by mouth. These include aluminum or magnesium antacids, laxatives, large amounts of bran, and the antibiotic neomycin. Elders may not be able to tolerate digitalis well due to loss of lean body mass and possible impaired kidney functioning. They are also prone to electrolyte imbalances, especially low potassium levels; thus it may be necessary to prescribe smaller dosages for this age group.

Nitroglycerin

Nitroglycerin is prescribed to dilate the blood vessels. Available in extended release tablets or capsules, sublingual tablets, lingual spray, transdermal ointment, or intravenously, it helps to improve blood flow through the coronary blood vessels. The sublingual tablets should be stored in the tightly closed original container and kept in a dry, cool place; a fresh supply should be purchased every 3 months. It is not advisable to ingest alcohol, antivasodilators, or antihypertensive drugs with nitroglycerin, nor should one suddenly discontinue its use. Side effects of nitroglycerin include headache, rash, flushing of the face and neck, nausea, vomiting, low blood pressure, and visual disturbances.

Diuretics

Diuretics (Hydro-Diuril, Aldactone, and Lasix, for example) are used to treat acute and chronic cardiovascular disease as well as hypertension and heart failure. There are three types: thiazide diuretics, loop diuretics, and potassium sparing diuretics. The first two deplete the body of potassium and require the ingestion of potassium-enriched food such as bananas, oranges, green leafy vegetables, or potassium supplements. Diuretics should be taken at the same time each day, preferably in the morning because they increase voiding and may interfere with sleep if taken in the evening. Side effects related to potassium loss include thirst, erratic or weak heart beat, mental changes, nausea, vomiting, weakness, fatigue, and muscle cramps. Other reactions to the drug include orthostatic hypotension (lowering of the blood pressure when moving from a lying to a standing position), bleeding, bruising, rash, increase in blood sugar levels, and excess uric acid in the blood. Electrolytes should be monitored regularly and weight taken daily. Furosemide (Lasix), for example, may be toxic to the ear (ototoxic) and result in deafness that is usually transient but can be permanent. Special care should be taken not to use these drugs if hearing is already impaired. Diuretics require close monitoring because they enhance the action of digitalis, lithium, oral diabetic medications, antihypertensives, skeletal muscle relaxants, and reduce the action of anticoagulants.

Beta-Adrenergic Blocking Drugs

Beta-adrenergic drugs, such as atenolol (Tenormin), propranolol (Indural), and others, lessen oxygen requirements of the heart by reducing the heart's workload with a resultant decrease in heart rate, force of contraction, cardiac output, and blood pressure. Older African-Americans and cigarette smokers are often resistant to these drugs' intended actions. They have, however, been proven effective for most older persons with hypertension, angina, arrhythmias, or post-myocardial infarction. Individuals with chronic lung disease or diabetes are not likely candidates for them because of their influence on blood sugar and lung functioning. Side effects include fatigue, insomnia, sexual dysfunction, slow heart rate, and decreased blood flow to the periphery of the body. Certain side effects particularly common in elders include hypotension, cardiac failure, low blood sugar, thyroid dysfunction, arthritic symptoms, and depression. They should not be withdrawn suddenly because angina, heart attack, or death could result.

Calcium Channel Blocking Drugs

Diltiazem (Cardizem, Cardizem CD) and nifedipine (Procardia) and other channel blocking drugs dilate blood vessels increasing blood flow both to peripheral blood vessels and to coronary blood vessels. They are used to lower blood pressure, decrease angina attacks, and control cardiac dysrhythmias. Side effects are usually mild with headache and constipation being the most common. Individuals who have asthma, peripheral vascular disease, or diabetes are given these drugs because they may not be able to tolerate beta-adrenergic blockers. They are often prescribed for older adults and African-Americans who may not respond to other classes of hypertensive drugs.

Angiotensin-Converting Enzyme Inhibitors

The ACE inhibitors such as ramipril (Altace), benazepril (Lotensin), and captopril (Capoten) are used to treat hypertension, myocardial infarction (MI), heart failure, and diabetic neuropathy, and to prevent strokes, MI, or death in individuals who are at high risk for developing cardiovascular attacks. Blood pressure may drop suddenly due to vasodilation after taking the first dose of an ACE inhibitor, thus caution should be observed when starting this drug and blood pressure levels should be carefully monitored. Five to ten percent of those taking ACE inhibitors experience a dry, irritating, persistent cough necessitating its discontinuance. It can also cause the kidneys to retain potassium, therefore those taking it should be advised not to take potassium supplements or use salt substitutes that contain potassium (Lehne, 2007).

Angiotensin Receptor Blockers

Angiotensin receptor blockers such as losartan (Cozaar), irbesartan, (Avapro), and valsartan (Diovan) are prescribed for hypertension, heart failure, MI, diabetic neuropathy, and to prevent strokes. They are usually well tolerated and often prescribed for individuals who cannot tolerate ACE inhibitors because they do not cause cough or high potassium levels (Lehne, 2007).

Aldosterone Antagonists

Aldosterone antagonists such as eplerenone (Inspra) and spironolactone (Aldactone) are used for hypertension and heart failure. Their major side effect is high potassium levels, so they should be monitored frequently and the older adult instructed not to take potassium supplements or use a salt substitute that contains potassium (Lehne, 2007).

Direct Renin Inhibitors

Direct renin inhibitors are a new class of drugs to lower blood pressure. There is only one drug in this class, alskiren (Tekurna), which may be prescribed alone or in combination with other antihypertensive drugs. Serum creatinine and potassium levels should be assessed every six months or yearly and urine checked for proteinuria every year (Wright, 2008).

Antihypertensive Drugs

Hypertension is a commonly occurring health problem among older adults. Aerobic exercises, weight loss, reduced fat and cholesterol intake, salt reduction, smoking cessation, and reducing stress all help to decrease blood pressure or maintain it within normal limits. In addition, the stepped-care approach, in which one drug is prescribed with various others added as time goes on to meet the goal of a normal blood pressure, may be used to treat hypertension. The first drug of choice is usually a diuretic with others, such as beta-adrenergic blockers, calcium channel blockers, angiotensin-converting enzyme (ACE) inhibitors, angiotensin 11 receptor blockers, or direct renin inhibitors, added as necessary.

The greatest risks with antihypertensive drugs involve reduced cardiac output, low blood pressure, dehydration, and orthostatic hypotension. Individuals on antihypertensive drugs should be instructed to rise slowly from a sitting or lying position and to monitor their blood pressure and pulse frequently. If the blood pressure is below 90/60 mm Hg or the pulse below 60, or if there is dizziness, confusion, weakness, lethargy, or hypotension, a health care professional should be contacted immediately.

Drugs for Disorders of Coagulation

Because older persons are at higher risk for blood clots, anticoagulant therapy may be prescribed. Warfarin (Coumadin or Panwarfin) and dicumarol are oral medications used to prolong bleeding time and prevent formation of blood clots. Heparin is given subcutaneously and intravenously to attain a high level of anticoagulation or prevent the formation of postoperative blood clots. Enoxaparin (Lovenox) given subcutaneously is used to prevent deep vein thrombosis, especially following knee or hip surgery. This age group has a higher risk for increased bleeding when given anticoagulants. Blood coagulation time should be regularly monitored because a major side effect is hemorrhage. Because of this dangerous side effect individuals may be anxious about taking the drug, thus careful monitoring and teaching are imperative. Doses should never be omitted and they must be taken specifically as prescribed.

Aspirin should not be taken with, or seven days before or after, warfarin therapy. Any drug containing aspirin can increase the effectiveness of anticoagulants and cause bleeding. Because eating foods high in vitamin K promotes blood clotting and decreases the effectiveness of anticoagulants, foods containing this vitamin are usually limited to four ounces per day. When on anticoagulants, elders should be advised never to take any new drug, by prescription or OTC, unless first checking with the primary care provider. All caregivers should be informed when an older person is on an anticoagulant.

Elders on anticoagulants should be cautioned about falling, cutting, or bumping themselves because these accidents may cause bleeding. Nose or gum bleeding, blood in the urine, stool, or phlegm may indicate an overdose, and a severe headache might signal intracranial bleeding. All must be reported immediately to the primary care provider or the closest medical service. The use of a medic alert identification bracelet or card is highly recommended for those on anticoagulant therapy.

Antiplatelet Agents

These drugs cause anticoagulation by interfering with a variety of processes involving platelet formation, especially platelet aggregation. They are used to prevent the formation of clots in the arteries. Aspirin, available over-the-counter, is often prescribed in a small dose such as 80 to 325 mg daily to prevent strokes or coronary heart attacks. Other drugs such as Plavix (clopidogrel), Persantine (dipyridamole), and ReoPro (abciximab) are antiplatlet agents. They increase bleeding time and may cause GI or other types of bleeding or bruising. Anyone taking these drugs should not ingest any medications containing aspirin. If bleeding or bruising occurs, a health care practitioner should be contacted immediately.

Thrombolytic Drugs

Streptokinase (Steptase), alteplase (tPA), and tenecteplase (TNKase) are among the drugs used to dissolve blood clots in the coronary vessels, in acute pulmonary embolism, and in deep vein thrombosis. Because these conditions demand immediate attention, thrombolytic drugs are usually administered in the emergency room. It is imperative if an individual is suffering from any of the above acute conditions they be taken to the hospital immediately because each drug must be administered within a strict time frame. Bleeding and its complications are among the most dominant side effects, but streptokinase may also cause an allergic reaction. These medications are being used to treat older individuals, but the cost is quite expensive. Contraindications include recent surgery, serious trauma, cerebrovascular disease, active internal bleeding, recent GI bleeding, and severe hypertension (Lehne, 2007).

Cholesterol-Lowering Drugs

Used to treat hyperlipidemia (greater than normal amounts of plasma cholesterol or plasma triglycerides), cholesterol-lowering drugs lower LDL cholesterol and triglycerides and raise HDL cholesterol. Drugs include HMG-CoA reductase inhibitors (statins), bile-acid sequestrants (Questran), nicotinic acid, and ezetimibe (Zetia). Statins are the most effective in lowering cholesterol and are widely prescribed, but if withdrawn, serum cholesterol will return to pre-treatment levels so they must be taken for a life time. Adverse effects include myopathy (injury to the muscle tissue) with symptoms of muscle weakness or aching. Such symptoms should be reported immediately to a primary care provider because it could progress to myositis (muscle inflammation) and to even more fatal muscle disintegration. Other adverse effects include liver toxicity, headache, constipation, abdominal pain, rash, and dyspepsia (Lehne, 2007; Adams, Holland, & Bostwick, 2008).

Drugs for Joint Disorders

Two of the most annoying and painful diseases associated with older age are osteoarthritis (degenerative arthritis) and rheumatoid arthritis. Although drugs of choice for these conditions vary, only those commonly prescribed will be discussed here.

Nonsteroidal Anti-Inflammatory Drugs (NSAIDs)

Aspirin (acetylsalicylic acid) is the most commonly used OTC drug for arthritis, but it is not without serious side effects such as GI bleeding and iron deficiency anemia. According to Clark, Queener, and Karb

(1990), about 10 to 30 ml of blood can be lost daily from long-term aspirin use. Enteric-coated aspirin is sometimes recommended because it is released in the small intestine rather than in the stomach and is less irritating to the stomach. Other adverse effects of aspirin include ringing in the ears, rashes, nausea, vomiting, confusion, and deafness. Salicylate toxicity-induced confusion is often undiagnosed and may occur even with normal therapeutic dosage. It is also important to recognize that many other OTC drugs contain aspirin, including Alka-Seltzer, Anacin, Excedrin, Pepto-Bismol, and Doan's Pills (Flemming-Courts, 1996). Alcohol should be avoided by those taking aspirin. Antacids increase the excretion of aspirin, which necessitates larger dosages of aspirin. The action of both oral antidiabetic and anticoagulant drugs is increased by aspirin; however, it lowers the blood levels of other NSAIDs. The blood levels of aspirin can be measured in the blood; side effects are not an accurate indicator of overdose.

NSAIDs are most frequently chosen for treating mild to moderate arthritis. Additionally, they may lower body temperature and reduce inflammation. Drugs in this category include indomethacin (Indocin), piroxicam (Feldene), tolmetin (Tolectin), and naproxen (Naprosyn), among others. They are likely to cause gastric irritation, bleeding, peptic ulcers, and water retention. Indocin may result in headaches, dizziness, nausea, vomiting, rash, and difficulty breathing. This group of drugs has a high incidence of adverse effects in older persons and should be used with caution. They should always be taken with milk or food, and careful monitoring is advised for those with heart, kidney, and liver disease.

Ibuprofen (Motrin, Advil, Nuprin) usually causes fewer gastrointestinal symptoms, but they do occur in some individuals. Adverse effects include nausea, vomiting, abdominal pain, gastrointestinal bleeding, headache, dizziness, and skin eruptions. Alcohol, oral anticoagulants, or aspirin should not be taken concurrently with ibuprofen.

Cox-2 inhibitors such as Celecoxib (Celebrex) are prescribed for severe arthritic conditions and for those who need a more effective anti-inflammatory drug. Gastric bleeding and peptic ulcers are possible when high dosages are used. There is considerable evidence that Cox-2 inhibitors increase the likelihood of developing a stroke, MI, or serious cardiovascular episode. Vioxx and Bextra have been taken off the market because the risk of cardiovascular events is highest with them. Celebrex should be prescribed in the lowest dose possible for the shortest possible time period and care taken not to prescribe this drug for individuals who have a cardiovascular disease (Lehne, 2007).

There are other drugs prescribed for arthritis, such as Acetaminophen (Tylenol). Acetaminophen is useful in controlling pain and lowering temperature, but it is not an antirheumatic or anti-inflammatory medication. Tylenol does not cause stomach irritation, but overdosing can cause liver damage (Lehne, 2007). Central acting drugs such as Clonidine (Catapres) or Tramadol (Ultram) may also be prescribed. Other antirheumatic drugs commonly prescribed include methotrexate (Mexate, Folex), leflunomide (Arava), penicillamine (Depen), and others. Individuals with arthritis may experience temporary relief from injections of intra-articular glucocorticoids. A newer type of drug, hyaluronate (Hyalgan), is sometimes injected into the knee joint to replace lessened hyaluronic acid due to arthritis (Adams, Holland & Bostwick, 2008).

Gold Salts

Gold salts, taken orally or by injection, are sometimes prescribed for arthritis, but supervision by a rheumatologist is strongly recommended. Numerous adverse reactions are possible during, or even a few months after, therapy. These include skin rashes or itching, mouth irritation, ulcers, diarrhea, bleeding of the gums, blood in the stool, jaundice, visual changes, fever, nausea and vomiting, kidney dysfunction, and cardiac or respiratory problems. This drug should be taken with food to avoid stomach irritation (Spratto & Woods, 1994).

Steroids

Glucocorticoids such as Deltasone, Meticorten, and Cortef may be prescribed for individuals with rheumatoid arthritis, but they should be used for short periods of time and only after other less potent drugs have been ineffective. They should never be discontinued abruptly, but be tapered off gradually. Side effects include nausea, gastric distress, ulcers, hemorrhage, sodium and water retention, euphoria, thinning skin, easy bruising, depression, impaired wound healing, and increased incidence of osteoporosis.

Drugs for Gout

Individuals with gout have above-normal uric acid levels that crystallize in joints, tendons, or bursae, causing extreme pain. Therapeutic goals are to terminate the acute attack and prevent further episodes.

Novacolchine Colchicine is used both for acute attacks and to prevent attacks. This drug requires careful monitoring, especially with older persons who have heart and kidney problems. Alcohol should be avoided when taking it. Side effects include nausea and vomiting followed by diarrhea, stomach pain, mental confusion, numbness, tingling, bleeding, bruising, weakness, and skin rash. Allopurinol (Zyloprim), also prescribed for gout, usually causes minimal side effects such as skin rash or itching, bruising, bleeding, weakness, or drowsiness, and should be taken with meals or a snack to avoid gastric irritation. Probenecid (Benemid) and sulfinpyrazone (Anturane) are also prescribed, but should be avoided by those with kidney stones or kidney failure. Occasionally, GI upset or allergic reactions may occur. It is advisable to drink 10 to 12 eight-ounce glasses of water daily and avoid aspirin or aspirin-containing substances. Regular monitoring of serum uric acid levels is recommended.

Drugs for Osteoporosis

As ovarian function decreases during menopause, estrogen production usually falls gradually, but it may cease abruptly following surgical removal of the ovaries. Lower estrogen levels are a major cause of osteoporosis. Because osteoporosis contributes to the disability or death of many older women, considerable research focuses on this health issue. Regular exercise, preferably walking, together with a diet high in calcium, are thought to reduce the likelihood of developing osteoporosis. Post-menopausal women need a calcium intake of about 1,500 mg daily, especially if they are not taking estrogen supplements. When purchasing calcium it is important to be aware that not all brands deliver the optimal amount of calcium. In addition, an intake of 400 to 800 IU of vitamin D is recommended to aid in the absorption of calcium.

Estrogens such as Premarin are prescribed to alleviate the symptoms of menopause and to retard post-menopausal bone loss. They are available in several forms; oral, transdermal patch, injection, and intravaginal estrogens. Adverse effects include breast cancer, fluid retention, MI, deep vein thrombosis, stroke, pulmonary embolism, and dementia. The Women's Health Initiative Study 2002 (Women's Health Initiative www.nhlbi.nih.gov/whi/) indicated that those taking Prempro had a greater risk for breast cancer, stroke, coronary artery disease, and venous thrombosis. Those women taking Premarin showed a slight but significant increase in the incidence of stroke, but no increase in heart disease or breast cancer; however, women age 60 and over were at higher risk.

As a consequence of this study thousands of women discontinued the use of hormone replacement therapy. Rather than remaining on hormone replacement therapy for years, consulting a health care provider is highly recommended. When used to treat menopausal symptoms, estrogens are usually prescribed on an individual basis with the lowest dosage, for the shortest time period (Adams, Holland, & Bostwick, 2008). Because of the risks involved in taking this drug, product labels must have the highest level of warning (boxed warning) describing its many risks.

Other drugs used to treat osteoporosis by inhibiting bone resorption include calcitonin (Cibacalein), which is available as an injection and as a nasal spray Calcitonin salmon (Miacalcin). The latter may cause rhinitis in about 10% of the users. Another group of drugs available are the selective estrogen receptor modulators (SERMs) such as raloxifene (Evista). Evista mimics estrogen in certain tissues of the body and its action reduces bone resorption; however it may cause hot flashes and, in some cases, leg cramps and venous thrombosis.

Bisphosphonates, another category of osteoporosis medications, slows bone metabolism and bone turnover, even building new bone and thus increasing bone density or bone mass by 50%. Examples include alendronate (Fosamax), risedronate (Actonel), and ibandronate (Boniva). Alendronate (Fosamax) is also used to treat osteoporosis in men. There is a slight tendency to develop osteonecrosis (bone destruction) of the jaw when taking Fosamax. The first two drugs are taken once a week, and Boniva is taken once a month. They should be taken in the morning on an empty stomach with a full glass of water. Other food or drink must not be ingested for a half hour and the individual must remain sitting or standing for at least 30 minutes. These drugs are usually well tolerated, but esophagitis, nausea, vomiting, and musculoskeletal pain can result. Zoledronic acid (Reclast) is the only FDA approved treatment for osteoporosis that is administered once a year by IV injection. Daily calcium and vitamin D are also encouraged to strengthen the bones.

Drugs for Parkinson's Disease

Parkinson's disease is a movement disorder in which the individual develops muscle rigidity, difficulty initiating any movement, and tremor. Certain drugs such as reserpine (Serpasil), norepinephrine (Levophed), and antipsychotic drugs also cause symptoms of Parkinson's disease. Early treatment involves the use of anticholinergic drugs such as benztropine (Cogentin) or biperiden (Akineton), but possible side effects include dry mouth, urinary retention, constipation, blurred vision, disorientation, insomnia, restlessness, and impairment of recent memory. Individuals with mental problems, narrow-angle glaucoma, urinary or intestinal obstruction, or those with a rapid heart beat should not take these drugs because they may worsen these conditions.

Dopaminergic drugs potentiate the individual's ability to carry out activities of daily living and are the first line of treatment for Parkinson's disease. They include levodopa (L-Dopa), amatadine (Symmetrel), and carbidopa-levodopa (Sinemet). Possible side effects include aggressiveness, dizziness, restlessness, nausea, vomiting, anorexia, agitation, orthostatic hypotension, GI bleeding, darkened urine, confusion, and blurred vision. Carbidopa-levodopa (Sinemet) seems to be better tolerated by older persons and has fewer side effects. Pramipexole (Miraplex) is prescribed early in the disease and used in combination with levodopa in the more advanced stages of Parkinson's disease (Lehne, 2007).

Psychotherapeutic Drugs

Anti-Anxiety (Anxiolytic) Drugs

Prior to prescribing anti-anxiety medications, older adults should be carefully assessed, including a physical examination, a history of personal losses, and other stresses in addition to drug, alcohol, OTC, nicotine, and caffeine use. It is preferable to counsel and teach the individual improved coping strategies prior to taking these medications. Benzodiazepines are the most likely drugs used in the treatment of anxiety. Medications with a short half-life include alprazolam (Xanax) and lorazepam (Ativan). They are eliminated from the body fairly quickly but may cause rebound anxiety and insomnia. Long-acting anti-anxiety drugs include chlordiazepoxide (Librium), clorazepate (Tranxene), and diazepam (Valium). These drugs are highly addictive yet effective in treating anxiety. Short-acting benzodiazepines are usually preferable in treating older adults; however elders tend to metabolize benzodiazepines less quickly resulting in drugs remaining in the blood stream for prolonged periods of time and causing toxic effects. Side effects that may continue for several days after the drug has been discontinued include dizziness, headache, daytime sedation, motor incoordination, confusion, memory impairment, agitation, cognitive impairment, and drug dependency. Older debilitated individuals require careful monitoring regarding safety issues, and some may be misdiagnosed because side effects can mimic dementia. Buspirone (BuSpar) is a nonbenzodiazepine anti-anxiety, non-sedating drug that does not cause dependence. Prescribed for chronic anxiety, it usually takes several days to weeks to become fully effective. Adverse effects include lightheadedness, nausea, headache, dizziness, and nervousness, but it is usually well tolerated (Lehne, 2007; Gulick & Jett, 2008).

Sedative-Hypnotic Drugs

Sedatives function by initiating sleep more rapidly and reducing the number of short awakenings during the night. Usually the effectiveness of these drugs is brief, and when they are stopped, former patterns of sleep resume. Certain characteristics of hypnotics, such as depression of the central nervous system, limit their use with older adults. Tolerance usually develops over a few days, making it necessary to increase the dosage. The half-life of many hypnotics is very long, and some, especially barbiturates, have a very narrow margin of safety between what constitutes a therapeutic dose and a toxic or fatal dose.

Barbiturates, used to induce sleep, are not considered appropriate for older persons because of the likelihood of dependence, their narrow margin of safety, and their considerable interactions with other drugs (Benjamin and Fletcher, 2006). Benzodiazepines such as flurazepam (Dalmane) and temazepam (Restoril) produce only limited suppressed REM sleep with no rebound (reoccurrence of the medication's effects after it has been stopped). On the other hand, benzodiazepines suppress deep sleep Stages 3 and 4, which are already appreciably reduced in the elderly. There is danger of accumulation in the body because the half-life of Dalmane may be 120 to 160 hours in older adults. It may be useful for individuals who require prolonged therapy, but side effects such as over-sedation, dizziness, and excitement are not unusual in this age group. Chloral hydrate (Noctec), a long-used hypnotic, does not seem to affect REM sleep, rarely causes a hangover, and is excreted from the body fairly rapidly. Zolpidem (Ambien) is used to treat insomnia but has potential for causing sedation and confusion. Melatonin, an OTC drug, has been used to promote sleep because sleep disorders in older adults are often linked to changes in the melatonin cycle (Kane et al., 1999).

Adverse effects of hypnotics include confusion, ataxia (uncontrolled movements), gastric irritation, excessive drowsiness during the day, and a severe "hangover" effect. They generally account for the stuporous behavior often observed in nursing home and hospital patients. Some sleeping medications contain scopolamine and should not be given to anyone with glaucoma. Acute poisoning can result when certain sedatives are ingested with alcohol. Rather than relying on sedatives it is best to first use nonpharmacologic approaches. Initially determine prior sleep patterns and the causes for not sleeping. Causes might be a full bladder or rectum, anxiousness, loneliness, fear, or grief. Discussing the tendency toward more numerous short awakenings in older age, and emphasizing that little overall sleep is actually lost might alleviate concerns over not sleeping. A glass of warm milk, a back rub, soothing music, and showing concern by listening can often accomplish better results than administering hypnotics. Daytime napping should be discouraged as much as possible.

Antidepressant Drugs

A large array of antidepressant drugs are available that are quite effective in treating depression, however it takes from 2 to 4 weeks for their action to be fully realized. Selective serotonin reuptake inhibitors (SSRIs) are most often the first choice for older adults and have replaced the tricyclic antidepressants and MAO inhibitors. The tricyclic antidepressants sometimes cause serious adverse reactions such as cardiac toxicity or memory problems. In addition, the half-life of several of these drugs is longer than 24 hours, which could cause serious life-threatening side effects. SSRIs may result in GI upset, drowsiness, dizziness, headache, confusion, agitation, and nervousness. Depression can usually be relieved with low dosages of these drugs (Deglin & Vallerand, 2007; Gulick & Jett, 2008).

Mood Stabilizers

Lithium carbonate (Carbolith, Eskalith) are prescribed for the treatment of bi-polar affective disorders to level out extreme shifts in emotions. They should be used with caution in older persons because of their narrow margin of safety and because serum levels must be continually monitored to prevent drug overdose. Side effects are multiple and involve major body systems. Among them are confusion, drowsiness, stupor, restlessness, muscle weakness, hypotension, aphasia, and many others. They should be used with caution in older adults and those with thyroid, diabetes, renal, and cardiac disease. It is advisable to take Lithium with meals and at specific times each day with no omissions or changes in dosage without contacting a primary care practitioner (Deglin & Vallerand, 2007).

Antipsychotic Drugs (Neuroleptics)

Prescribed to control psychotic, agitated, or violent behavior, antipsychotic drugs are often quite effective, yet most produce serious side effects. Specifically they are used to control symptoms such as paranoia, disordered thinking, hallucinations, delusions, aggressive, and disordered behavior. Haloperidol (Haldol) is a high potency medication that should be used cautiously with older individuals. Other drugs used are phenothiazines, such as chlorpromazine (Thorazine, sparine), and thioridazines (Mellaril). Side effects and adverse reactions of neuroleptics can be severe depending upon the drug used and the dosage prescribed. The lowest possible dosage for the shortest length of time is recommended. An array of adverse reactions are possible when taking these drugs, including tardive dyskinesia (chronic involuntary movements of the tongue, lips, and face, as well as agitated movements of the feet, hand, fingers, and toes). Extrapyramidal effects have been found in 50% of older adults who use antipsychotics and include tremor, agitation, and a shuffling gait, all of which mimic Parkinson's disease. Other side effects include akinesia (a fixed, flat expression), apathetic manner, dulled speech, hypotension, restlessness, photosensitivity, constipation, jaundice, difficult urination, cardiovascular effects, cognitive impairment, delirium, and dementia (Deglin & Vallerand, 2007).

Neuroleptic drugs are to be taken with food or milk and carefully monitored regarding dosage and times taken. Individuals should be advised to rise slowly from a lying or sitting position because hypotension may occur. These drugs are not to be ingested with alcohol or other CNS depressants, or within an hour of antacid or antidiarrheal medication. Haldol has a narrow margin of safety regarding dosage, and the blood levels must be carefully monitored.

A newer group of atypical antipsychotic drugs have been developed that influence the serotonin and dopamine receptors. Among these are clozapine (Clozaril), risperidone (Risperdal), and quetiapine (Seroquel). They have fewer extrapyramidal side effects than others, but they may cause diabetes, weight gain, elevated lipids, and stroke, especially among older individuals (Benjamin & Fletcher, 2006; Deglin & Vallerand, 2008).

Of all the drug classes, neuroleptic drugs are the most overused and misused with older adults. They are not to be prescribed for relatively minor behavior problems. Careful assessment is paramount in determining the cause of the presenting behavior because it could well mask the presence of a urinary tract infection, electrolyte imbalance, dehydration, adverse drug reaction, or sudden environmental change (Bullock & Saharan, 2002).

Antibiotics

Antibiotics are a major group of drugs frequently prescribed for older adults to treat infections. Drug-drug interactions and adverse reactions to them are more common in older adults than in younger persons. Included among the anti-infective drugs are penicillins, cephalosporins, tetracyclines, aminoglycosides, macrolides, fluoroquinolones, sulfonamides, and selected others. There are also antiviral and antifungal drugs. Broad-spectrum antibiotics are effective against many different pathogens, whereas narrow spectrum antibiotics are appropriate for only one or a special group of pathogens. Identifying the pathogen (culture and sensitivity testing) prior to initiating anti-infective therapy is important because taking an inappropriate drug may result in developing resistance or causing the pathogen to progress further in the body. Usually one anti-infective drug is prescribed, but at times two or more may be necessary. Organisms can become resistant to all available antibacterial drugs and death might occur. Care must be taken to avoid allergic or adverse reactions between medications as well as foods that may either enhance or reduce medication effectiveness (LeFever-Kee & Hayes, 2000). The tetracyclines (such as Vibramycin or Terramycin) enhance the effects of anticoagulants and aminoglycosides. Gentamicin sulfate (Garamycin) may cause deafness and damage the kidneys, and cephalosporin (Cephalexin) may result in bleeding disorders. Because these drugs are mostly excreted in an unchanged form by the kidneys, kidney functioning must be carefully monitored. Doses should be far enough apart to allow for delayed excretion. Essential to effective treatment is taking the full course of medications, the correct dosage at the right time, avoiding certain identified foods or other medications, and drinking sufficient fluids.

Antidiabetic Drugs

Diabetes mellitus, a chronic illness, increases in prevalence after age 50. It is characterized by elevated blood glucose levels with a decrease in the body's ability to respond to insulin and/or the absence (or decrease) of insulin produced in the pancreas. Although some older individuals have insulin-dependent diabetes (IDDM), most have non-insulin dependent diabetes (NIDDM). Insulin injections act as a replacement for insulin normally secreted by the beta cells in the pancreas. Insulin is available in several forms short acting, intermediate acting, and long acting, as well as combinations of these and as insulin analogs. The type of insulin prescribed is based upon blood sugar levels and other factors. Unopened insulin should be refrigerated, but insulin currently being used may be stored at room temperature. Insulin may be administered by injection intravenously, subcutaneously, by inhalation (Exubera), and by an insulin pump.

Careful instructions are necessary in teaching older persons how to check blood sugar levels and give themselves insulin injections. Understanding the signs and symptoms of hypoglycemia and hyperglycemia and taking appropriate corrective actions are very important. Demonstrations and practice sessions, together with oral, audiovisual, computer, and written information are helpful teaching techniques. Special types of injectors to administer insulin are available as well as other assistive devices for those who are visually or otherwise disabled.

Non-insulin dependent diabetics manage their diabetes on a regulated regimen of diet and regular exercise. Others require oral hypoglycemic agents to lower the blood sugar. There are six different classes of oral hypoglycemic agents that may be prescribed as a single drug class or two different drug classes if necessary. They utilize various mechanisms to lower blood sugar. Failure of two drugs to control blood sugar levels usually indicates a need for insulin. Some drugs are combined into one tablet to achieve the desired effect. Several newer drugs have been approved to treat diabetes including Januvia, Byetta, and Symlin (Adams, Holland, & Bostwick, 2008). Antidiabetic medications may cause hypoglycemia (low blood sugar) and sensitivity to direct sunlight. Careful monitoring of blood sugar levels is necessary as well as attention to possible complications. It is advisable to carry some form of carbohydrate in case of a hypoglycemic reaction. Weight and stress reduction, regular exercise, following the prescribed diet, and avoiding alcohol are highly advised.

Laxatives

After viewing television and reading the many advertisements for laxatives, it might seem that individuals cannot function without them. Older individuals often abuse the use of laxatives and stool softeners. Laxatives cause dependency, dehydration, loss of muscle tone in the intestines, loss of important salts and minerals, and reduced absorption of vitamins A and D. Anyone using laxatives regularly should consult a primary care practitioner to determine the actual cause of the problem. Keep in mind that some drugs taken by elders cause constipation. Rather than resorting to laxatives, eating a diet with adequate fiber, drinking plenty of water, and exercising can be most helpful in preventing constipation.

ATTITUDES TOWARD "PILL POPPING"

Attitudes toward taking medications are highly varied among older adults. Some believe that all medicines are worthless and do not take their prescribed medications. Others use prescribed pills when critically ill, but discard them as soon as some improvement occurs. Still others hold fixed, inaccurate ideas about what a particular pill will do for them.

Quackery is an ever-present threat to appropriate health care. Certain medications, treatments, and cures appear on the market from time to time, especially on television and via the written word. They promise instant cures for a wide variety of ailments including arthritis, diabetes, cancer, GI, and other problems. Not only are they expensive, but their use may cause a delay in seeking appropriate medical treatment and could even result in death.

PREVENTION OF DRUG ACCIDENTS

Lack of accurate information about medications is common in the older age group. Some believe if one pill helps, two will be sure to cure. Medications are forgotten, the treatment regimen is not understood, or the medications are not taken at the proper time or in the proper amount, especially if multiple medications are prescribed. When five or six or more pills are prescribed to be taken at different times, even a young person would be challenged. Setting the alarm clock to ring when medications are due or using pill containers with seven or more compartments may encourage compliance. There are several specialized electronic pill reminders available to assist individuals in taking their medications appropriately. These include computer-generated reminder charts and electronic medication compliance aids. Seeking the assistance of a relative or friend might also be helpful. Prescriptions may not be refilled, often because of cost. Sometimes pills are swapped with a friend, a common but dangerous practice. At other times they are taken along with herbs or supplements with which they may be incompatible.

Health care professionals have an obligation to ensure elders understand the purpose of each medication, how and when to take it, and its side effects or adverse reactions. Written information is included with all prescriptions filled in most pharmacies. Reviewing the information with the older adult would help ensure proper understanding and increase compliance. Use of the computer or resource books are also valuable sources of information. Those with visual impairments may benefit from large print instructions, color coding, and improved illumination. Older adults should be encouraged to ask questions and obtain information about all prescribed and OTC medications they are taking.

SUMMARY

Medications are of tremendous value to many older adults whose very lives depend upon them. An understanding of age-related factors that influence absorption, distribution, metabolism, and excretion, as well as side effects, adverse reactions, actions, and interactions of drugs is imperative. To ensure optimal physical, psychological, and social well-being, drug dosages should be as low as possible, the number of drugs taken should be minimal, and their effectiveness and adverse reactions and interactions should be evaluated on a regular basis. With a thoughtful treatment plan, medications will prevent disease, permit healthy living, and promote longevity.

REFERENCES

Adams, M. P., Holland, L. N., & Bostwick, P. M. (2008). *Pharmacology for nurses* (2nd ed.). Upper Saddle River, NJ: Prentice Hall.

Amoako, E. P., Richardson-Campbell, L., & Kennedy-Malone, L. (2003). Self-medication with over-the-counter drugs among elderly adults. *Journal of Gerontological Nursing, 29*(8), 10–15.

Avorn, J., & Gurwitz, J. H. (1997). Principles of pharmacology. In C. K. Cassel, H. J. Cohen, E. B. Larson, D. E. Meier, N. M. Resnick, L. Z. Rubenstein, & L. B. Sorensen (Eds.), *Geriatric medicine* (3rd ed., pp. 55–70). New York: Springer-Verlag.
Benjamin, C., & Fletcher, K. (2006). Pharmacologic management. In S. E. Meiner, & A. G. Lueckenotte (Eds.), *Gerontologic nursing* (3rd ed., pp. 447–467). St. Louis: Mosby Elsevier.
Bullock, R., & Saharan, A. (2002). Atypical antipsychotics: Experience and use in the elderly. *International Journal of Clinical Practice, 56*(7), 515–525.
Clarke, J. B., Queener, S. F., & Karb, V. B. (1990). *Pharmacological basis of nursing practice* (3rd ed.). St. Louis: Mosby.
Culberson, J. W. (2006). Alcohol use in the elderly: Beyond the edge. *Geriatrics, 6*(10), 22–27.
Cuozzo, C. A. (2007). How medications are born. *Advance for Nurses, 8*(26), 31–32.
Deglin, J. H., & Vallerand, A. H. (2007). *Davis' drug guide for nurses* (10th ed.). Philadelphia: F.A. Davis.
Ditrapano, C., & Peoples, M. (2008). Generic vs. brand name drugs. *Advance for Nurses, 9*(10), 33–34.
Fick, D. M., Cooper, J. W., Eade, W. E., Waller, J. L., Maclean, J. R., & Beers, M. H. (2003). Updating the Beers criteria for potentially inappropriate medication use in older adults. *Archives of Internal Medicine, 163*, 2716–2724.
Fleming, M. F. (2002). Identification and treatment of alcohol use disorders in older adults. In A. M. Gurnack, R. Arkinson, & N. Osgood (Eds.), *Treating alcohol and drug abuse in the elderly* (pp. 85–108). New York: Springer.
Flemming-Courts, N. (1996). Salicylism in the elderly: "A little aspirin never hurt anybody!" *Geriatrics, 17*, 55–62.
Gulick, G. G., & Jett, K. (2008). Geropharmacy. In P. Ebersole, P. Hess, T. A. Touhy, K. Jett, & A. S. Luggen (Eds.), *Toward healthy aging* (7th ed., pp. 295–322). St. Louis: Mosby Elsevier.
Healthy People 2010. *Understanding and improving health* (2000). Boston: Jones & Bartlett.
Kane, R. L., Ouslander, J. G., & Abrass, I. B. (1999). *Essentials of clinical geriatrics.* New York: McGraw-Hill.
LeFever-Kee, J., & Hayes, E. R. (2000). *Pharmacology: A nursing process approach* (3rd ed.). Philadelphia: Saunders.
Lefkovitz, A., & Zarowitz, B. (2007). Top 10 lists-medications associated with adverse events and medications involved with errors. *Geriatric Nursing, 28*(5), 276–279.
Lehne, R. A. (2007). *Pharmacology for nursing care* (6th ed.). St. Louis: Saunders.
Lin, S. H., & Lin, M. S. (1993). A survey on drug-related hospitalization in a community teaching hospital. *International Journal of Clinical Pharmacology, Therapy, and Toxicology, 31*, 66–69.
Maiese, D. R. (2002). Healthy people 2010—leading health indicators for women. *Women's Health Issues, 12*, 155–164.
Mauk, K. (2006). *Gerontological nursing.* Sudbury, MA: Jones & Bartlett.
Melman, K. L., Morrelli, H. F., Hoffman, B. B., & Nierenberg, D. W. (1993). *Melman and Morrelli"s clinical pharmacology: Basic principles in therapeutics* (7th ed.). New York: McGraw-Hill.

Merrick, E. L., Horgan, C. M., Hodgkin, D., Garnick, D. W., Houghton, B. S., Panas, L., Saitz, R., & Blow, F. (2008). Unhealthy drinking patterns in older adults: Prevalence and associated characteristics. *Journal of the American Geriatric Society, 56*(2), 214–223.

Miller, C. (2009). *Nursing for wellness in older adults* (5th ed.). Philadelphia: Wolters Kluwer/Lippincott Williams & Wilkins.

Nurses drug handbook (2003). Blue Bell, PA: Blanchard & Loeb.

Pepper, G. A. (1999). Drug use and misuse. In J. T. Stone, J. F. Wyman, & S. A. Salisbury (Eds.), *Clinical gerontological nursing* (2nd ed., pp. 537–552). Philadelphia: Saunders.

Petrone, K., & Katz, P. (2005). Approaches to appropriate drug prescribing for the older adult. *Primary Care: Clinics in Office Practice, 32,* 755–775.

Physician"s Desk Reference. (2009). (63rd ed.). Montvale, NJ: Thomson Reuters.

Rolita, L., & Freedman, M. (2008). Over-the-counter medication use in older adults. *Journal of Gerontological Nursing, 34*(4), 8–17.

Schwartz, J. B. (1999). Clinical pharmacology. In W. R. Hazzard, J. P. Blass, W. H. Ettinger, J. B. Halter, & J. G. Ouslander (Eds.), *Principles of geriatric medicine and gerontology* (4th ed., pp. 303–332). New York: McGraw-Hill.

Shorr, R. I. (2007). *Drugs for the geriatric patient*. Philadelphia: Saunders Elsevier.

Spratto, G. R., & Woods, A. L. (1994). *RN's NDR 94: Nurses drug reference*. Albany, NY: Delmar.

Vestal, R. E. (1990). Clinical pharmacology. In W. R. Hazzard, R. Andres, E. L. Bierman, & J. P. Blass (Eds.), *Principles of geriatric medicine and gerontology* (2nd ed., pp. 201–211). New York: McGraw-Hill.

Wilson, I. B., Schoen, C., Newman, P., Strollo, M., Roger, W., Chang, H., & Safran, P. (2007). Physician-patient communication about prescription medication nonadherence: A 50-state study of America's seniors. *Journal of General Internal Medicine, 22*(1), 6–12.

Wright, W. L. (2008). Hypertension update. *Advance for Nurse Practitioners, 16*(12), 37–42.